ETHICAL ISSUES IN WOMEN'S HEALTHCARE

ETHICAL ISSUES IN WOMEN'S HEALTHCARE

Practice and Policy

Edited by Lori d'Agincourt-Canning

Carolyn Ells

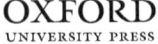

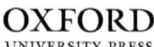

Oxford University Press is a department of the University of Oxford. It furthers the University's objective of excellence in research, scholarship, and education by publishing worldwide. Oxford is a registered trade mark of Oxford University Press in the UK and certain other countries.

Published in the United States of America by Oxford University Press
198 Madison Avenue, New York, NY 10016, United States of America.

© Oxford University Press 2019

All rights reserved. No part of this publication may be reproduced, stored in a retrieval system, or transmitted, in any form or by any means, without the prior permission in writing of Oxford University Press, or as expressly permitted by law, by license, or under terms agreed with the appropriate reproduction rights organization. Inquiries concerning reproduction outside the scope of the above should be sent to the Rights Department, Oxford University Press, at the address above.

You must not circulate this work in any other form
and you must impose this same condition on any acquirer.

CIP data is on file at the Library of Congress
ISBN 978–0–19–085136–1 (pbk.)
ISBN 978–0–19–085137–8 (hbk.)

This material is not intended to be, and should not be considered, a substitute for medical or other professional advice. Treatment for the conditions described in this material is highly dependent on the individual circumstances. And, while this material is designed to offer accurate information with respect to the subject matter covered and to be current as of the time it was written, research and knowledge about medical and health issues is constantly evolving and dose schedules for medications are being revised continually, with new side effects recognized and accounted for regularly. Readers must therefore always check the product information and clinical procedures with the most up-to-date published product information and data sheets provided by the manufacturers and the most recent codes of conduct and safety regulation. The publisher and the authors make no representations or warranties to readers, express or implied, as to the accuracy or completeness of this material. Without limiting the foregoing, the publisher and the authors make no representations or warranties as to the accuracy or efficacy of the drug dosages mentioned in the material. The authors and the publisher do not accept, and expressly disclaim, any responsibility for any liability, loss, or risk that may be claimed or incurred as a consequence of the use and/or application of any of the contents of this material.

CONTENTS

About the Cover Art   ix
Preface   xi
Acknowledgments   xv
Contributor Biographies   xvii

1. Women's Healthcare Through a Feminist Ethics Lens
   —LORI D'AGINCOURT-CANNING AND CAROLYN ELLS   1

SECTION I: *Locations, Migrations, and Access to Healthcare*

2. Indigenous Women, Health, and Healthcare
   —CHARLOTTE LOPPIE AND ALEXANDRA KENT   21

3. Caring for Refugees, New Immigrants, and Uninsured Women: Social Responsibility and Access to Healthcare
   —PAUL CAULFORD AND SUMATHY RAHUNATHAN   45

4. Rural Women: Place, Community, and Accessing Healthcare
   —CHRISTY SIMPSON AND FIONA MCDONALD   63

SECTION II: *New and Emerging Themes*

5. Drivers and Dilemmas of Female Genital Cosmetic Surgery
   —DOROTHY SHAW AND NICOLE TODD   87

6. Ethical Issues in the Care and Support of Women Living with HIV
—RUBY RAJENDRA SHANKER, ANGELA UNDERHILL, VALERIE NICHOLSON, LOGAN KENNEDY, DENISE JAWORSKY, AND MONA LOUTFY 107

7. Ethical Issues in Healthcare for Women in the Context of Violence—ROCHELLE EINBODEN AND COLLEEN VARCOE 129

8. Sex Work, Ethics, and Healthcare—VICTORIA BUNGAY AND LAUREN CASEY 149

9. Primary Healthcare for Queer Women and Trans People: Confronting Heteronormativity and Cisnormativity —ERIN FREDERICKS AND KELLY BAKER 167

SECTION III: *Reproductive Healthcare*

10. The Moral Agency of Abortion Providers: Conscientious Provision, Dangertalk, and the Lived Experience of Doing Stigmatized Work—LISA HARRIS 189

11. Perinatal Mental Health: The Lens of Relational Ethics —LORI D'AGINCOURT-CANNING AND DEIRDRE RYAN 209

12. Technology and the Ethical Practice of Reproductive Care: A Woman-Centered Lens—LAURA A. STURGILL, SARA G. SHIELDS, AND LUCY M. CANDIB 233

13. Women with Disabilities: Ethics of Access and Accommodation for Infertility Care—LESLIE FRANCIS, ANITA SILVERS, AND BRITTANY BADESCH   259

14. Research with Pregnant Women: A Feminist Challenge
    —MARGARET OLIVIA LITTLE, MARISHA N. WICKREMSINHE, ELANA JAFFE, AND ANNE DRAPKIN LYERLY   279

Index   299

ABOUT THE COVER ART

First Nations people of the Northwest coast observe the Dragonfly to be a creature of the wind and also of the water. It represents a symbol of change in the view of self-understanding and the kind of change that has its source in mental and emotional maturity and the insight of the deeper meaning of life. The Dragonfly's swift flight and its ability to move in all six directions radiate a sense of power and poise, something that comes only with age and experience. The female dragonfly in this painting can be seen with its tail in the water laying her eggs, which represents resilience and hope for the future and signifies the birth and creation of new life across the land.
Artist: Khrystal Harper

PREFACE

My reasons for pursuing this collection stemmed from my experience as a practicing healthcare ethicist. Feminist epistemology and feminist ethics had greatly influenced my thinking as a doctoral student. These perspectives provided the theoretical framework for my empirical research and later analysis of ethical issues pertaining to genetic testing for hereditary breast/ovarian cancer. However, once in practice—first at a cancer agency and then at a women's and children's health center—I saw a disjuncture between academic/theoretical writing and what occurred in real life. The questions we privileged as feminist bioethicists and academics were often a far cry from the pain, anxiety, confusion, and deep sadness I saw at the bedside. The connect between the world of abstract theory and the world of clinical engagement was hazy, and I worried that what we were writing about didn't really touch or affect women's everyday lives. I was dismayed by what I perceived to be the often over-simplified critique of healthcare practice and medical practitioners by some of my mentors. The words of Payam Akhavan, a human rights lawyer, struck me deeply: "The knowledge that mattered most, I realized, could only be found on the ground, in the intimate trenches of human struggle, not by observing the world at thirty thousand feet."[1(p67)]

Yet, at the same time feminist ethics provided a valuable framework for understanding many of the ethical tensions I saw in healthcare. The tendency to judge patients devoid of context was real and dangerous, as was the tendency to view medical knowledge as the only truth or to be unaware of the power one held as a provider. Moving back and forth between a pediatric hospital and a woman's hospital put into sharp relief how we think about children and women in isolation of each other. On one side of the house, pediatric patients were viewed as entities within themselves and parents more as a means to an end than anything else. On the other, women's "autonomous" choices took strict precedence. Yet, in reality, most mothers (fathers and all parents) would do anything for their children but might face constraints—physical, cognitive, social, familial, economic—that did not allow them to exercise their preferred "choice." Feminist ethics, together with what I saw in practice, reminded me again and again that we cannot separate women's (or anyone's) health and well-being from the contexts, systems, and institutional structures in which we live.

Yet, while theoretical terrain is always intriguing, I am drawn to the practical applications of bioethics and feminist approaches. From the ground as a practicing ethicist, I saw women's healthcare poorly addressed in a bioethics literature that fixated on reproduction but little else related to women's health. Thus, I wished to help address that gap. The best way to do this, I thought, was to bring voices from clinical practice into conversation with those in academia to illuminate connections, fissures, and perhaps future directions for research. I invited a colleague to help explore this terrain with me. I knew Carolyn also had a keen interest in the lived experience of people (patients, health professionals, directors) in healthcare settings. She too thought that despite the attention feminist bioethicists have given to issues relevant to women's health, there has not been enough attention to issues and solutions at the clinical level.

What unfolded was a complicated discussion about clinical practice, real-world experiences, and ethics. Most of our contributors will not be recognized by the feminist bioethicist community, but they bring a wealth of practical, clinical, and personal experience. In doing so, they identify ethical issues pertaining to women's healthcare that have gone unrecognized and offer recommendations to ethical practice in these complex situations.

For instance, some contributors take up feminist ethics and relational theory to identify new approaches to the ethical treatment of women experiencing violence and those living with HIV or with mental illness, or in rural communities. These authors step outside the world of abstract theory to show how feminist bioethics can inform service delivery and practice, recognizing that the structures shaping practice are multiple and complex. Other chapters describe ethical challenges associated with healthcare access for marginalized groups of women, including Indigenous women, refugees and undocumented immigrants, women engaged in sex work, queer women and trans people, and those with disabilities. Other chapters focus on harms to women caused by unnecessary medical procedures (cosmetic genital surgery) and others by the lack of research (exclusion of pregnant women from clinical trials). And still others expand on lived experience to discuss women-centered reproductive care and create new ways of conceptualizing issues pertaining to feminist ethics. Lisa Harris's description of "dangertalk" is extremely instructive in this regard as she reminds us that—even as feminists—we may not allow some to state their truths.

Ultimately, this collection is an attempt to bridge divides. By making connections between practice and theory and theory and practice, the goal has been not just to *write* about making women's lives better but to identify strategies and pursue reflections that can be *enacted* in practice and policy. Some authors also seek to connect theory and practice with users of the health system by including women's voices in their research. We benefit greatly from hearing women's reflections and insights on their real-world experiences.

In selecting topics for the book, it is worth mentioning there were many issues that we could not address due to page limitations set by the publisher. Among the topics we saw affecting women in need of critical reflection are ethical issues related to obesity, aging, and international women's health. Another regret is that we were not able to include more international writers to bring a more global perspective.

In closing, however, I'd like to pose a question to ethicists, clinicians, and other readers of this essay—one that I first heard when learning about qualitative research: What questions do we fail to ask in our own research or practice that contribute to the erasure of those we study? Who do we fail to include in our theoretical discussions or exclude from our academic and clinical silos that also dismisses women from our view? Drawing from Paul Farmer's insights about structural violence, do we also do violence to women by writing from our theoretical perspectives in isolation? The evolution of recent movements is significant here. Indigenous nations in Canada now rightfully insist that "Nothing About Us Without Us" is essential to moving past the effects of colonization and facilitating self-determination and sustainable change with Indigenous people. Greater Involvement of People Living with HIV/AIDS (GIPA) and Meaningful Involvement of People Living with HIV (MIPA) (see Chapter 6) are principles and processes respectively aimed at ensuring that people living with HIV are central to the creation of policies, funding, services, research, and initiatives that affect them. As we think about the future of feminist bioethics, should we or how do we apply this thinking to our work? As McBride and Schostak[2] observe, when practitioners carefully study their own work, they nearly always find inconsistencies, problems, and new possibilities.

It seems that we are in the middle of an exciting time of self-reflection, learning, and action. Collaborative practice is a hallmark of feminist thinking. There will always remain farther to go.

Lori d'Agincourt-Canning

References

1. Akhavan P. *In Search of a Better World: A Human Rights Odyssey* (CBC Massey Lectures). Toronto: House of Anansi Press; 2017.
2. McBride R, Schostak J, Professional development. http://www.enquirylearning.net/ELU/Issues/ Research/Res1Ch8.html. Accessed March 30, 2012.

ACKNOWLEDGMENTS

A collection like this requires the expertise and commitment of its contributors. As editors, we extend our thanks most of all to those who participated in our project and honor their amazing work.

At Oxford University Press, we thank Lucy Randall and Hannah Doyle for their guidance and encouragement. OUP engaged two of the world's finest feminist bioethics scholars to provide external peer review. Jackie Leach Scully and Susan Dodds reviewed our book proposal and Susan again reviewed a full draft of the set of book chapters. Each offered insights and suggestions that strengthened the collection.

Carolyn Ells acknowledges her academic home in the Faculty of Medicine, McGill University. It is a stimulating environment for a philosopher engaged with theory, practice, and research in bioethics. I have been fortunate to learn from and work with extraordinary faculty and students who boldly favor innovation and development that nurtures patient-centered, relationship-based healthcare, through teaching, faculty development, healthcare practice, and research. My reflections on ethics in relationships of healthcare have been influenced by discussions with many patients, family members, health professionals, and others at the Jewish General Hospital, who shared their perspectives and insights (often deeply personal) about the ethical challenges they faced. I thank you all. The proposal for this book was developed while I was Visiting Scholar at the University of Toronto Joint Centre for Bioethics. I thank my parents, who ground me and cheer from a distance as I pursue my life and career in Montreal. I share my life and love with Terry Element. I thank you, Terry, for your unwavering support, patience, and enthusiasm as I worked on this project.

Lori d'Agincourt-Canning would like to thank her colleagues at BC Women's Hospital, where the idea for this book was first articulated. This collection is the product of discussions and reflections with coworkers, and patients themselves, about the complexity of women's healthcare. I would like to particularly acknowledge the influence of Dorothy Shaw, Medical Director, and Cheryl Davies, Chief Operating Officer, at BCW, whose advocacy and commitment to ethical care for women are second to none. Among my academic colleagues with whom I discussed the project, I want to particularly thank Christy Simpson for her support and encouragement. I am grateful, as ever, to my daughters, Rachel and Erin, for their understanding. Finally, an enormous thanks goes to Peter Canning, whose faith, love, and humor sustained me through this work.

Carolyn and Lori acknowledge the Indigenous lands within which we live, play, and work. Carolyn's place of work, McGill University, is located within the traditional and unceded territory of the Kanien'kehá:ka, a place that has long served as a site of meeting and exchange among nations. The University of Toronto is located within the traditional territory of the Wendat, the Anishnaabeg, Haudenosaunee, Métis, and the Mississaugas of the New Credit First Nation. Lori's place of work is within the unceded and traditional territory of the Musqueam, Tsleil-Waututh, and Squamish Coast Salish peoples. We are grateful to have the opportunity to work on these lands.

CONTRIBUTOR BIOGRAPHIES

Brittany Badesch, MD, is currently a fourth-year resident physician in the Johns Hopkins Combined Internal Medicine-Pediatrics residency program. She completed her undergraduate education at Vanderbilt University with a major in Education Studies—Special Education. She then obtained her medical degree from the University of Colorado School of Medicine. She plans to pursue a career in medicine focused on caring for children and adults with disabilities and complex healthcare needs.

Kelly Baker, PhD, is an anthropologist and photographer based in Fredericton, New Brunswick, Canada. She teaches courses in the areas of urban ethnography, visual anthropology, and qualitative research methods. Her research and artistic work examine diverse meanings of place and space with a particular focus on sexuality and race in gentrifying space. Her most recent project combines photovoice with portraiture to examine meanings of home and self among people experiencing housing insecurity in Fredericton.

Victoria Bungay, PhD, RN, is an Associate Professor at the School of Nursing at the University of British Columbia and holds a Canada Research Chair in Gender, Equity and Community Engagement. As the Director of the Capacity Research Unit at UBC, her work focuses on addressing inequities that negatively affect people's health and well-being, including the devastating effects of stigma, discrimination, and violence. She is interested in how research partnerships can positively impact communities that are regularly excluded in health and social policy and programming that affect their lives and how community-based interventions support real-world evidence. Her current research and partnerships are tackling such issues as research ethics in practice, equity-oriented care, gender-based violence, and evidence-informed recommendations to promote and protect the health, safety, and human rights of people engaged in the sex industry.

Lucy M. Candib, MD, is a Professor of Family Medicine and Community Health, at the University of Massachusetts Medical School, and practiced family medicine, including obstetrics, at the Family Health Center of Worcester for 40 years. Throughout her career she drew attention to the needs and concerns of women trainees and practitioners. In her book *Medicine and the Family: A Feminist Perspective* (Basic, 1995) she focused on gender issues in medical theory and practice. She co-edited with her colleague Dr. Sara Shields *A Woman-Centered Care in Pregnancy and Childbirth* (Radcliffe, 2010). Today she continues teaching about sexual abuse and violence against women and about refugees and asylum seekers.

Lauren Casey, PhD, RN, has worked with several regional, national, and international organizations committed to reducing health inequalities in society and, more particularly, among sex work populations. She has created, developed, and delivered successful government-funded harm reduction programs and has received several awards for her contribution to the betterment of health and well-being of persons involved in the sex industry. She has been the co-lead on several important Canadian sex work projects, including the CIHR-funded project entitled "Supervising Sex Work: Challenges to Workplace Safety and Health" (2011–2017) that examined managers' experiences in the sex industry with the goal of learning about their perspectives on health, safety, and well-being in their workplaces.

Paul Caulford, MSc, MD, CCFP, FCFP, is an Assistant Professor, Department of Family and Community Medicine, University of Toronto. He is a practicing family physician with a focus on primary migration healthcare in Scarborough, Toronto, Canada. In 1999, he co-founded a community volunteer health clinic for uninsured refugees, immigrants, and undocumented migrants denied access to healthcare. More recently, in 2015, he co-founded the Canadian Centre for Refugee and Immigrant Health Care with volunteer nurses, doctors, dentists and community members.

Lori d'Agincourt-Canning, PhD, is a Clinical Associate Professor, Department of Pediatrics, University of British Columbia and an Adjunct Professor in the UBC School of Nursing. She also serves as an ethics and healthcare consultant for several organizations. Her primary responsibilities include ethics consultation, ethics education, and service development. Prior to working as an independent consultant, Lori was lead ethicist at BC's Women's and Children's Hospitals for 10 years. Here she acquired direct exposure to ethical quandaries in women's healthcare, which included many issues that had not captured the attention of academic bioethicists.

Rochelle Einboden, PhD, RN, is currently a postdoctoral researcher and lecturer at the University of Sydney, Australia in the Faculty of Medicine and Health. She is a registered nurse with a clinical background in pediatrics, including emergency and youth health, and has held academic roles in Canada and Australia. Her doctoral work studied nursing responses to child neglect and abuse using critical discursive analysis. Her research interests focus on using critical social theory and methods to explore health policy, programs, and everyday nursing practices, with the aim of enhancing ethical practice and social justice.

Carolyn Ells, RRT, PhD, is an Associate Professor, Department of Medicine and Biomedical Ethics Unit, McGill University and Research Associate, Lady Davis Institute for Medical Research, both in Montreal, Canada. For 11 years, Carolyn was Clinical Ethicist at the Jewish General Hospital, a large McGill teaching hospital emphasizing specialized and ultra-specialized care, for a religiously and culturally diverse population. A former respiratory therapist with graduate studies in philosophy (medical ethics), Carolyn's research and service interests in bioethics flow through the practices and policies of healthcare delivery and research ethics review. Her current research contributes to the theory and implementation of patient-centered care.

Leslie Francis, JD, PhD, is Distinguished Alfred C. Emery Professor of Law and Distinguished Professor of Philosophy, University of Utah, US. Past president of the Pacific Division of the American Philosophical Association, Leslie has recently edited the *Oxford Handbook of Reproductive Ethics* (OUP, 2017). She writes widely on ethical issues in healthcare, reproductive ethics, and disability ethics and law.

Erin Fredericks, PhD, is an Associate Professor, Department of Sociology at St. Thomas University in Fredericton, New Brunswick, Canada. She teaches courses in the areas of sociology of gender, sociology of health, queer sociology, and research methods. Her research examines the healthcare, illness, and wellness experiences of those marginalized by gender and sexual orientation. Erin's current research explores the imagined futures of queer, trans, and two-spirit youth.

Lisa Harris, MD, PhD, is an Associate Professor, Obstetrics & Gynecology at the University of Michigan, US. Her research examines issues at the intersection of clinical obstetrical and gynecological care and law, policy, politics, ethics, history, and sociology. She conducts interdisciplinary, mixed-methods research on many issues along the reproductive justice continuum, including abortion, miscarriage, contraception, in vitro fertilization (IVF), infertility and birth, and racial, ethnic, and socioeconomic disparities in access to reproductive health resources.

Elana Jaffe, BA, is a Research Project Manager in the Department of Social Medicine and the Center for Bioethics at the University of North Carolina at Chapel Hill, US.

Denise Jaworsky, MD, is a general internal medicine physician in the community of Terrace in Northwestern British Columbia, Canada, where she provides HIV care in additional to general internal medicine care. She is also the co-site director of the local Integrated Community Clerkship undergraduate medical education program and a PhD student in Clinical Epidemiology and Health Care Research at the University of Toronto.

Logan Kennedy, RN, MN, is a Research Associate at Women's College Hospital, Toronto, Canada. Her clinical and academic work focuses on women's sexual and reproductive health, celebrating diversity, and challenging social inequity. This has led to expertise in the field of women and HIV. Logan completed her nursing education at Ryerson University, where she is a lecturer. She intends to pursue doctoral education to facilitate developing a program of research that critically explores sexual and reproductive health issues of importance to young women.

Alexandra Kent, MPH, PhD(c), is a doctoral student in Simon Fraser University's Faculty of Health Sciences. Alex's research interests include determinants of Indigenous health equity as well as enhancing the accessibility of healthcare and health systems. Her current research explores anti-racism education and cultural safety training for Master of Public Health students in Canadian universities. Alex situates herself in this work as a non-Indigenous allied researcher of British and Dutch ancestry.

Margaret Olivia Little, BPhil, PhD, is a Senior Research Scholar at the Kennedy Institute of Ethics (KIE) and Professor of Philosophy at Georgetown University in Washington, DC, US. She served 9 years as Director of the KIE Director of Ethics Lab and continues to serve as Director of its Ethics Lab. A Fellow of the Hastings Center, Maggie has twice served as visiting scholar in residence at the National Institutes of Health Department of Bioethics. Together with Ruth Faden and Anne Lyerly, she co-founded the Second Wave Initiative, which works to promote responsible research into the health needs of pregnant women.

Charlotte Loppie, PhD, is a Professor in the School of Public Health and Social Policy at the University of Victoria, Canada, and the former Director of the university's Centre for Indigenous Research and Community-Led Engagement (CIRCLE) (2012–2018). The center provides a supportive environment for students, researchers, and communities to engage respectfully in research activities aimed at addressing the health disparities experienced by First Nations, Inuit, and Métis peoples in Canada. Charlotte partners with First Nation communities, regional and national Indigenous organizations, health charities, and government bodies on a range of projects. Her research interests include Indigenous health inequities, Indigenous HIV/AIDS, barriers to accessing the social determinants of health, racism and cultural safety, cancer among Indigenous peoples, research capacity building, and the sexual and reproductive health of Indigenous women, among others. Charlotte served as Editor of the *Journal of Indigenous Health Research* from 2012 to 2017; she was accepted as a member of the RSC College of New Scholars, Artists and Scientists in 2017, when she was also awarded CIHR's Gold Leaf Award for Transformation: Patient Engagement.

Mona Loutfy, MD, FRCPC, MPH, is a Professor, Infectious Diseases Specialist, and Clinician Scientist at the University of Toronto and Women's College Hospital in Toronto, Canada. She founded the Women and HIV Research Program at the Women's College Research Institute in 2006. Mona is passionate about using community-based research and anti-oppression in all her work. Her goal is to contribute to a world where there is no judgment, stigma, or discrimination in any regards and all can actualize their full potential.

Anne Drapkin Lyerly, MD, MA, is a Professor of Social Medicine and Associate Director of the Center for Bioethics at the University of North Carolina at Chapel Hill, US. An obstetrician-gynecologist and bioethicist, she has published widely on complex issues in reproduction, including her book *A Good Birth: Finding the Positive and Profound in Your Childbirth Experience* (Penguin Group, 2014). Together with Ruth Faden and Maggie Little, she co-founded the Second Wave Initiative, and is Principal Investigator of the NIH-funded PHASES (Pregnancy and HIV/AIDS: Seeking Equitable Study) Project.

Fiona McDonald, JSD, is an Associate Professor with the School of Law and the Co-Director of the Australian Centre for Health Law Research at the Queensland University of Technology, Australia. She is an Adjunct

Associate Professor in the Department of Bioethics at Dalhousie University, Canada. She is the co-author of *Rethinking Rural Health Ethics* (Springer, 2017) and *Ethics, Law and Health Care: A Guide for Nurses and Midwives* (Palgrave McMillan, 2014) and a co-editor of *Health Law in Australia* (3rd ed.) (Thomson Reuters, 2018) and *Health Workforce Governance* (Ashgate, 2012). Her research encompasses issues related to health governance and has three broad themes: the governance of health institutions and systems (including rural health), the governance of health professionals, and the governance of health technology and innovation.

Valerie Nicholson is an Elder and an Indigenous Warrior woman living with HIV. She is a Peer Navigator with Positive Living BC and also works in community-based research. She is the Chair of the Board of Directors of the Canadian Aboriginal AIDS Network and board member of AIDS Vancouver. She is a trainer with the Positive Leadership Development Institute, is honored to mentor HIV-positive youth, and is a Peer Elder for YouthCo's Camp Moomba and Yuusnewas.

Sumathy Rahunathan, BSc (honours), MPH, is the Clinic Coordinator and Research Lead at the Canadian Centre for Refugee and Immigrant Health Care, Scarborough, Canada. She completed an Honours Bachelor of Science at the University of Toronto in Integrated Biology, Health Studies, and Anthropology, followed by a Master's of Public Health at New York University.

Deirdre Ryan, MB, FRCP(C), is a Clinical Associate Professor of Psychiatry, University of British Columbia, and Medical Director for the BC Reproductive Mental Health Program, Canada. She leads a team of specialized and multidisciplinary professionals that has many years of clinical and research experience working with women dealing with mental health challenges or disorders and emotional difficulties related to reproduction.

Ruby Rajendra Shanker, MBBS, MHSc, is a Healthcare Ethicist at the University Health Network, and Women's College Hospital, Toronto, Canada. She comes from Medicine with experience in community medicine. Ruby completed her Master's degree, and Fellowship in Clinical & Organizational Bioethics at the University of Toronto's Joint Centre for Bioethics, where she is an Adjunct Lecturer. She is currently pursuing doctoral studies in Health Professions Education Research at the University of Toronto, and is passionate about social justice education and culturally dexterous approaches to practice. Ruby is a board member of the Canadian

Bioethics Society and the Canadian Association for Practicing Healthcare Ethicists.

Dorothy Shaw, OC, MBChB, FRCSC, is a Clinical Professor in Obstetrics and Gynaecology and Medical Genetics at the University of British Columbia, Vancouver, Canada. She is well known globally for advocacy and policy work on women's sexual and reproductive health and rights, and harmful traditional practices, including female genital mutilation. She has published widely and is a frequent invited speaker. She served as President of the Society of Gynecologists and Obstetricians of Canada and was the first woman to be President of the International Federation of Gynecologists and Obstetricians.

Sara G. Shields, MD, MS, is a Professor of Family Medicine and Community Health at the University of Massachusetts and the Family Health Center, Worcester, Massachusetts, US. She received her AB from Harvard-Radcliffe and her MD from the University of California at San Francisco, followed by Residency at the University of Rochester and a Fellowship in Maternal and Child Health and an MS in Community Health at Brown University. She and her colleague Lucy Candib co-authored *Woman-Centered Care in Pregnancy and Childbirth* (Radcliffe Press, 2010).

Anita Silvers, PhD, is a Professor of Philosophy at San Francisco State University and an affiliate of the SFSU Health Equity Institute, California, US. Her current research is in bioethics, social philosophy, and philosophy and disability. Anita was awarded the Phi Beta Kappa Society's Lebowitz Prize for philosophical achievement and contribution, the American Philosophical Association Quinn Prize for service to philosophy and philosophers, the California State University System's Wang Outstanding Faculty Excellence Award, and the inaugural Human Rights Award from the California Faculty Association.

Christy Simpson, PhD, is an Associate Professor and Head of the Department of Bioethics in the Faculty of Medicine, Dalhousie University in Nova Scotia, Canada. As a member of the Department's Ethics Collaborations Team, she provides ethics support for the IWK Health Centre, the Nova Scotia Health Authority, and the Nova Scotia Health Ethics Network. She is an Adjunct Professor with the Australian Centre for Health Law Research at the Queensland University of Technology, Australia. Christy is co-author of *Rethinking Rural Health Ethics* (Springer, 2017). She has also published on a range of clinical, organizational, and health policy ethics issues, including the role of hope in healthcare, professionalism for practicing healthcare ethicists, and pediatric ethics.

Laura A. Sturgill, MD, MEd, is an Assistant Professor of Family Medicine and Community Health at the University of Massachusetts Medical School, US. Prior to entering medicine, she studied medical and nutritional anthropology and worked in elementary and early childhood education. Laura's primary clinical setting is the Family Health Center of Worcester, where she serves as Assistant Education Director and practices and teaches woman- and family-centered primary care with a focus on reproductive health and care of the young family. She provides inpatient care for women and newborns at the University of Massachusetts Memorial Medical Center.

Nicole Todd, MD, is a Clinical Assistant Professor in Obstetrics and Gynaecology at the University of British Columbia. She completed a fellowship in Pediatric and Adolescent Gynaecology through the University of Ottawa and was a catalyst in the creation of subspecialty multidisciplinary clinics for complex contraception, thrombosis, and oncofertility. Nicole is a tireless advocate for at-risk youth and marginalized populations, and her clinical and research work focuses on providing high-quality reproductive and pregnancy care to these populations.

Angela Underhill, MSc, PhD(c), completed her Master of Science degree in the Family Relations and Human Development program at the University of Guelph, Canada, where she is now working toward her doctorate degree. She is a research coordinator for the Women and HIV Research Program at Women's College Hospital, Toronto, Canada, and a research associate of Re•Vision: The Centre for Art and Social Justice, Guelph, Canada. Angela is passionate about sexual and reproductive differences and related, critical feminist perspectives and community-based research approaches.

Colleen Varcoe, PhD, RN is a Professor in the School of Nursing at the University of British Columbia, Canada. Her research focuses on violence and inequity, with an emphasis on both structural and interpersonal violence. Her completed research includes studies of the risks and health effects of violence, including for rural and Indigenous women. Her current research includes studies to promote equity (including cultural safety, harm reduction, and trauma- and violence-informed care) in primary healthcare and emergency departments, and studies of health interventions for women who have experienced violence, most recently for Indigenous women.

Marisha N. Wickremsinhe, MSc, is a Research Associate at the Kennedy Institute of Ethics in Washington, DC, US.

1
WOMEN'S HEALTHCARE THROUGH A FEMINIST ETHICS LENS

Lori d'Agincourt-Canning and Carolyn Ells

This book is the result of the editors working for over 25 years combined as practicing healthcare ethicists, one in a women's hospital and the other in a tertiary hospital serving a culturally diverse population. It reflects ethical dilemmas seen in day-to-day practice, as well as conversations and debates held with other ethicists and health practitioners who share a passionate interest in women's healthcare. The collection also features the experiences of clinicians who are at the forefront in delivering care to women. In the past, clinicians—namely physicians—received well-deserved critique for paternalistic practices that medicalized women, undermined their autonomy, and ignored many of the health concerns women raised. Some of these practices continue. However, we are also seeing change for the better. From our vantage point in Canada, paternalistic practices are abating and there is greater interest in listening and responding to the experiences and needs of patients, including women. Though we have some ways to go, it is encouraging to see unequal power relations being challenged and imbalances becoming less extreme. Many clinicians are at the vanguard of addressing women's needs and serving the broader goals of social justice. Their contributions to women's healthcare, and understandings of what ethical care requires, are central to our book.

Bioethics has always had a lot to say about ethical issues related to women's reproductive capacities. Genome editing of eggs and embryos, uterine transplantation, sex selection, surrogacy and postmenopausal pregnancy are just some of the topics that garner attention today. Yet, bioethics has been slow to address the broader range of ethical issues pertaining to women's healthcare. Feminists have contributed much to bioethics theory and scholarship, including a steady broadening of the range of issues that ethically impact women's lives and healthcare. Feminists in clinical settings, or engaged with policy work, have demonstrated the usefulness of feminist approaches in these domains and have been undaunted by the complex realities that shape our societies. Yet, feminists could contribute so much more to women's healthcare. As ethicists and practitioners, we have to question what dominant discourses on women's healthcare leave out.

This book helps to address that gap by highlighting areas related to women's healthcare that have received little attention from bioethicists to date. We do not work alone. Collaboration among stakeholders is crucial for identifying, understanding, critiquing, and responding to ethical issues in women's healthcare. Women, particularly women who have been marginalized and practitioners involved with their care, are partners with us in this endeavor. Imagine what we can achieve together when we consider healthcare practices from the perspective of women seeking care for health needs important to them, or that they identify.

Indeed, many of the topics for this book emerged from conversations with clinical colleagues about ethical situations faced in practice. Some of these—ethical issues pertaining to care of refugees, female genital cosmetic surgery, and healthcare for sex workers—are decidedly absent from the bioethics and feminist ethics literature. Other chapters expand on topics previously discussed in the literature but yield new insights by addressing the clinical realities of these situations—such as a case-finding approach to women exposed to violence, gender and the human immunodeficiency virus (HIV), perinatal mental health, and the felt, moral agency of being an abortion provider. We also invited contributors who, through both clinical work and academic scholarship, contribute strategies toward improving women's health in the real world, particularly for those who are under-represented or marginalized (Indigenous women, rural women, queer women, and trans people). Recognizing that pregnancy and birth are still relevant to women's experiences, we asked other contributors to address ethical gaps they saw in practice (technology and reproductive care, infertility care for women with disabilities, research with pregnant women), each of which required addressing theory and policy as well.

The volume starts from the premise that gender is central to the evaluation of healthcare and healthcare practices. Feminist perspectives influenced our selection of topics for the book, but not all chapters are feminist in orientation. Recognizing that some readers will be new to feminist ethics, in this introduction we review a few themes that are central to this work and pertinent to the analyses in this book. These themes include relational components of moral life, justice and oppression, women-centered care, implications of sex and gender distinctions, and examining issues through an ethics lens.

Relational Components of Moral Life

One of the key contributions of feminist ethics has been to articulate the relational components of moral life and how these are affected by the social, political, and economic structures in which women live. Falling under the general umbrella of relational theories, these approaches acknowledge a more holistic conception of persons that highlights the importance and complexity of relationships and their impact on individuals' identities and choices. Relational theorists are attuned to the gendered distribution of power, which structures and impacts women's access to resources and opportunities, including healthcare.

There is a tendency in healthcare practice to reduce autonomy to informed consent and view it as a patient's free and informed choice, selected from a restricted set of options.[1] This formulation of the principle fails to recognize the crucial role that relationships play in shaping and exercising choice. Relational theorists reject the notions that individuals can be abstracted from their context and that choices are made in a social vacuum. Rather, feminist writings emphasize the interdependent and situated aspects of relational life, and their role in development and expression of autonomy. Relational autonomy emerges from the recognition that we are socially embedded and interdependent. Jennifer Nedelsky (2011) puts it this way:

> I see autonomy as the core of a capacity to engage in the ongoing, interactive creation of our selves—our relational selves, our selves that are constituted, yet not determined, by the web of nested relations within which we live ... Autonomy exists on a continuum. As we act (usually partially) autonomously, we are always in interaction with the relationships (intimate and social-structural) that enable our autonomy. Relations are then constitutive of autonomy rather than conditions for it.[2(p45-46)]

Relational theorists embrace an understanding of autonomy that is grounded in the complex experiences of relational life. Autonomy, they argue, is not simply a reflection of unencumbered choice but is constructed in and through complex networks of personal (intimate) relationships and social interactions. The choices and decisions we make are bound up with the choices and decisions of others. Thus, healthcare providers must become sensitive to the ways in which relationships affect who people are and the decisions they make.

In a related vein, feminist writings bring an awareness of the effects of class, ability, ethnicity, sexual orientation, and the intersections of these and other social determinants on the distribution of power and ultimately the choices available to women.[1,3] Feminist ethics parallels other forms of critical scholarship in that it embraces the view that issues pertaining to women's healthcare cannot be understood in isolation from the social and political structures of which medicine is a part. Women live in a world that (too often) presents constraints to their health as "natural" when they are due less to individual ill health than to established institutional structures and practices. Ideally, the structures of any given society would be equitable, creating systems that would allow anyone to access resources and derive benefits, including access to appropriate healthcare. Yet, structural determinants and institutional practices have served to oppress groups of people based on social or political identity. Feminist and critical theorists stress that healthcare disparities are not simply a reflection of individual circumstances. Rather, they are best understood as the outcome of (historically constructed) structural determinants that hinder or promote health through social, political, cultural, and economic systems. Deeply connected to racism, discrimination, and other inequitable social practices, systems and institutional structures create and recreate harms.

Justice and Oppression

Given these concerns, feminist theorists have pushed hard on the front of justice and social and political change. Iris Marion Young was one of the first philosophers to frame justice not in terms of resource distribution alone but instead in terms of broader social conditions. In a landmark essay entitled "Five Faces of Oppression," she proposes an "enabling" conception of justice that takes into account conditions necessary for "the development and exercise of individual capacities."[4(p39)] She asserts that oppression is a "structural concept"[4(p40)] that places restrictions on social groups in five distinct ways: exploitation, marginalization, powerlessness, cultural imperialism (the culture and experience of a dominant group is taken to be the norm), and violence. Young acknowledges that within social groups who experience oppression, not all are oppressed in the same way or to the same degree. She uses this analysis to identify how injustice becomes embedded in political and social structures, systematically excluding and limiting life opportunities and courses of action open to those who are oppressed. According to her approach, the goal of justice would be to prevent social conditions that interfere with people developing and exercising their capacities.

Feminists referring to "oppression" often have in mind one or more of the five distinct "faces" of oppression that Young identified. Acting to end sexist oppression is a central commitment of feminist movements. Yet, recognizing that oppression does not always have a sexist motivation, many feminists are broad in their commitment to look at and end oppression in all its forms and all its motivations (including sexism, racism, ableism, and classism).

Drawing on the experience of people with disabilities, Elizabeth Purcell[5] proposes three additional forms of systematic oppression: stigma (a social misrepresentation and devaluing of people through stereotypes), questioned personhood (the dignity and value of human life is assumed to be based on an individual's capacities, rather than on being human), and societal incapacity (physical and learning environments privilege "able" bodies and "dis-able" others). Purcell raises the concern that these additional forms of oppression are not easily addressed in models of justice oriented around "primary goods" or "material needs." Accordingly, she suggests a role for innovation in theorizing about the relation of justice and oppression. Stigma, in particular, is a theme that emerges and reemerges throughout this collection, causing significant hardship for many women (see Chapters 6, 8, 9, 10, and 11). Questioned personhood (see Chapters 7 and 9) and societal incapacity (see Chapters 9 and 13) are also reflected in the collection, suggesting that these forms of oppression may extend beyond the experience of people with disabilities, and may supplement the five forms of oppression described by Young.

In a similar vein, scholars and advocates from a variety of disciplines have developed a deeper understanding of structural violence and its relation to health and social justice.[6-9] Their work, like Young's, emphasizes the need to shift moral focus away from isolated acts or choices of individuals to evaluation of the context and systems shaping such acts. In population and global health, structural violence is understood as a major cause of social and health inequities. It refers to disadvantage and health disparities that arise from policies, institutional practices, and social arrangements that are innately unjust.[7] "The arrangements are structural because they are embedded in the political and economic organization of our social world; they are violent because they cause injury to people."[7(p1686)]

Farmer and colleagues[7] critique clinical medicine for taking a predominantly biomolecular approach to illness. They argue that scientific inquiry tends to ask mainly biological questions about phenomena that are far more complex in nature. Indeed, treatment effectiveness—both in individuals and populations—is shaped by social and environmental factors such as poverty, gender inequality, racism, and pollution, not by biological factors alone. These authors use HIV as a compelling example of how structural violence becomes embodied as excess mortality and premature death in socially disadvantaged groups. Like Young, Farmer and colleagues call on practitioners to recognize the connections between social, economic, and political factors and health inequalities. Thus, what relational theorists and those interested in structural violence have in common is a commitment to frame ethical problems and their redress in a form that is avowedly contextual and systems-based.

Woman-Centered Care

The importance of relational features of people's lives is becoming more apparent in healthcare policy and practice, including in the widely endorsed ideal of patient-centered care. The Institute of Medicine (IOM) defines patient-centered care as "providing care that is respectful of and responsive to individual patient preferences, needs and values and ensuring that patient values guide all clinical decisions."[10] Although the IOM did not originate the concept of patient-centered care, by presenting it in a major guidance document as essential to quality care, healthcare institutions and health professions in the United States and beyond took note. Recognizing that structural- and institutional-level practices contribute to quality individualized patient care, patient-centered care gives prominence to the setting within which healthcare is provided, the policies that guide practices, actual patient experiences to guide evaluation of programs, as well as a clinical method that puts the patient at the center of individualized care planning, in partnership with health professionals. Bioethics scholars are beginning to contribute an ethics perspective to theorizing about patient-centered care and its implications.[11,12] It has been argued that relational autonomy is an essential component of patient-centered care.[13]

Where the healthcare in question is specific to women, we can speak specifically of "woman-centered care." Using this term acknowledges that there are features of being a woman that merit specific attention when individualizing care, and structuring health systems and institutional environments, to be responsive to the specific needs, interests, and values of patients who are women.

Currently, those advocating and implementing woman-centered care typically consider it with respect to prenatal care, sexual and reproductive health, and women's rights as they affect these areas of healthcare.[14,15] See Chapter 12 of this book for key features of this model and an example of how women-centered clinicians use it to guide, in this case, ethical techno-maternity care. See Chapter 6 to learn about how a group of Canadian researchers, clinicians, and women living with HIV are collaborating to develop and operationalize a model of women-centered HIV care. Women's healthcare considered broadly could learn much from these approaches.

We propose that adopting a conception of women-centered care that mirrors the breadth of patient-centered care may have merit in guiding and critiquing women's healthcare across the full range of healthcare that women seek. Perhaps this book could be a test of this idea. As we turn our critical ethics lens to the healthcare needs, interests, and values of women who are situated differently in our communities, women who are socially marginalized, and women whose sex or gender has (unmet) implications for the healthcare they seek, let us consider the patient at the center of, and in partnership with, her circle of care as a woman, with her own particular relational reality shaping her identity, experiences, responsibilities, and vulnerabilities. What would the ideal model of care be for this woman, each woman?

As observed elsewhere, women are the main users of healthcare.[16] Even when they are not themselves patients, women frequently make decisions about others' use of healthcare based on their role as mothers, daughters, friends, and intimate partners. Women are also relied on for successful continuity of care and patient navigation within healthcare systems and institutions, both for their loved ones and for themselves. Taking an explicitly woman-centered perspective of the main users of healthcare would include taking these roles and responsibilities into account to develop and facilitate best practices.

Sex and Gender Distinctions Have Implications for Women's Healthcare

"Sex" and "gender" have distinct meanings, although they are often confused. Lack of clarity in how these terms are understood, used, and measured results in missed opportunities to understand and improve health in women, men, and gender-diverse people. "Sex" refers to a set of biological attributes, including reproductive/sexual anatomy, hormone levels, chromosomes, and gene expression, and how they function. Often categorized by the two poles of "female" and "male," there is a spectrum of variation in the physical, physiological, and genetic attributes of sex.[17]

"Gender" refers to the "socially constructed roles, behaviours, expressions and identities of girls, women, boys, men, and gender diverse people."[17(n.p.)] As a psychosocial construct, gender influences how people perceive themselves and each other, how they act and interact, and the distribution of power and resources in society. Beyond the binaries of girl/woman and boy/man, there is considerable diversity in how individuals and groups understand, experience, and express gender.[17]

It is now widely acknowledged that the distinctions between "sex" and "gender" matter in healthcare, health research, and other domains. Especially with respect to sex differences, evidence has undermined assumptions that what is learned about males can be generalized to females. Regarding drug safety for example, in 2001 the US General Accounting Office reported that most drugs withdrawn from the US market between 1997 and 2000 had greater health risks for women than for men.[18] Not long after, the US Food and Drug Administration issued a safety warning to cut the dose of anti-insomnia drugs containing zolpidem in half for women. It was determined that the drug is eliminated more slowly from women's bodies than men's and that women are more susceptible to next-morning impairment than men.[19] This was the first time a regulatory agency recommended lowering a dosage for women for a drug already on the market. Other agencies followed. A telling example from preclinical chronic pain research reveals that male and female mice have different pain pathways (i.e., hypersensitivity is mediated by microglial cells in male mice and by T cells in female mice).[20] The implications are stunning: male mice should not serve as proxies for female mice in research where sex distinctions matter. The same implications extend to research involving human and non-human animal cells.

It is important (both scientifically and ethically) to take sex and gender into account in research that involves, or applies to, humans. Though sex differences in health research have gained attention in recent years, research that focuses on gender and the impact of gender on health has not kept pace. This is an area of research that requires redress.

Thanks to an international effort led by the Gender Policy Committee of the European Association of Science Editors, we now have an excellent resource in the "Sex and Gender Equity in Research (SAGER) Guidelines" to elevate the quality of reporting sex and gender information in study design, data analyses, results, and interpretation of findings.[21] These guidelines apply to all research with humans, animals, or materials originating from humans or animals, and disciplines whose results will be applied to humans (e.g., engineering, mechanics).[21]

For further parsing of the concepts of "sex" and "gender" and a critical reflection on biases and assumptions of what is "normal," see Chapter 9, where this leads to recommendations for providing quality care to queer women and trans people. For discussion about how gendered social structures and norms, including behavior expectations of women and men, create the foundation and justification for violence against women, see Chapter 7. For a sobering review of the pernicious healthcare consequences of avoiding research with pregnant women, and systemic and scientific challenges to overcome this evidence gap, see Chapter 14.

Ethical Analysis

This introduction provides some background context for ethical reflection and analysis about issues in women's healthcare. We draw on themes and approaches common to feminist ethics. At the same time, it is important to acknowledge that other ethics theories have relevance for addressing ethical issues in women's healthcare. These include the "four principles" approach of Beauchamp and Childress, utilitarianism, virtue ethics, ethics of care, and narrative ethics, to name a few. Ethics theories (and ethics scholarship more broadly) can help to explore deeper nuances and complexity of real-world issues. They can be used to help distinguish features of an issue under consideration, the values at stake, and potential processes to support ethical action. In bioethics, we need theories that are informed by the real world and that can have application in the real world.[22] They help us to assess issues from different perspectives, thereby gaining both breadth and depth in our analyses. See Chapter 6 of this book for an example of how one theory (feminist theory) can inform new conceptions of important concepts (specific principles) that are more prominent in another theory (the four principles approach).

Likewise, we recognize that ethics is not solely the domain of philosophers. Its practitioners come from a variety of disciplinary backgrounds—clinical, academic, and the lay public.[23] Ethical problems in women's health arise everywhere. Drawing from Ruth Behar's comments about ethnography, for feminist bioethics to matter in a multicultural world, "it needs to reach a wider range of audiences both in and beyond the academy."[24(p21)] As such, ethical analysis is informed by and benefits from multiple and diverse perspectives.

Chapter Overviews

Recognizing that attention to women's health often focuses on issues of reproduction, this book expands discussions of women's healthcare to topics that include but go beyond reproduction. Most importantly, it brings voices from clinical practice (voices of patients, health professionals, and ethics consultants) together with those of academic researchers to reflect on the diverse realities of women's lives and their implications for healthcare. Contributors take seriously the multilayered aspects of relationality as a means of understanding women's health and the need to push forward and contextualize these concepts to identify gaps and possible solutions. In doing so, contributors bring greater attention in particular to socially marginalized groups of women.

Subsequent chapters are divided into three sections, each of which challenge readers to reflect on the intersections between ethics, healthcare, social practices, institutional structures, and policy.

The impact on access to healthcare of attachment to place and culture, or of being displaced from one's community or country of origin, is the dominant theme running through Section I, *Locations, Migrations, and Access to Healthcare*.

In Chapter 2, "Indigenous Women, Health, and Healthcare," Indigenous scholar Charlotte Loppie and ally Alexandra Kent address an area that remains largely under-represented in the feminist ethics literature: the historical and contemporary impact of colonial forces upon the health of Indigenous women and peoples. Integrating Indigenous approaches with the social determinants of health, the *Xpey' Relational Environments Framework* serves as a model for exploring Indigenous women's encounters in healthcare, including the relational, systemic, and structural contexts that shape these encounters. The authors critically examine how complex jurisdictional inequities, culturally unsafe environments, and gendered racial discrimination form a toxic milieu in which Indigenous women must attempt to access care for themselves and their families. Using the metaphor of a tree to describe the relationships between different environments, they describe strategies aimed to enhance wellness and Indigenous health equity at these different levels. This chapter yields key insights into the marginalizing influences that mainstream structures and institutions continue to have on Indigenous people.

Many of these learnings extend into Chapter 3, "Caring for Refugees, New Immigrants, and Uninsured Women: Social Responsibility and Access to Healthcare." Strangely, bioethicists have largely stayed silent about this issue, despite the growth in asylum seeker and migrant numbers globally.

Here, Paul Caulford and Sumathy Rahunathan consider ethical, legal, political, and healthcare perspectives related to care of women who are refugees, new immigrants, or uninsured. A high proportion of new women to Canada are pregnant, without antenatal care access. Access to sexual health screening, preventive care, and health literacy opportunities is also problematic. Drawing from their experiences providing and advocating for healthcare for these populations, they argue that even in a country like Canada with a "universal" public healthcare system and a public commitment to opening its doors to refugees and immigrants, inconsistent and fragmented policies leave large gaps in healthcare access for refugees and immigrant women. These, in turn, result in harms to the health, safety, and potential life opportunities for women new to the country. In revealing these gaps through poignant case studies, the authors insist that healthcare access must become a central part of the broader conversation on social responsibility to refugees, women, and their families.

In Chapter 4, "Rural Women: Place, Community, and Accessing Healthcare," Christy Simpson and Fiona McDonald focus on ethics and healthcare access for rural women, a group who may face a "double disadvantage" due to their gender and rural place of residence. A critique of feminist bioethics has been that it represents mainly the interests of white, educated Western (urban-based) women, neglecting the viewpoints of those who occupy different social or minority locations.[25-27] As a counterpoint to these concerns, Simpson and McDonald urge readers to think about the effects of geographic location on healthcare for women. They draw from their earlier work on rural health ethics to argue that gendered and place constructions of "good" rural women can create stereotypes, which have positive and negative implications for rural women and rural communities more generally. They examine the ways in which rural women's access to health services involve multiple dimensions, including availability, affordability, accessibility, acceptability, and accommodation. Their insights into gendered and place constructions of women's roles, together with values of place, have importance in shaping the design and delivery of health services to rural communities.

In Section II, contributors consider several distinctive *New and Emerging Themes* in women's healthcare that deserve greater attention in bioethics and clinical practice. Themes of ethics, practice, and policy flow through each chapter. Some chapters focus their issue on clinical practice and draw on theory or policy and/or empirical research to critique and make recommendations. Other chapters highlight some aspect of ethical theory or policy, and then show how their work relates to certain practices.

In Chapter 5, "Drivers and Dilemmas of Female Genital Cosmetic Surgery" (FGCS), Dorothy Shaw and Nicole Todd demonstrate that there is considerable pressure for FGCS, which raises complex ethical issues that are under-described in the bioethics literature and in medical training. The increasing requests for such cosmetic procedures by women occur in a context of lack of knowledge of normal anatomic variation and sexual response. Shaw and Todd review ethical concerns regarding informed consent, autonomy, and beneficence, as well as conflicts of interest pertaining to these surgeries. Critiquing cultural and social "norms" regarding female genital appearance, they argue that an ethical approach to FGCS requires much more than naively agreeing to a request for surgery on the basis of personal autonomy.

In Chapter 6, "Ethical Issues in the Care and Support of Women Living with HIV," Ruby Shanker, Angela Underhill, Valerie Nicholson, Logan Kennedy, Denise Jaworsky, and Mona Loutfy reflect on the intersection between social and structural determinants, gender, and policy when exploring ethical issues related to HIV care. They add an unusual level of complexity to our understanding by describing ethical issues encountered by women living with HIV not at one point in time but across the lifespan, from prepubescence and adolescence, to youth and midlife, to older years. Critical to their analysis are the reflections and experiences of a woman living with HIV, who, as a peer research associate and knowledge keeper, and through her Indigenous identity, lends crucial insight to the discourse. The authors draw on both principle-based theory and feminist ethics to explore the ethical challenges related to HIV disclosure, treatment adherence, pregnancy and breastfeeding, and health issues associated with aging. Importantly, this chapter offers a model of how collaborative texts can be created when community members join with clinicians and academic voices to explore ethical issues affecting their health.

Ethical issues involved in providing healthcare to women who have experienced intimate partner violence or sexual assault is the theme of Chapter 7, "Ethical Issues in Healthcare for Women in the Context of Violence." Challenging individualistic approaches that frame most responses to violence against women, authors Rochelle Einboden and Colleen Varcoe place the intersecting themes of ethics, policy, and practice at the center of their analysis. Such an analysis includes attention to context, power relations within which women live and within which healthcare is provided, and the structural conditions of women's lives. The authors also address the complex ethical issues that must be considered when children witness violence against their mothers. Recognizing that current healthcare approaches to violence may actually disenfranchise women experiencing violence, these authors advocate for "case finding" instead of routine screening, and culturally safe and trauma- and violence-informed care for women.

Working empirically with participants rather than with abstract considerations, Victoria Bungay and Lauren Casey address a rarely mentioned issue, that of barriers to healthcare for women engaged in consensual sex work. Many of those who work in the sex industry experience serious health problems, including violence, mental illness, sexually transmitted infections, and HIV. Yet, as seen in Chapter 8, "Sex Work, Ethics, and Healthcare," these women tell harrowing stories of disrespect when seeking healthcare. Understanding risk factors predisposing women to sex work, as well as risk factors and health issues associated with sex work itself, requires a focus on structural conditions and contextual factors of race, gender, and class. As one of several chapters to draw attention to stigma, Bungay and Casey show how stigma normalizes violence against sex workers at a structural level to the extent it becomes embedded in systems and practices, including the larger healthcare system. Presenting results from qualitative research, and the voices of women engaged in sex work, their chapter illustrates that stigma and devaluation create the foundation of access barriers, as well as lead to neglect of sex workers by healthcare providers. The chapter closes with evidence-informed recommendations that are women-centered and support sex workers' active engagement in health policy, programming, and health practices that affect their everyday life.

Erin Fredericks and Kelly Baker also engage with the theme of stigma in Chapter 9, "Primary Health Care for Queer Women and Trans People: Confronting Heteronormativity and Cisnormativity." Drawing on social science research, they argue that healthcare provision for these patients must be approached with an understanding of how healthcare has contributed to the systematic and historical oppression that queer women and trans people have experienced. They show how the clinic environment, as well as interactions with health providers and clinic staff, often institutionalizes heterosexuality and being cisgender (i.e., one's gender identity corresponds with one's sex assigned at birth) as the "norm" and implies that queer and trans people are "abnormal," which contributes to their erasure and to discrimination and stigma. The authors provide concrete suggestions (structural and relational) for how primary care providers can make their clinics and practices more welcoming and safer for these patients, and how they can build more trusting patient–provider relationships with them, thereby increasing access to quality healthcare for this community. Readers familiar with patient-centered care and with professional codes of ethics and standards for ethical practice (including need for humility, importance of trust, and other factors in fostering and sustaining a therapeutic relationship) will see how these ethical commitments align with this social science analysis. Likewise, although the authors do not explicitly connect their analysis to ethics, readers are encouraged to consider the analysis in this chapter in light of ethics concepts and discussions in other chapters (e.g., relational ethics, primary care in rural settings and with other women facing oppression).

Section III, *Reproductive Healthcare*, focuses on ethical issues relevant to pregnancy and birth. Authors address important themes previously identified as well as have us confront issues in women's healthcare that many prefer to avoid. They encourage readers to think about the effects of stigma on some women's reproductive healthcare, and on the conscientious provision of stigmatized care. The values, prejudices, policies, and practices of our larger society are ever-present in this final section of the book. We are reminded that the quality and availability of women's reproductive care are deeply and troublingly affected by social conditions.

Lisa Harris takes up another issue that is rarely addressed in bioethics, that of the lived experience and moral agency of being an abortion provider. In Chapter 10, "The Moral Agency of Abortion Providers: Conscientious Provision, Dangertalk, and the Lived Experience of Doing Stigmatized Work," Harris draws from research and her own experiences to explore the nuances of how caregivers make decisions to provide or not provide abortion care. She critiques bioethics for its narrow focus on conscientious objection, highlighting instead the moral agency of caregivers who engage in the conscientious *provision* of stigmatized services. Harris also takes up the problem of pro-choice/pro-life rhetoric. She broadens our understanding of the lived experience of being an abortion provider to include openness to the moral ambiguities and complexities of abortion. The ability to hold this "tension of opposites," she argues, may provide a model for civic engagement on a number of contested issues.

Chapter 11, "Perinatal Mental Health: The Lens of Relational Ethics," provides a discussion of ethical concerns pertaining to the treatment of pregnant women and new mothers with mental illness. Lori d'Agincourt-Canning and Deirdre Ryan apply feminist relational theory to provide unique perspectives on current issues in maternal reproductive mental health. They reject traditional bioethics analyses, which have treated mother and fetus as two separate beings, and argue instead that the interests and well-being of mother and fetus are intimately intertwined. The authors also highlight how

5. Purcell E. Oppression's three new faces: rethinking Iris Young's "Five Faces of Oppression" for disability theory. In: Seth N, Asumah SN, Nagel M, eds. *Diversity, Social Justice, and Inclusive Excellence*. Albany: SUNY Press; 2014:185–205.
6. Farmer P. Medicine and social justice. *America*. 1995;173(2):13–17.
7. Farmer P, Nizeye B, Stulac S, Keshavjee S. Structural violence and clinical medicine. *PLoS Med*. 2006;3(10):1686–1691.
8. Taylor S. Structural violence, oppression, and the place-based marginality of homelessness. *Can Soc Work Rev*. 2013;30(2):255–273.
9. Browne AJ, Varcoe C, Lavoie J, et al. Enhancing health care equity with Indigenous populations: evidence-based strategies from an ethnographic study. *BMC Health Serv Res*. 2016;16(544):1–17.
10. IOM Committee on Quality of Health Care in America, Institute of Medicine. *Crossing the Quality Chasm: A New Health System for the 21st Century*. Washington, DC: The National Academies Press; 2001. https://doi.org/10.17226/10027. Accessed March 27, 2018.
11. Clarke S, Ells C, Thombs B, Clarke D. Defining elements of patient-centered care for therapeutic relationships: a literature review of common themes. *Eur J Pers Cent Healthc*. 2017;5(3):362–372.
12. Hunt MR, Ells C. A patient-centered care ethics analysis model for rehabilitation. *Am J Phys Med Rehab*. 2013;92(9):818–827.
13. Ells C, Hunt MR, Chambers-Evans J. Relational autonomy as an essential component of patient-centered care. *Int J Fem Approaches Bioeth*. 2011;4(2):79–101.
14. World Health Organization's consolidated guideline on sexual and reproductive health and rights of women living with HIV. http://www.who.int/reproductivehealth/publications/gender_rights/Ex-Summ-srhr-women-hiv/en/. Published in 2017. Accessed March 27, 2018.
15. Shields SG, Candib LM, eds. *Woman-Centered Care of Pregnancy and Birth*. Oxford: Radcliffe Medical Press; 2010.
16. Wolf SM. *Feminism and Bioethics: Beyond Reproduction*. New York: Oxford University Press; 1996.
17. Canadian Institutes of Health Research. What is gender? What is sex? http://www.cihr-irsc.gc.ca/e/48642.html. Modified October 30, 2014. Accessed March 27, 2018.
18. GAO-01-286R Drug Safety: Most Drugs Withdrawn in Recent Years Had Greater Health Risks for Women. United States General Accounting Office. Washington DC; January 19, 2001. https://www.gao.gov/assets/100/90642.pdf. Accessed March 27, 2018.
19. FDA. Questions and Answers: Risk of next-morning impairment after use of insomnia drugs; FDA requires lower recommended doses for certain drugs containing zolpidem (Ambien, Ambien CR, Edluar, and Zolpimist); 2013. https://www.fda.gov/Drugs/DrugSafety/ucm334041.htm#q10. Updated February 13, 2018. Accessed March 27, 2018.

20. Sorge RE, Mapplebeck JCS, Rosen S, et al. Different immune cells mediate mechanical pain hypersensitivity in male and female mice. *Nat Neurosci*. 2015 Aug;18(8):1081–1083.
21. Heidari S, Babor TF, De Castro P, Tort S, Curno M. Sex and Gender Equity in Research: rationale for the SAGER guidelines and recommended use. *Res Integr Peer Rev*. 2016;1(2):1–9.
22. Benjamin M. Between subway and spaceship: practical ethics at the outset of the twenty-first century. *Hastings Cent Rep*. 2001;31(4):24–31.
23. Scully J, Banks S, Shakespeare T. Chance, choice and control: lay debate on prenatal social selection. *Soc Sci Med*. 2006;63:21–31.
24. Behar R. Introduction: out of exile. In: Behar R, Gordon DA. *Women Writing Culture*. Berkeley: University of California Press; 1995:21.
25. Lugones M, Spelman E. Have we got a theory for you! Feminist theory, cultural imperialism, and the demand for "the women's voice." *Women's Stud Int Forum*. 1983;6(6):573–581.
26. Collins PH. *Black Feminist Thought: Knowledge, Consciousness, and the Politics of Empowerment*. New York: Routledge.
27. Fitzpatrick P, Scully JL. Introduction to feminist bioethics. In: Scully JL, Baldwin-Ragaven L, Fitzpatrick P. *Feminist Bioethics: At the Center, On the Margins*. Baltimore, MD: Johns Hopkins University Press; 2010:1–10.

LOCATIONS, MIGRATIONS, AND ACCESS TO HEALTHCARE

2 INDIGENOUS WOMEN, HEALTH, AND HEALTHCARE

Charlotte Loppie and Alexandra Kent

Introduction

Within the Canadian healthcare context, Indigenous women encounter relational, systemic, and structural environments, the characteristics of which can support as well as undermine their wellness and capacity to obtain essential services. Several authors have explored the healthcare experiences of Indigenous peoples generally[1-3] and Indigenous women specifically.[4,5] Yet, the majority of these studies focus on face-to-face encounters between healthcare providers and Indigenous people, with relatively few focusing on the diverse contexts that shape these encounters. The *Xpey' Relational Environments Framework* serves as a model for exploring Indigenous women's encounters in healthcare, as it facilitates identification of key opportunities and challenges within relational, systemic, and structural environments.

Indigenous Peoples and Cultures

Globally, there are more than 370 million Indigenous peoples,[6] who hold ancestral connections to lands, languages, and cultural traditions. Within the Canadian context, the term *Aboriginal* is often used to represent Inuit, Métis, and First Nations peoples,[7] who are culturally distinct from one another but share a common experience of colonization, land dispossession, and colonial oppression.[8] The term Aboriginal was included in the Constitution Act of Canada (Section 35, 2)[9] devoid of prior consultation with Indigenous peoples. More recently and with increasing frequency, the term *Indigenous* is being used as a more inclusive term to refer to First Peoples. Across Canada, Indigenous cultures, languages, and practices are as diverse as any throughout the world (e.g., Europe, Africa, South America) and are likewise shaped by the traditional territories upon which specific Indigenous peoples have historically lived.

Indigenous worldviews conceptualize health holistically, encompassing mental, physical, spiritual, and emotional dimensions,[10] so that wellness and illness are not viewed as necessarily opposing or purely physiological phenomena. Balance is sought among multiple dimensions as well as within individuals, families, communities, and nations, which are also considered integrally connected to one another and to the natural world. The social, economic, political, historical, cultural, and medical contexts within which Indigenous women experience healthcare, as well as the substance and quality of their relationships with care providers, settings, institutions, and policies, shape the degree to which they are able to maintain wellness and balance.[11]

Indigenous Women's Health and Wellness

The lived experiences of Indigenous women are conspicuously absent from the historical record. As well, in the not-too-distant past, health literature tended to describe "Indigenous health" in isolation of gender—assuming the same reality for men and women. Where it does exist, literature on the health of Indigenous women tends to concentrate on a disproportionate burden of illnesses or social disadvantage, leading to poor health. While these statistics paint a grim and often misleading picture, it is nevertheless important to understand the health issues facing Indigenous women, as these issues often prompt individuals to engage with healthcare environments.

According to the *First Nations Regional Health Survey*, among First Nations women, the most pressing health concerns, in descending order, include diabetes, allergies, arthritis, and osteoporosis. Just over 50% of First Nations women report at least one chronic health condition, 20% of whom report having more than four.[12] Among Métis women, the most commonly reported chronic health conditions, in descending order, include arthritis, high blood pressure, asthma, stomach problems or intestinal ulcers, and diabetes. Four percent of Métis women report being diagnosed with a chronic condition, 28% of whom report two or more.[13] Among Inuit women the chronic conditions most commonly reported, in descending order, include high blood pressure, arthritis, asthma, mood disorders, and diabetes. Thirty-seven percent of Inuit women report chronic health conditions, half of those with one condition, 26% with two, and 25% with three or more.[12]

Among First Nations and Métis women, Pap testing rates are similar to that of non-Indigenous women, irrespective of age; however, Pap testing rates are lower among Inuit women. Among Métis women over 40, 74% have received a breast exam and 86% (age 50 to 69) have had a mammogram, while First Nations and Inuit women have lower rates of breast self-examination and mammography screening. Indigenous people represent over 4% of the Canadian population yet make up 8% of all existing human immunodeficiency virus (HIV) infections and 12.5% of all new infections. Indigenous women account for 50% of HIV infections among Indigenous people in Canada, with the highest rate increases among women age 15 to 29.[12]

External stressors represent a substantial health challenge for Indigenous women. Low socioeconomic status and experiences of racism have been associated with moderate to high distress among First Nations and Inuit women.[12] Additionally, Indigenous women 15 years and older are 3.5 times more likely to experience violence than non-Indigenous women. Homicide rates among Indigenous women are also disproportionately high, and Indigenous women account for the majority of missing and murdered women in Canada.[12]

The most recent National Household Survey (NHS) reports the birth rate among Indigenous women as 2.2 children per woman, compared with 1.6 children for non-Indigenous women.[14] Research also indicates that Indigenous women experience higher rates of problematic birth outcomes (e.g., stillbirth, preterm birth), which are linked to gestational diabetes and lack of adequate prenatal care.[15] These statistics suggest that Indigenous women are engaging with perinatal health providers more often and in more extreme circumstances.

The NHS also reports that Indigenous children represent 28% of the Indigenous population, while non-Indigenous children represent 16.5% of that population.[14] About 35% of Indigenous children live in a lone-parent (mostly mothers) family, compared to 17.5% of non-Indigenous children.[14] Sheppard and colleagues also report that Indigenous mothers tend to be younger, unmarried, and less likely to have attended university.[15] These demographics indicate that Indigenous women are caring for more children, and younger children, and are often shouldering this responsibility alone, at a younger age and in conditions of low income.[16]

The cultural and structural barriers to accessing formal care, particularly for Indigenous elders, often means that the responsibility for informal caregiving is left to Indigenous mothers, daughters, sisters, and aunts, many of whom are also caring for children and/or grandchildren. With over half of First Nations women living off reserve, while a higher proportion of the elderly still live on reserve,[13] women are often traveling to engage in these caregiving responsibilities.

Context of Indigenous Women's Health and Wellness

The physical, emotional, mental, and spiritual wellness of Indigenous women is influenced by a range of determinants beyond lifestyle behaviors, including relationships and interactions with family, community, the environment, and society. The World Health Organization (WHO) describes these social determinants of health as

> the conditions in which people are born, grow, live, work and age . . . shaped by the distribution of money, power and resources at global, national and local levels. The social determinants of health are mostly responsible for health inequities—the unfair and avoidable differences in health status seen within and between countries.[17(n.p.)]

Several decades of research clearly links wellness to socioeconomic status, demonstrating that people with the most resources experience the best health.[16,18] Due to ongoing colonial forces,

> Aboriginal [Indigenous] people are at the bottom of almost every available index of socioeconomic well-being [, including] educational levels, employment opportunities, housing conditions, per capita incomes or any of the other conditions that give non-Indigenous Canadians one of the highest standards of living in the world.[8]

Poverty not only creates barriers to meeting basic needs,[19] but it also hinders one's capacity to address health issues when they arise. These challenges have immediate impacts on health as well as cumulative effects on wellness over the lifespan.[20]

Making the Connections: Xpey' Relational Environments

Informed by the WHO framework for social determinants of health,[21] along with critical Indigenous theory,[22] Indigenous researchers Drs. Charlotte Loppie and Jeannine Carriere developed an Indigenous relational framework to facilitate exploration of immediate, systemic, and structural environments within healthcare.[23] The framework is adapted from a tree

Indigenous Women • 25

metaphor previously developed by Loppie to represent proximal, intermediate, and distal determinants of Indigenous health.[20] After consultation with Shauna Underwood, Indigenous Advisor at the University of Victoria, the Hul'q'umi'num term *Xpey'*—meaning western red cedar—was adopted for its cultural significance as a sacred medicine. While not distinct to Indigenous cultures, the tree metaphor offers a holistic and interconnected model:

> We typically think of trees as possessing three interconnected elements: the crown (leaves and branches), the trunk, and the roots. Each part of the tree is dependent not only upon the other parts for sustenance and support, but also upon the environment that nourishes and sometimes damages them.[24(p4)]

Within the Xpey' framework, relational environments are conceptualized as the three elements of the tree: stem, core, and roots (Xpey' Relational Framework Fig. 2.1). Stem environments represent explicit and direct relationships and conditions,[24] such as interpersonal encounters between nurses and patients. Having a more tacit effect, core environments represent the bureaucracies within which Indigenous peoples access care, including local systems, healthcare management and leadership, arrangement of authorities, as well as institutional policies. Finally, root environments represent the historical, political, social, and cultural structures from which all

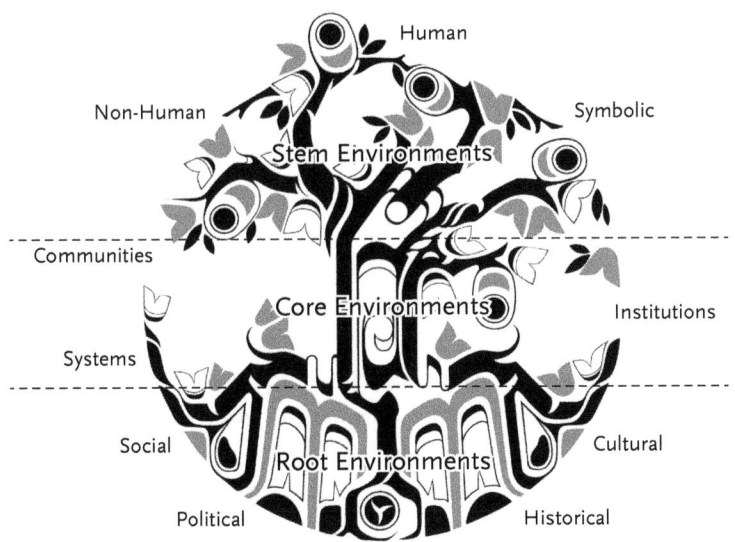

FIGURE 2.1 Xpey' Relational Framework

other environments evolve.[20] Loppie explains, "Just as maladies observed in the leaves are generally not the cause of unhealthy trees, inequities in human health frequently result from corruption or deficiencies in the unseen but critical root system."[24(p5)] Within Indigenous contexts, these roots might also be represented by historical and intergenerational experiences, political and social relationships, as well as cultural connections.

Stem Environments

Stem environments represent human interactions as well as non-human settings and symbols that can have a direct and immediate impact on individuals' wellness. Perhaps the most powerful stem environments are the encounters and relationships between Indigenous clients and care providers, which are shaped by cultural perspectives and social positions, including racialization. In this section, we will explore stem environments that might be considered toxic to Indigenous wellness as well as those that can nurture wellness.

Toxic Stem Environments

According to the *First Nations Regional Health Survey* (2008–2010), approximately one-third of all First Nations adults reported experiencing at least one instance of racism in the past 12 months.[12] Although there have been no national Canadian surveys that directly report on racism against Métis and Inuit peoples, research reveals experiences of racism within these populations.[25] In the context of healthcare, racism can critically influence the provision of services to Indigenous peoples.[26] In some cases, Indigenous patients are covertly rendered invisible through neglect, as analyses of health database reveal that Indigenous people receive fewer referrals to specialists.[27,28] In other cases, overt discrimination and disempowerment is practiced, as Indigenous people describe longer wait times as well as outright dismissal and disrespect in clinical settings.[29] Indigenous women seeking cancer care and HIV treatment likewise report inequities in their access to appropriate treatment as well as psychosocial support.[30–33]

The term *cultural safety* is increasingly being used to indicate the degree to which racialized discrimination is evident in healthcare. Cultural safety is "an environment . . . [that] is spiritually, socially and emotionally safe, as well as physically safe for people; where there is no assault challenge or denial of their identity, of who they are and what they need. It is about shared respect, shared meaning, shared knowledge and experience of learning together."[34(p213)]

Healthcare encounters can only be deemed "culturally safe" by the recipients of care, based on their experience.

Despite the diversity of Indigenous peoples and cultures, many non-Indigenous Canadians continue to erroneously presume a single "pan-Indigenous" experience. Within the context of healthcare, this misunderstanding can detrimentally impact patient–provider relationships as well as clinical practice. In particular, Indigenous-focused stereotyping (e.g., alcohol and drug addiction, unemployment, and violence) by health professionals undoubtedly hinders the development of healthy relationships.[35-37] For example, health and social service providers are often uninformed about the high rate of alcohol *abstinence* among Indigenous peoples. They are likewise unaware that high incidences of problematic drug and alcohol use occur among a relatively small number of Indigenous people. Consequently, in emergency departments, Indigenous people are often assumed to be "under the influence" of drugs or alcohol when seeking care.[38] Such stigmatizing stereotypes, which operate in subtle and overt, but often unquestioned, ways in the discourse and practice of providers, can create overwhelming barriers to accessing health services for Indigenous peoples.

In the case of Indigenous women, how they are treated by healthcare providers is central to their perceptions of clinical encounters,[26] particularly with respect to trust in healthcare professionals and clinical practices.[39] Trust is eroded when Indigenous women face racist assumptions about drug and alcohol abuse, irresponsible sexual activity, and lack of adherence to treatment regimens.[31,32,40] Among Indigenous mothers, fear that these assumptions might lead to child apprehension can deter them from seeking healthcare for themselves.[5] Indeed, multiple forms of racism are so pervasive within healthcare that Indigenous people typically feel compelled to develop strategies to navigate toxic relational environments or avoid seeking care entirely.[41]

Nurturing Stem Environments

By virtue of the disproportionate burden of illness and comorbidities experienced by Indigenous peoples,[20] the necessity for encounters with healthcare providers is multiplied, and thus the need for culturally safe and responsive care is critical. Nurturing stem environments are composed of individuals who are well informed about the social determinants of First Nations, Inuit, and Métis peoples' health;[42] who possess an empathic understanding of how colonization, colonialism, and residential schools have contributed to health inequities; and whose practice aligns with the recommendations of the Truth and Reconciliation Commission (TRC).[33,35,43-45] Healthcare professionals who take the time to learn about local Indigenous cultures, protocols, and priorities often develop respectful relationships with Indigenous peoples and communities. When they also seek to understand the historical and contemporary socioeconomic and political determinants that shape Indigenous peoples' health and encounters within multiple healthcare environments, they are better able to provide helpful, culturally safe care, treatment, and support.

Studies show that when healthcare professionals engaged in empathetic, nonjudgmental relationships, Indigenous women perceived care to be more enjoyable and effective.[45,46] Pregnant First Nations women have identified trust, cultural understanding, and context-specific services as key features of successful prenatal care. Feelings of safety enhance not only Indigenous women's physical health but also their perceptions of emotional and social wellness.[26] Engaging in genuine relationships and learning from Indigenous patients is preferred over simply obtaining cultural sensitivity training,[45] but ultimately, when healthcare professionals are responsive to Indigenous women's unique sociocultural contexts and care is flexible, inclusive, and accessible, improved health outcomes are more likely.[45,47] Nurses play an especially important role in shaping stem environments through not only promoting respectful relationships but also educating colleagues about the unique determinants of Indigenous peoples' health, countering negative stereotypes, and supporting self-determination among Indigenous women.[48,49]

Context is a critical component in the provision of care and support for Indigenous women. When healthcare providers find ways to deliver appropriate information that links women to culturally safe formal or informal supports, women's experiences of screening, treatment, and care are enhanced.[33] For example, sexual assault is more likely to be experienced by Indigenous women at a younger age, by a perpetrator in a position of power.[50] Healthcare providers must therefore be prepared to address distinctly related psychosocial outcomes, including increased anxiety, depression, substance use, and future posttraumatic stress disorder. Studies in this area reveal the urgent need for contextually responsive interventions that address the complexity of risk and opportunities for healing among Indigenous women.[51]

As a consequence of the widespread silence around cancer within Indigenous communities, women's access to crucial resources, supports, and services is limited.[33] Thus, cervical cancer education and screening initiatives that are destigmatizing and reflect the cultural and socioeconomic contexts of diverse Indigenous women are seen as contributing to women's reproductive self-determination.[49,52] Similarly, for Indigenous women who must travel away from home to give birth, the provision of culturally appropriate initiatives such as hospital-based doula programs and/or visits in the hospital by urban Indigenous Elders have helped to achieve balance between clinical and cultural safety.[53]

Sharing decision-making power with Indigenous women is a critical component of nurturing stem environments. Collaborative decision making can contribute to reduced health inequities by enhancing Indigenous women's sense of control over their bodies as well as the treatment and support they receive.[54,55] Indigenous women exercise greater control when practitioners engage in genuine partnerships as well as strength-based and participatory approaches to decisions about women's healthcare.[39,46,54] This is demonstrated when practitioners respect women's control over birth experiences in terms of how and where they deliver their babies.[42,48,56] Similarly, practitioners who attend to physical and emotional discomfort regarding pelvic exams and the privacy of test results, by offering self-sampling over physician-conducted Pap screening, are enhancing Indigenous women's choice and control.[57]

Core Environments

Core environments are represented by the policies and organization of health systems, as well as the management of healthcare services within institutions. Enhancements in Indigenous healthcare cannot be realized without institutional leadership and administrators who are mindful of the dominance of Western worldviews and biomedical knowledge within core environments.[23] Equally relevant within these environments is the positioning of Indigenous worldviews, knowledges, and practices.[27]

Toxic Core Environments

Indigenous peoples in Canada receive healthcare through a complex arrangement of federally and provincially funded programs and services differentially available to people living off and on reserve. Directed by provisions in the Canada Health Act, management and delivery of health services is primarily the responsibility of each province or territory. These "insured" services are defined as physician, hospital, and surgical-dental services,[58] but provinces and territories have the option to provide certain groups (e.g., children, seniors) with additional health benefits, programs, and services such as dental care and prescription drugs. This extra coverage is not made available to many Indigenous people because Health Canada offers the Non-Insured Health Benefits (NIHB) program to (1) status First Nations, legally designated as "Indians" under the Indian Act,[59] and (2) Inuk people, as recognized by an

Inuit land claim organization.[60] This program provides funding for a range of health, dental, and vision services as well as pharmaceutical drugs and medical transportation.[60]

Although the NIHB program is intended to reduce the barriers Indigenous people face in accessing healthcare, there is persistent discord between federal and provincial/territorial governments about their respective responsibilities for Indigenous health, particularly for services outside those governed by the Canada Health Act. As a result, Indigenous women seeking care are often caught in a "jurisdictional quagmire."[61] As an example, the escalating closure of health facilities in rural areas as well as the lack of nursing stations in remote and northern communities means that most Indigenous women living in these communities must travel to urban centers to give birth.[47,62] While provincial governments are responsible for providing safe birthing facilities (i.e., hospitals), funding for on-reserve First Nations' healthcare is a federal responsibility. Hence, although the NIHB program will support women's transportation to birthing services, it does not fund transportation for midwives to practice in First Nations communities.[42,63,64] This results in several complications for Indigenous women, as their extended absence from home can have detrimental impacts on their cultural and emotional wellness, family responsibilities and cohesion, as well as newborn infant health.[48,49,53,65] Similarly, structural barriers linked to transportation and a scarcity of Indigenous community-based healthcare providers reduces cervical cancer screening among Indigenous women.[66]

Despite advances in integrated models of healthcare, a siloed approach to service provision remains common across Canada. Consequently, Indigenous women, particularly those living with multiple health conditions, are at heightened risk of falling through gaps in the system.[26] In addition to limiting links to care, disconnected health services restrict health education opportunities for Indigenous women living with chronic conditions.[67] Of particular concern are young and economically disadvantaged Indigenous women, who already face complex socioeconomic barriers to accessing appropriate healthcare and support.[40]

Nurturing Core Environments

The presence of equity is revealed when the most disadvantaged in a given society have access to the highest attainable standard of health, as measured by the health status of the most advantaged.[68] An essential feature of nurturing core environments is policies that ensure equitable access to essential services, such as perinatal care and the treatment of chronic illness.[27,42,64] Equitable access further requires the provision of services that are responsive to population needs. Healthcare policies within core environments also have the potential to address the insidiousness of racism within stem environments.[5,37] Policies shape the extent and quality of the education healthcare professionals receive about the role of power and privilege within healthcare environments,[69] the effects of racism on the health of Indigenous peoples, and the importance of culturally safe approaches to care.[5]

Beyond conventional healthcare settings, core environments also encompass community settings, many of which are nurturing to Indigenous women's wellness. Core environments that facilitate community leadership, peer-based learning, flexible programming, as well as outreach services and mobile resources not only facilitate good relationships with Indigenous communities but can also increase opportunities for Indigenous women to obtain care in cultural and contextually safe ways.[27,40,42,63] Indigenous women also report the most positive and beneficial experiences when there is continuity between institutional and community care.[63]

Nurturing core environments are those that support collaborative institutional and community programs that align with local Indigenous priorities,[33,42,70] including the opportunity for women living in remote Indigenous communities to receive not only midwifery care but also midwifery training.[62,64] In 1986, the Inuulitsivik Health Centre represented the first birthing center in Nunavik. Following an Indigenous community approach, the center was shaped through prolonged engagement with Elders and traditional midwives, as well as childbearing and young women. With a commitment to integrate Western healthcare approaches with community development and reclaim traditional birth and midwifery, the center offers sexually transmitted infection prevention, contraception education and distribution, and cancer screening, in addition to prenatal and perinatal care throughout pregnancy and birth as well as postnatal care. Through this work, Inuulitsivik midwives have reduced the number of births in southern hospitals.[71]

In an effort to enhance community capacity, a midwifery training program in Nunavik has successfully adapted the clinical content of midwifery education programs in southern Canada to northern realities, including community-based care. Although traditional practices such as storytelling and oral methods of teaching are central to the curriculum, this program ensures that students are recognized as midwives by the ministry of Health of Quebec, so they can practice in their communities.[70]

Indigenous community-based birthing with Indigenous midwives represents a restoration of strength, capacity, and healing. "Participating in birth builds family and community relationships and intergenerational support and learning, through promoting respect for traditional knowledge, and through teaching transcultural skills both within the local community and with nonlocal healthcare providers."[70(p390)] When Indigenous communities feel a sense of ownership and investment in their care, women are more apt to actively participate. This was demonstrated in Indigenous infant–toddler health promotion programs in which local community investment and ownership, as well as sustained community participation and leadership, were linked to positive changes in access to prenatal and postnatal care, birth outcomes, breastfeeding, infant nutrition, dental health, and child development.[70]

Root Environments

Root environments represent the deeply entrenched social, political, and economic foundations of a given society that can either promote or hinder healthy core and stem environments. Within the context of Canadian healthcare, these roots manifest as historical and contemporary colonial relationships and traumas, "political relationships and arrangements, social and material inequities, and cultural connection or loss."[23(p400)] Alternatively, root environments that support Indigenous individuals, families, and communities to address social inequities (e.g., racism, poverty) have a profoundly beneficial impact on health.[20,29]

Toxic Root Environments

Within Canada and elsewhere, Indigenous peoples have endured centuries of oppression through geographic and cultural dispossession, economic marginalization, and racialized discrimination.[36,72] Indigenous cultures, worldviews, and knowledge systems have also been marginalized through assimilative efforts and the dominance of Western knowledge, with its origins in classical Greek and Roman culture, the Christian religion, and the scientific method.[73] Unfortunately, the roots of this oppression are also those that have shaped the institutions, policies, and practices of the Canadian healthcare system.[29,48]

One of the primary goals of early Indigenous health policy was medical assimilation. The practice of Indigenous healers (including midwives) was outlawed by governments as well as ridiculed and undermined by healthcare providers.[74] For instance, early intrusion of Western medicine led to the stigmatization of Indigenous birthing traditions and pressure to medicalize birth.[49,62,75] The earliest approach to settler-based maternity care came in the form of English midwife nurses, who were meant to replace, not collaborate with, Indigenous midwives. As recently as the past four decades, policies that favor Western obstetrical approaches have virtually replaced traditional Indigenous birthing practices.[42,48] Beginning in the 1970s, Indigenous women living in remote and northern communities were routinely evacuated to hospitals in distant urban centers, where the majority continued to spend several weeks away from family and community support networks.[48,75,76]

Most Canadians are now familiar with the physical, emotional, and sexual trauma inflicted on Indigenous children who were forced to attend residential schools between the early 1800s and the late 1900s,[77] as well as the current overrepresentation of Indigenous children in foster care.[78] Approximately 19.5% of all First Nations adults report having attended a residential school; 52.7% had one or more parents who attended; and 46.2% had one or more grandparents who attended.[12] Lifelong and intergenerational trauma resulting from a range of abuses (e.g., childhood sexual abuse) within these settings increases the likelihood that Indigenous women will experience teen pregnancy, substance abuse, and sex work, as well as reducing the likelihood that they will seek healthcare.[79-81] As well, Indigenous women's odds of being sexually assaulted in adulthood are significantly higher among those with at least one parent who attended a residential school.[51] The legacy of sexual abuse, gender segregation, and religious-based sexual shaming practiced within residential schools[77] represents an additional barrier to accessing care among Indigenous women, who may experience a strong sense of shame about their body, sexuality, and sexually transmitted infections.[82]

During the late 1800s and early 1900s, the federal government provided minimal and sporadic medical services to First Nations people, by doctors who accompanied Indian Agents to reserves.[82] With the exception of Treaty 6 territory, where Indigenous peoples negotiated a "Medicine Chest" clause in their treaty with the federal government, the government maintained that health services were provided to Indigenous peoples for humanitarian reasons as well as to protect settler populations from the spread of disease.[83] However, the decimation of Indigenous populations from communicable illnesses such as smallpox and tuberculosis prompted the federal government to establish the Department of Indian Affairs in 1904, with the purpose of developing health programs and services for Indigenous people identified as status Indians. Like residential schools, racially segregated sanitariums and "Indian hospitals" were poorly funded in terms of infrastructure, equipment, provisions, and staff.[84] These hospitals were also sites of unethical experiments on infants, children, and adults.[85]

After World War II, outpatient lung surgery and antimicrobial treatment for tuberculosis patients signaled the end of prolonged hospital stays. Yet, Indigenous patients, generally perceived as incapable of managing illness, had no choice but to remain in these institutions for months or years because a 1953 amendment to the Indian Act

> made it a crime for Indigenous people to refuse to see a doctor, to refuse to go to hospital, and to leave hospital before discharge. The RCMP [Royal Canadian Mounted Police] arrested patients and returned them to hospital or sent them to jail. However, the government would not return those who died at Indian hospitals to their communities unless the family paid the costs. Many were buried at the nearest cemetery in unmarked graves, forever lost to their families.[86(b, para.9)]

For Indigenous women, gender intersects with colonization to create multiple, complex challenges.[80] Although each woman's experience is shaped by local contexts, the impacts of colonization and medical domination have been profoundly harmful.[43,76,56] Indigenous beliefs about health and wellness are rooted in a worldview that diverges from Western science in fundamental ways,[47] thus hindering the development of culturally appropriate and safe healthcare environments. Similarly, colonial ideologies and medical paternalism have devalued Indigenous women's helping roles, pathologized their bodies, and dishonored their healing traditions.[75,80]

Nurturing Root Environments

Over the past two decades, the Canadian government has undertaken a number of processes intended to enhance Indigenous health equity. Appointed by the federal government in 2001, the Romanow Commission on Canadian Health Care identified a poorly established system of healthcare and funding mismanagement as the central causes of Indigenous health inequity. The report recommended meaningful restructuring of Indigenous healthcare, requiring collaboration between Indigenous communities and all levels of government.[87]

In 2008, the government established the TRC of Canada to document the experiences of Indian residential school survivors. For six years, the commission held national and regional events as well as community hearings across Canada, gathering over 6,750 statements from survivors and family members. The TRC report included 94 calls to action, several of which relate to ensuring the cultural safety of Indigenous peoples within healthcare environments.[77]

One of the best examples of efforts to create nurturing root environments is the establishment of the British Columbia First Nations Health Authority (FNHA) (2011), which evolved from the British Columbia Tripartite Framework Agreement on First Nations Health Governance (BCTFA). This 10-year arrangement between Health Canada, the provincial Ministry of Health, and the First Nations Health Society transferred control over decision making, and in some cases delivery, of federally funded health programs and services to FNHA.[88] Similarly, the 1999 formation of the Nunavut government ensured representation of Inuit culture, values, language, and traditions in many northern healthcare environments.[89]

Albeit long overdue, in 2016, Canada signed the United Nations Declaration on the Rights of Indigenous People (UNDRIP), which, among other things, states that

> Indigenous peoples have the right, without discrimination, to the improvement of their economic and social conditions, including, inter alia, in the areas of education, employment, vocational training and retraining, housing, sanitation, health and social security.[90]

Despite ongoing debates about the interpretation and implementation of the UNDRIP, many people are hopeful that it will inform the development or revision of federal policies that will create equity in health and other domains of life for Indigenous peoples.

In the spirit of decolonization and reconciliation, healthcare systems across Canada are beginning to support the concept of cultural safety by implementing initiatives designed to enhance the involvement of Indigenous peoples in the design of health programs and services, as well as address the spiritual and cultural healing needs of Indigenous clients, increase employment opportunities for Indigenous peoples, and mandate cultural safety training for health professionals.[91] Since 2006, the Provincial Health Services Authority of British Columbia has delivered a facilitated, online program (San'yas) providing healthcare professionals with cultural safety training that includes education about colonization, racism, residential schools, and the inequities experienced by Indigenous peoples. Participants also engage in interactive activities to develop their skills in providing culturally safe care.[92]

Nurturing root environments also include Indigenous peoples' deep cultural foundations that, despite centuries of attempted genocide, continue to shape collective identities, kinship relationships, community responsibilities, and ties to the land.[24] For Indigenous women, this connection is represented and strengthened through community development, cultural restoration, and colonial resistance.[65] Some authors have suggested that when Indigenous women choose to be assisted by a community midwife, they are practicing self-determination and resistance to the Western medicalization of their bodies.[48,75] Local Indigenous wellness practices such as community-based, midwife-assisted birthing are seen as a reassertion of women's traditional caregiving and knowledge-sharing roles,[52,70] as well as being strongly linked to Indigenous identity and traditional beliefs about wellness.[29]

Conclusions

Indigenous women's encounters within healthcare environments cannot be understood in isolation from their unique racialized and colonial realities. Just as the individual circumstances of Indigenous women's lives vary considerably (e.g., culture, location, income), so too do their experiences interacting with stem, core, and root healthcare environments. The roots of inequities expressed at the individual and collective levels are also those that have shaped the institutions, policies, and practices of the Canadian healthcare system. Colonialism has produced widespread inequities among Indigenous peoples, all of which justifiably hinder trust in colonial systems, even those meant to provide care. A restructuring of this relationship must begin before we can combat the health disparities facing Indigenous women. In colonized countries like Canada, poverty, social exclusion, and multiple forms of violence against Indigenous women are widespread. Yet, those who design healthcare policies, as well as administer and deliver services, often fail to acknowledge the significance of these intergenerational and gendered traumas.

In responding to intersecting health inequities experienced by Indigenous women, structural drivers must be carefully considered. Root environments characterized by racist ideologies, ethnocentrism, and cultural oppression have shaped the distribution of political, social, and economic power and resources, which in turn influence virtually every societal system, including health. Without attention to these interconnected structures and systems, those who design, administer, and deliver healthcare will continue to facilitate environments that are at best irrelevant and inaccessible and at worst unsafe for Indigenous women.

Health care is relational. It is characterized not only by clinical practices but by social processes, which are shaped, enacted, and experienced by people. Racism plays a powerful role in diffuse and targeted stigma within healthcare environments; thus, the resocialization of non-Indigenous people must be prioritized. This begins with learning about and acknowledging the existence and extent of racism, followed by engaging empathetically with the pain of rejection that racism produces. Within stem environments, health professionals must engage with Indigenous women on their own cultural and contextual terms, which means moving beyond superficial understandings of cultural diversity toward entrenching practice within reconciliation.

Ultimately, healthcare policymakers, administrators, and practitioners must consider the profound inequities experienced by Indigenous women, who face intersecting and racialized social, economic, and political injustices. If we neglect to consider how deep these injustices are entrenched in the core and root of our healthcare environments, we not only ignore what is now a critical mass of evidence, but we become complicit in the perpetuation of colonialism.

References

1. Lavoie JG, University of Manitoba. Centre for Aboriginal Health Research, Canadian Electronic Library. Indigenous Primary Health Care Services in Australia, Canada and New Zealand: Policy and Financing Issues. Winnipeg, Manitoba: Centre for Aboriginal Health Research, University of Manitoba; 2003.
2. Browne AJ, Varcoe C, Lavoie J, et al. Enhancing health care equity with Indigenous populations: evidence-based strategies from an ethnographic study. *BMC Health Serv Res.* 2016;16(1):544.
3. Carriere G, Bougie E, Kohen D, Rotermann M, Sanmartin C. Acute care hospitalization by Aboriginal identity, Canada, 2006 through 2008. *Health Rep.* 2016;27(8):3–11.
4. Fiske J-A, Browne AJ, British Columbia Centre of Excellence for Women's Health. *Paradoxes and Contradictions in Health Policy Reform: Implications for First Nations Women.* Vancouver: British Columbia Centre of Excellence for Women's Health; 2008.
5. Denison J, Varcoe C, Browne AJ. Aboriginal women's experiences of accessing health care when state apprehension of children is being threatened. *J Adv Nurs.* 2014;70(5):1105–1116.
6. United Nations. Human Development Report 2016: Human Development for Everyone. 2016. Retrieved from http://hdr.undp.org/sites/default/files/2016_human_development_report.pdf

7. Indigenous peoples and communities. Indigenous and Northern Affairs Canada website. https://www.aadnc-aandc.gc.ca/eng/1100100013785/1304467449155. Updated December 4, 2017. Accessed March 27, 2018.
8. Royal Commission on Aboriginal Peoples. *Report of the Royal Commission on Aboriginal Peoples (RCAP)*. Government of Canada; 1996.
9. Government of Canada. Constitution Act, 1867–1982. 1867. http://laws-lois.justice.gc.ca/eng/const/. Accessed January 30, 2018.
10. Weaver HN. Perspectives on wellness: journeys on the Red Road. *J Sociol Social Welfare*. 2002;29:5–15.
11. Wright A, Wahoush O, Gabel C, Jack S. Access to primary health-care services for urban-dwelling, Canadian Indigenous women of childbearing age: an integrative review. International Journal of Qualitative Methods. Thousand Oaks: Sage Publications Inc; 2017;16.
12. The First Nations regional health survey: Phase 2—2008–10 selected results. First Nations Information Governance Centre. http://fnigc.ca/sites/default/files/RHS%20Phase%202%20Results%20-%20HC%20presentation%20Sept%2027%202012%20FINAL%20FOR%20PUBLICATION.pdf. Published September 27, 2012. Accessed January 30, 2018.
13. First Nations, Métis and Inuit women. Statistics Canada website. http://www.statcan.gc.ca/pub/89-503-x/2010001/article/11442-eng.htm. Updated November 30, 2015. Accessed January 30, 2018.
14. 2011 national household survey: Data tables: Aboriginal peoples. Statistics Canada website. http://www12.statcan.gc.ca/nhs-enm/2011/dp-pd/dt-td/Lp-eng.cfm?lang=e&apath=3&detail=0&dim=0&fl=a&free=0&gc=0&gid=0&gk=0&grp=0&pid=0&prid=0&ptype=105277&s=0&showall=0&sub=0&temporal=2013&theme=94&vid=0&vnamee=&vnamef=. Updated January 7, 2016. Accessed March 27, 2018.
15. Sheppard AJ, Shapiro GD, Bushnik T, et al. Birth outcomes among First Nations, Inuit and Metis populations. *Health Rep*. 2017;28(11):11–16.
16. van Rossum CTM, Shipley MJ, van de Mheen H, Grobbee DE, Marmot MG. Employment grade differences in cause specific mortality: a 25-year follow-up of civil servants from the first Whitehall study. *J Epidemiol Comm Health*. 2000;54:178–184.
17. Social determinants of health. World Health Organization website. http://www.who.int/social_determinants/sdh_definition/en/. Modified 2018. Accessed March 27, 2018.
18. Wilkinson RG, Marmot M, World Health Organization Regional Office for Europe, WHO Healthy Cities Project, University College London. International Centre for Health and Society. *Social Determinants of Health: The Solid Facts*. 2nd ed. Copenhagen: WHO Regional Office for Europe; 2003.

19. Diderichsen F, Evans T, Whitehead M. *The Social Basis of Disparities in Health: Challenging Inequities in Health—From Ethics to Action.* New York: Oxford University Press; 2001.
20. Reading CL, Wien F. Health inequalities and social determinants and life course health issues among First Nations people in Canada. National Collaborating Centre for Aboriginal Health. 2009. http://www.nccah-ccnsa.ca. Accessed November 30, 2016.
21. World Health Organization Commission on Social Determinants of Health. A conceptual framework for analysis and action on the social determinants of health. 2010. http://www.who.int/sdhconference/resources/ConceptualframeworkforactiononSDH_eng.pdf. Accessed March 27, 2018.
22. Moreton-Robinson A. Introduction: critical Indigenous theory. *Cult Stud Rev.* 2009;15(2):11–12.
23. Kent A, Loppie C, Carriere J, MacDonald M, Pauly B. Xpey' Relational Environments: an analytic framework for conceptualizing Indigenous health equity. *Health Promot Chron Dis Prev Can.* 2017;37(12):395–402.
24. Reading C. Structural determinants of Aboriginal peoples' health. In: Greenwood M, De Leeuw S, Lindsay NM, Reading C, eds. *Determinants of Indigenous Peoples' Health in Canada: Beyond the Social.* Toronto: Canadian Scholars' Press; 2015:3–15.
25. Wilson D, de la Ronde S, Brascoupé S, et al. Health professionals working with First Nations, Inuit, and Métis consensus guideline. *J Obstet Gynaecol Can.* 2013;35(6):S1–S4.
26. Ghosh H, Benoit C, Bourgeault I. Health service needs for urban indigenous women with co-occurring health concerns. *Fourth World J.* 2017;15(2):5–25.
27. McCall J, Browne AJ, Reimer-Kirkham S. Struggling to survive: the difficult reality of Aboriginal women living with HIV/AIDS. *Qual Health Res.* 2009;19(12):1769–1782.
28. Vukic A, Jesty C, Mathews SV, Etowa J. Understanding race and racism in nursing: insights from Aboriginal nurses. *ISRN Nursing.* 2012; 2012:1–9.
29. Poudrier J, Mac-Lean RT. "We've fallen into the cracks": Aboriginal women's experiences with breast cancer through photovoice. *Nurs Inq.* 2009;16(4):306–317.
30. Hawkins K, Reading CL, Barlow K. *Our Search for Safe Spaces: A Qualitative Study of the Role of Sexual Violence in the Lives of Aboriginal Women Living with HIV/AIDS.* Vancouver, BC: Canadian Aboriginal AIDS Network; 2009.
31. Goodman A, Fleming K, Markwick N, et al. "They treated me like crap and I know it was because I was Native": the healthcare experiences of Aboriginal peoples living in Vancouver's inner city. *Soc Sci Med.* 2017;178:87–94.
32. Gould J, Sinding C, Mitchell TL, et al. "Below their notice": exploring women's subjective experiences of cancer system exclusion. *J Cancer Educ.* 2009;24(4):308–314.

33. Hammond C, Thomas R, Gifford W, et al. Cycles of silence: First Nations women overcoming social and historical barriers in supportive cancer care. *Psychooncology*. 2017;26(2):191–198.
34. Williams R. Cultural safety—what does it mean for our work practice? *Aust N Z J Public Health*. 1999;23:213–214.
35. Browne AJ. Clinical encounters between nurses and First Nations women in a western Canadian hospital. *Soc Sci Med*. 2007;64(10):2165–2176.
36. de Leeuw S, Kobayashi A, Cameron E. Difference. In: Del Casino VJ, Del Casino VJ, eds. *A Companion to Social Geography*. 1st ed. Malden, MA: Wiley-Blackwell; 2011.
37. Lawrence HP, Cidro J, Isaac-Mann S, et al. Racism and oral health outcomes among pregnant Canadian Aboriginal women. *J Health Care Poor Underserved*. 2016;27(1 Suppl):178–206.
38. Tang S, Browne A. "Race" matters: racialization and egalitarian discourses involving Aboriginal people in the Canadian healthcare context. *Ethnicity Health*. 2010;13:109–127.
39. Kelly J. Decolonizing sexual health nursing with Aboriginal women. *Can J Nurs Res*. 2013;45(3):50–65.
40. Shannon K, Rusch M, Shoveller J, Alexson D, Gibson K, Tyndall MW. Mapping violence and policing as an environmental-structural barrier to health service and syringe availability among substance-using women in street-level sex work. *Int J Drug Policy*. 2008;19(2):140–147.
41. Browne AJ, Smye VL, Rodney P, Tang SY, Mussell B, O'Neil J. Access to primary care from the perspective of Aboriginal patients at an urban emergency department. *Qualit Health Res*. 2011;21(3):333–348.
42. Couchie C. A report on best practices for returning birth to rural and remote aboriginal communities. *J Obstet Gynaecol Can*. 2007;29(3):250–254.
43. Badry D, Felske AW. An examination of the social determinants of health as factors related to health, healing and prevention of foetal alcohol spectrum disorder in a northern context—the Brightening Our Home Fires Project, Northwest Territories, Canada. *Int J Circumpolar Health*. 2013;72(1):21140. doi:10.3402/ijch.v72i0.21140
44. Di Lallo S. Prenatal care through the eyes of Canadian Aboriginal women. *Nurs Womens Health*. 2014;18(1):38–46.
45. Oster RT, Bruno G, Montour M, et al. Kikiskawawasow—prenatal healthcare provider perceptions of effective care for First Nations women: an ethnographic community-based participatory research study. *BMC Pregnancy Childbirth*. 2016;16(1):216.
46. Smith DA, Edwards NC, Martens PJ, Varcoe C. "Making a difference": a new care paradigm for pregnant and parenting Aboriginal people. *Can J Public Health*. 2007;98(4):321–325.
47. Douglas VK. Converging epistemologies: critical issues in Canadian Inuit childbirth and pregnancy. *Alaska Med*. 2007;49(2 Suppl):209–214.

48. Varcoe C, Brown H, Calam B, Harvey T, Tallio M. Help bring back the celebration of life: a community-based participatory study of rural Aboriginal women's maternity experiences and outcomes. *BMC Pregnancy Childbirth*. 2013;13:26.
49. Wright AL. Role of the nurse in returning birth to the North. *Rural Remote Health*. 2015;15:3109.
50. Du Mont J, Kosa D, Macdonald S, Benoit A, Forte T. A comparison of Indigenous and non-Indigenous survivors of sexual assault and their receipt of and satisfaction with specialized health care services. *PLoS One*. 2017;12(11):e0188253.
51. Pearce ME, Blair AH, Teegee M, et al. The Cedar Project: historical trauma and vulnerability to sexual assault among young aboriginal women who use illicit drugs in two Canadian cities. *Violence Against Women*. 2015;21(3):313–329.
52. Wakewich P, Wood B, Davey C, Laframboise A, Zehbe I. Colonial legacy and the experience of First Nations women in cervical cancer screening: a Canadian multi-community study. *Crit Public Health*. 2016;26(4):368–380.
53. O'Driscoll T, Kelly L, Payne L, et al. Delivering away from home: the perinatal experiences of First Nations women in northwestern Ontario. *Can J Rural Med*. 2011;16(4):126–130.
54. Jull J, Giles A, Boyer Y, Lodge M, Stacey D. Shared decision making with Aboriginal women facing health decisions: a qualitative study identifying needs, supports, and barriers. *AlterNative Int J Indigenous Peoples*. 2015;11(4):401–416.
55. Marmot MG. Mastering the control factor. Part 2, e-health report. Radio National, 2007.
56. Darroch FE, Giles AR. Health/service providers' perspectives on barriers to healthy weight gain and physical activity in pregnant, Urban First Nations women. *Qual Health Res*. 2016;26(1):5–16.
57. Zehbe I, Wakewich P, King AD, Morrisseau K, Tuck C. Self-administered versus provider-directed sampling in the Anishinaabek Cervical Cancer Screening Study (ACCSS): a qualitative investigation with Canadian First Nations women. *BMJ Open*. 2017;7(8):e017384.
58. Canada Health Act. Government of Canada website. https://www.canada.ca/en/health-canada/services/health-care-system/canada-health-care-system-medicare/canada-health-act.html. Modified November 9, 2017. Accessed March 27, 2018.
59. Government of Canada. Indian Act (R.S.C., 1985, c. I-5). 1985. http://laws-lois.justice.gc.ca/eng/acts/i-5/index.html. Modified March 23, 2018. Accessed March 27, 2018.
60. Non-insured health benefits for First Nations and Inuit. Government of Canada website. https://www.canada.ca/en/health-canada/services/non-insured-health-benefits-first-nations-inuit/who-is-eligible-non-insured-health-benefits-program.html. Modified February 21, 2018. Accessed March 27, 2018.
61. First Nations Health Council. *Implementing the Vision: BC First Nations Health Governance: Reimagining First Nations Health in BC*. Vancouver, BC: Author; 2011.

62. James S, O'Brien B, Bourret K, Kango N, Gafvels K, Paradis-Pastori J. Meeting the needs of Nunavut families: a community-based midwifery education program. *Rural Remote Health*. 2010;10(2):1355.
63. Corcoran PM, Catling C, Homer CSE. Models of midwifery care for Indigenous women and babies: a meta-synthesis. *Women and Birth*. 2017;30(1):77–86.
64. Olson R, Couchie C. Returning birth: the politics of midwifery implementation on First Nations reserves in Canada. *Midwifery*. 2013;29(8):981–987.
65. Kornelsen J, Kotaska A, Waterfall P, Willie L, Wilson D. The geography of belonging: the experience of birthing at home for First Nations women. *Health Place*. 2010;16(4):638–645.
66. Maar M, Burchell A, Little J, et al. A qualitative study of provider perspectives of structural barriers to cervical cancer screening among First Nations women. *Womens Health Iss*. 2013;23(5):e319–325.
67. Tait Neufeld H. Patient and caregiver perspectives of health provision practices for First Nations and Metis women with gestational diabetes mellitus accessing care in Winnipeg, Manitoba. BMC Health Serv Res. 2014;14:440.
68. Sparks M. A health promotion approach to addressing health equity. *Glob Health Promot*. 2010;17(1):77–82.
69. Baba L. *Cultural Safety in First Nations, Inuit and Métis Public Health: Environmental Scan of Cultural Competency and Safety in Education, Training and Health Services*. National Collaborating Centre for Aboriginal Health; 2013.
70. Van Wagner V, Epoo B, Nastapoka J, Harney E. Reclaiming birth, health, and community: midwifery in the Inuit villages of Nunavik, Canada. *J Midwif Womens Health*. 2007;52(4):384–391.
71. Centre de santé Inuulitsivik. Midwives. Healthcare and Health Services. Inuulitsivik website. http://www.inuulitsivik.ca/healthcare-and-services/healthcare/midwives. Published 2011. Accessed January 31, 2018.
72. Loppie S, Reading C, de Leeuw S. *Aboriginal Experiences and Effects of Racism*. Prince George, BC: National Collaborating Centre for Aboriginal Health; 2014.
73. *Western Civilization; Ideas, Politics, and Society*. 10th ed. Reference & Research Book News. Portland, OR: Ringgold, Inc; 2012;27.
74. Kelm M. *Colonizing Bodies: Aboriginal Health and Healing in British Columbia, 1900–1950*. Vancouver: University of British Columbia Press; 1998.
75. Shaw JC. The medicalization of birth and midwifery as resistance. *Health Care Women Int*. 2013;34(6):522–536.
76. Brown H, Varcoe C, Calam B. The birthing experiences of rural Aboriginal women in context: implications for nursing. *Can J Nurs Res*. 2011;43(4):100–117.
77. Truth and Reconciliation Commission of Canada. *Final Report of the Truth and Reconciliation Commission of Canada: Honouring the Truth, Reconciling for the Future*. 2nd printing. Toronto: James Lorimer & Company Ltd., Publishers; 2015.
78. Trocmé N, Knoke D, Blackstock C. Pathways to the overrepresentation of Aboriginal children in Canada's child welfare system. *Soc Serv Rev*. 2004;78(4):577–600.

79. McCall J, Lauridsen-Hoegh P. Trauma and cultural safety: providing quality care to HIV-infected women of Aboriginal descent. *J Assoc Nurses AIDS Care*. 2014;25(1 Suppl):S70–78.
80. Oliver V, Flicker S, Danforth J, et al. "Women are supposed to be the leaders": intersections of gender, race and colonisation in HIV prevention with Indigenous young people. *Cult Health Sex*. 2015;17(7):906–919.
81. Hawkins K, Reading CL, Barlow K, Canadian Aboriginal AIDS Network. *Our Search for Safe Spaces: A Qualitative Study of the Role of Sexual Violence in the Lives of Aboriginal Women Living with HIV/AIDS*. Vancouver, BC: Canadian Aboriginal AIDS Network; 2009.
82. Waldram JB, Herring DA, Young TK. *Aboriginal Health in Canada: Historical, Cultural, and Epidemiological Perspectives*. Toronto: University of Toronto Press; 1995.
83. Health of Indigenous Peoples in Canada. Canadian Encyclopedia website. https://www.thecanadianencyclopedia.ca/en/article/aboriginal-people-health/. Published February 7, 2006. Updated May 15, 2015. Accessed March 27, 2018.
84. Lux MK. Care for the "racially careless": Indian hospitals in the Canadian West, 1920–1950s. *Can Hist Rev*. 2010;91(3):407–434.
85. Friesen JW, Meijer Drees L. Healing histories: stories from Canada's Indian hospitals. *Can Ethnic Stud J*. 2015;47:181.
86. Indian hospitals in Canada. Canadian Encyclopedia website. https://www.thecanadianencyclopedia.ca/en/article/indian-hospitals-in-canada/. Published July 11, 2017. Modified January 31, 2018. Accessed March 27, 2018.
87. Commission on the Future of Health Care in Canada, Building on Values: The Future of Health Care in Canada: Final Report, Roy J. Romanow, Commissioner. Saskatoon, Sask: Privy Council; 2002. http://publications.gc.ca/pub?id=9.686360&sl=0 Accessed March 27, 2018.
88. Government of Canada. *British Columbia Tripartite Framework Agreement on First Nations Health Governance*. Ottawa, ON: Aboriginal Affairs and Northern Development Canada; 2011.
89. Canadian Council on Social Determinants of Health. *Roots of Resilience: Overcoming Inequities in Aboriginal Communities*. Canadian Council on Social Determinants of Health; 2013.
90. United Nations Declaration on the Rights of Indigenous Peoples. United Nations; 2008. http://www.un.org/esa/socdev/unpfii/documents/DRIPS_en.pdf. Accessed March 27, 2018.
91. Reading C. *Policies, Programs and Strategies to Address Aboriginal Racism*. Prince George, BC: National Collaborating Centre for Aboriginal Health; 2014.
92. San'yas Indigenous cultural safety training. Provincial Health Services Authority website. http://www.phsa.ca/health-professionals/education-development/sanyas-indigenous-cultural-safety-training. Updated 2018. Accessed March 27, 2018.

3 CARING FOR REFUGEES, NEW IMMIGRANTS, AND UNINSURED WOMEN

SOCIAL RESPONSIBILITY AND ACCESS TO HEALTHCARE

Paul Caulford and Sumathy Rahunathan

... the protection of refugees is not only the responsibility of neighbouring States of a crisis; it is a collective responsibility of the international community.

—ANTONIO GUTERRES, *UN Secretary General*

Introduction

It is well established that refugees are one of the most vulnerable populations. Many have left home because of conflict or hopeless poverty and have had no access to healthcare. Others fleeing war and persecution are making arduous journeys in poor living conditions where overcrowding and lack of basic sanitation, water, and food cause a myriad of health problems. Compounding their difficulties is the fact that many refugees are not granted public health insurance in the countries that receive them, so they are left with no means to pay for needed healthcare after relocation.[1] The complex vulnerability of these groups is largely absent from the health ethics literature, despite the growth in asylum seekers and migrant numbers globally. In this chapter, we discuss ethical concerns related to caring for refugees, new immigrants, and uninsured immigrant women in Canada. Case examples from our clinic illustrate systemic barriers many refugees and uninsured immigrant women face when attempting to access healthcare. We show how systemic barriers to healthcare result in delayed diagnosis, underdiagnosis, and inappropriate use of emergency services by refugees and undocumented immigrants. We also reflect on the moral obligations of host countries and healthcare providers to refugee and uninsured women and their families. We begin our discussion, however, with an overview of the broader context shaping migration and refugee patterns today.

World Numbers: Unprecedented

Since earliest times, people have moved around. Some people move to search for new economic opportunities and to build better lives. "Others move to escape armed conflict, poverty, food insecurity, persecution, terrorism, or human rights violations and abuses. Still others do so in response to the adverse effects of climate change, natural disasters (some of which may be linked to climate change), or other environmental factors. Many move, indeed, for a combination of these reasons."[2]

Yet, according to the United Nations, more people than ever before live in a country other than the one in which they were born. Migrants are present in all countries in the world. During the period from 2000 to 2017, the total number of international migrants increased from 173 to 258 million persons, an increase of 85 million (49%).[3] Most concerning, however, is that within this population are roughly 65 million forcibly displaced persons, including over 21 million refugees, 3 million asylum seekers, and over 40 million internally displaced persons.

The terms *migrant, refugee, displaced person,* and *undocumented immigrant* are often used interchangeably. For the purpose of this chapter, we use the following definitions summarized from the United Nations[3] and the International Organization for Migration.[4] Host countries accepting new arrivals may create additional categories as well.

> *Migrants:* People who move from their home country to another with a view to being employed and/or achieving a better life for themselves and their families. Movement is in keeping with the laws and regulations governing exit of the country of origin and travel, transit, and entry into the destination or host country.
>
> *Refugees:* Persons who have left their country of origin and crossed an international border for fear of persecution due to race, religion, nationality, membership of a particular social group, or political opinions. Refugees may also include people who have been compelled to leave their country owing to conflict, generalized violence, or other circumstances that have seriously disturbed public order and who, as a result, require international protection.
>
> *Internally displaced people (IDPs):* Persons or groups of persons who have been forced or obliged to flee or to leave their homes or places of

habitual residence, in particular as a result of or in order to avoid the effects of armed conflict, situations of generalized violence, violations of human rights, or natural or human-made disasters, and who have not crossed an internationally recognized state border.

Undocumented immigrants: Persons who have traveled to a host country outside the regulatory norms of the sending, transit, and receiving countries. From the perspective of destination countries, it is entry, stay, or work in a country without the necessary authorization or documents required under immigration regulations.

Asylum seekers: Persons who seek safety from persecution or serious harm in a country other than their own and await a decision on the application for refugee status under relevant international and national laws. In case of a negative decision, the person must leave the country and may be expelled, as may any non-national in an irregular or unlawful situation, unless permission to stay is provided on humanitarian or other related grounds.

In 2017 the United Nations High Commission for Refugees (UNHCR) reported that 65.6 million individuals were forcibly displaced worldwide as a result of persecution, conflict, violence, or human rights violations.[5,6] That was an increase of 300,000 people over the previous year, and the world's forcibly displaced population is at a record high. The majority of forced displacement has been driven by the conflict in Syria: 12 million people at the end of 2016, which included 5.5 million refugees, 6.3 million IDPs, and nearly 185,000 asylum seekers. Crises in sub-Saharan Africa (Burundi, the Central African Republic, Democratic Republic of the Congo, South Sudan, and Sudan) have contributed as well. Tragically, there has also been a significant rise in unaccompanied youth. In 2016, 75,000 unaccompanied or separated children lodged asylum applications in 70 countries, but the figure is assumed to be an underestimate.[5] There are also 10 million stateless people (not considered a national by any state) who have been denied a nationality and access to basic rights such as education, healthcare, employment, and freedom of movement.[6]

Where Do Refugees Go?

The vast majority of refugees go to low-income developing countries, particularly those that are proximate to their countries of origin. According to the

UNHCR,[5] countries that have the fewest resources are among the greatest affected. In 2016, a small number of developing nations hosted 84% of the world's UNHCR refugees and 66% of the overall forcibly displaced migrants. More than 5.9 million refugees under UNHCR's mandate reside in countries where the GDP per capita is below $5,000 (USD).[7] Turkey recorded the largest refugee population, hosting some approximately 3.1 million refugees and asylum seekers. In 2016, the second largest country of asylum was Jordan, hosting around 2.9 million refugees, followed by Palestine (2.2 million), Lebanon (1.6 million), and Pakistan (1.4 million).[3]

Women as Migrants and Refugees

In 2016 the UNHCR reported that women and girls constitute almost half of the refugee population, and the proportion who are under age 18 is 51%.[5] The number of migrant women has also been increasing steadily, reaching 52% of all immigrants in the developed world and approximately 44% of all migrants in developing regions.[8] The flow of migrating women is the result of their significant economic contribution to their families and communities. It is becoming increasingly evident that many women enter migration as the main economic providers for their families.[9]

Yet, women migrants encounter gender-based barriers and challenges.[9,10] For one, gender roles in most cultures create the expectation that women should be the direct caregivers for their children. This means that most mothers who migrate still face the direct pressure of caring for their children. These women are under enormous pressure to settle quickly so that they can bring their children to the host country. Further, women who migrate from low-income countries often do not leave their children with their fathers, but rather in the care of other family members. This creates additional pressure to get their children to join them.[10]

Women who are displaced because of conflict or war usually move with their children. Because they are the primary caregivers, they bear the responsibility of getting their children food and other necessary resources, even though they may have no means of earning an income.[10]

Trafficking and Violence Against Women

Another dimension of migration is human trafficking and forced labor. In the Global Report on Trafficking in Persons, sexual exploitation was noted as by far the most commonly identified form of human trafficking (79%), followed by forced labor (18%).[11] Women make up the vast majority of the detected victims who are trafficked for sexual exploitation. Some women become victims because of financial desperation or lax and complicit policing, while others are deceived and then transported to other countries and forced to work to stay alive.[10]

Stress and poverty in camps appreciably increases female partner violence, with 80% of women reporting being beaten by their husbands.[12–14] Low availability of access to protection, counseling, and mental health supports and the reluctance of women to step forward after abuse contribute to declines in mental and physical health status.

Lakshmi Puri, UN Assistant Secretary-General and Deputy Executive Director of UN Women, underscores the gender-based accumulation of vulnerabilities:

> As both migrants and refugees, women have specific needs and vulnerabilities. They are often forced to move by root causes such as conflict, poverty and inequality, and face a series of challenges, which include psycho-social stress and trauma, health complications, physical harm and risk of exploitation. They often become separated from their families, and refugee women and adolescent girls can find themselves unexpectedly as head of a household.
>
> Displaced and migrant women and girls are commonly subject to multiple and intersecting forms of discrimination. On top of gender-based discrimination, they may be targeted on additional grounds such as race, disability or belonging to a minority group. This discrimination limits women's access to basic services and to decision-making processes, affecting their interactions within their households or communities, in the labor market, as well as their mobility—within and outside their countries of origin. Their voice and participation are frequently constrained and the risk of sexual and gender-based violence, an ever-present reality for all women worldwide, significantly increases.[15]

LGBTQ Migrants

Lesbian, gay, bisexual, transgendered, and queer (LGBTQ) persons face targeted persecution and violence in many countries worldwide and significant disparities to healthcare access.[16] Asylum-seeking journeys generate additional gender-based health risks. Ninety-eight percent of asylum-seeking lesbian, gay, and bisexual survivors report experiencing persecution due to their sexual orientation. Eighty percent experienced torture. Many report efforts against them to change their sexual orientation, often through forced marriage. Women were more likely to be forced to move from place to place and to experience rape/sexual assault and threats. Men were more likely to be publicly persecuted. All report depression and anxiety.[16]

LGBTQ persons are appearing within forced migration populations in increasing numbers. New anti-LGBTQ legislation, torture, and the spread of terrorist networks have forced LGBTQ persons to flee to Eastern Europe.[17] Inadequate healthcare access and culturally non-competent healthcare are described by LGBTQ migrants crossing into the United States from Central America.[18]

In our Toronto clinics, LGBTQ government-assisted refugees began appearing for care in growing numbers, particularly since February 2017 when Canada formally developed policies for adjudicating LGBTQ refugee claims. We were surprised when gender-based social isolation and shunning was directed toward the arriving LGBTQ migrants by Syrian refugees cohabitating at the Toronto shelter. LGBTQ migrants reported that this exacerbated preexisting posttraumatic stress disorder symptoms of fear, anxiety, chronic pain, insomnia stemming from prior torture, lashings, beatings, imprisonment, and state-sponsored murders in their home countries.

Systemic Challenges

Against this background, it is no surprise that refugees have poorer health status than those of other immigrant groups.[19] Refugee women and girls are among the most negatively impacted. Access to public health is sporadic or nonexistent in camps. Deficiencies in reproductive, maternal and newborn care, communicable and noncommunicable diseases, and cancer screening and treatment are commonly reported.[5,10,20,21] Health status also deteriorates from neglected treatment of chronic diseases such as diabetes and hypertension.[22] Gender-based violence and sexual human trafficking adds to the health deficits. Syrian and other refugees arriving to our refugee clinics showed advanced oral decay.

Yet, as Graetz and colleagues observe—and our experience confirms—one of the biggest challenges refugees, undocumented immigrants, and new immigrants face in their host countries is the access to health services.

"Although the human right to health has been set out in the 1948 Constitution of the World Health Organization (WHO), as well as in subsequent international legal documents, in practice migrants often face formal and informal barriers in accessing health services."[23(p6)]

Haya's story helps illustrate challenges faced by those lacking insurance. We saw her at the Canadian Centre for Refugee and Immigrant Health Care (CCRIHC) in Scarborough, Toronto. Started in 1999, the CCRIHC provides health and dental care to refugee claimants and uninsured persons through volunteers offering multidisciplinary clinics.

> Haya is 74. She arrived at our clinic with chest pain that made it difficult to look after her grandchildren while her children worked. Haya's journey began 3 years ago in Syria. Her house was blown up in the war, killing her husband. Her children brought her to Canada. Her refugee claim in 2014 was rejected. This made Haya an undocumented 74-year-old forced migrant fleeing war with no status in her receiving country, and no access to public healthcare.

Despite Canada's universal healthcare system, many who reside here struggle to acquire public health insurance and accordingly needed healthcare. A recent study by Mahon and colleagues[24] reported that migrants from all immigrant categories face barriers accessing care in Canada; however, refugees and asylum seekers experience even greater difficulties. Systemic challenges may be differentiated into (1) legal-policy barriers and (2) social/cultural barriers.[25] We will explore each in turn.

Legal-Policy Barriers

McKeary and Newbold summarize the barriers related to Canadian policy succinctly: "Health care access is affected by the complexities and challenges of health insurance for refugees, which reflects a bureaucracy that impacts on health access as various levels of government are responsible for different components."[25(p535)] In Canada, some refugees may be eligible for provincial health insurance plans, based on their refugee status and (typically) on a minimum residency period in the province of up to 90 days. Refugee claimants may also be eligible for healthcare under a federal program called the Interim Federal Health (IFHP) insurance program. However, while the IFHP provides limited, temporary coverage of healthcare benefits, enrollment is not automatic; each refugee must file an application with the appropriate provincial authorities. The mix of government levels, programs, and eligibility requirements is confusing for refugees. Delays in receiving coverage are common, dangerous, and expensive. Further issues including fear, mistrust, and abject poverty mean that many new refugees may fall through the gaps.

In 2016, for example, a new and totally unexpected population began seeking care at the CCRIHC. African refugees, almost exclusively women and children, undertook dangerous crossings smuggled in the back of trucks in winter from the United States into Canada. All had originally fled life-threatening conditions in Africa and first made asylum claims in the United States, but then feared deportation under the Trump administration. After crossing, many were abandoned in snowy fields in the early hours of the morning. Oma's story is typical.

> Immigration and Customs Enforcement (ICE) agents in Texas were coming to medical clinics looking for pregnant immigrant women seeking healthcare. It got too dangerous to go for my pregnancy visits. I knew other women who were deported. Going back to Nigeria was no option. They wanted to cut my daughter.
>
> So I paid a smuggler. We climbed into the back of his unheated truck. There were five other men inside. Three days later the driver made the others get out after we crossed at Buffalo (New York). An hour later the truck stopped again. The man forced us out in a field. It was 4 a.m. No one was around. He told us to wait for another man. It was very cold. My children cried. Our clothes were not warm. The truck drove away. We waited. No one came. I never knew about cold like that. We started walking. A stranger driving by saw us and put us in his car. He bought us warm soup. Then he took us to a shelter. He saved our lives. I love Canada. Our fingers were painful and turned black.

Those with frostbite hid their injuries by wearing gloves at the shelter. They feared Canada would send them back to the United States if they sought health care. Delayed public health coverage access led to delays in seeking vital limb-saving care. Some of these women had fled to Italy first, but gangs forced them and other women into sexual trafficking. Oma showed us her scars from the machete wounds she suffered when she tried to escape. Other women told us of similar experiences. One told us, "The gangs are here now, doctor!"

While care was ultimately provided, this quote highlights why confusing administrative policies would pose a major obstacle to traumatized refugees and undocumented migrants needing healthcare. According to Newbold and McKeary,[19] insurance is included as a systemic barrier, but it is ultimately the complexity, cost, burdensome paperwork, and unclear eligibility rules that create obstacles for refugees.

Persons who are denied refugee status have a choice to either alter their application pathway (e.g., humanitarian) or seek legal support and appeal the refugee status rejection. If this in turn fails and the person receives a written notification of his or her removal date, the person then faces the choice of (a) leaving the country, (b) going into hiding, or (c) seeking legal support in an attempt to overturn the order removal.[26] The "choices" refugee claimants and others face occur typically in a context of poverty.

Sociocultural Barriers

Sociocultural factors frequently pose another barrier to accessing care. These include poor healthcare literacy (meaning inadequate knowledge of local healthcare systems), language and insufficient interpreter support, lack of access to transportation, confusion about entitlement to services among service providers, and cultural insensitivity among front-line health workers.[27,28] "In other words, learning how to navigate a complex system in a new country where service providers and patients do not share fluency in the same language or cultural customs likely makes it hard for patients to access that system."[27(p704)] At our CCRIHC clinics most refugees have never experienced an organized, primary care–based healthcare system. They express trepidation when confronting Canada's complex and daunting health system after gaining healthcare coverage. "What is a drugstore?" one young Syrian mother asked when we provided her a prescription for her daughter's earache. "How do I find a drugstore? Is it a woman who I talk to?" Beliefs about the need for healthcare or health services, based on the person's country of origin, may also affect access.[22]

Calls for more culturally competent care have been on the rise.[29] There is growing awareness of the need to educate health providers and help them to reflect on their own and others' cultural attitudes, beliefs, behavior, and communication strategies and to promote practice that fosters quality, nondiscriminatory care.[30] Currently, many health services are alienating to individuals who do not hold Western values.[4,29]

Systemic Barriers: Poorer Health Outcomes

Given systemic barriers, evidence shows—and our experience confirms—that refugees and uninsured immigrants avoid or delay seeking care until the situation is urgent.[29] A review of emergency visits in Ontario shows that while the uninsured are sicker than the insured, they are less likely to be admitted, more likely to leave without treatment, and more likely to die than those with insurance.[31] A case from our clinic highlights how intersecting vulnerabilities and lack of healthcare lead to significant harm.

Aisha, aged 18 years, from Grenada, was entering college when she experienced another in a series of sickle cell crises and sought medical care. Her condition was beyond primary care. We referred her to the hospital emergency department. At first, she refused to go, having experienced previous requests for upfront payment before receiving care. The doctor reassured Aisha that this would not happen. This was an emergency, we told her, providing her with a referral letter and calling ahead to the emergency department.

At the emergency department Aisha was told she had to pay $350 before they would provide care. She was told her current condition was not an emergency. Not having the money, Aisha explained that her sickle cell crisis would soon leave her unconscious; it had before. Emergency department admitting staff told her that if she became unconscious, they would take her in and treat her without demanding payment first. Aisha seated herself near the triage station in full view of the nurses and waited. When she collapsed, she was taken in. After 3 days in the hospital she received a bill for more than $5,000.

Aisha was a sponsored youth in Canada, sent for by her father and stepmother at age 12. Her parents later separated and left Canada. Her sponsorship lapsed. Aisha was left to fend for herself without health insurance. She managed to get a part-time job, find a room to rent, complete high school, and enter college in Scarborough. Her hospital bill ended her education.

Aisha's care experience seemed more like torture and assault than competent medical care. Being born in a developed country with a national health service should not be akin to winning a healthcare lottery.

Research also shows differences in pregnancy care and perinatal outcomes for uninsured immigrants and refugee claimants new to Canada compared to insured women.[32,33] For example, uninsured mothers experienced a higher percentage of cesarean sections due to abnormal fetal heart rates and required more neonatal resuscitations.[32] In our clinics 80% of undocumented migrants and failed refugee claimants report either absent or incomplete antenatal care.

In 2018 Jen arrived at our clinic for her first prenatal visit because of severe headaches. She was 37 years old and 34 weeks pregnant. Her symptoms were from a life-threatening obstetrical emergency. Jen immigrated to Canada 8 years ago as a foreign domestic worker. She had been steadily employed for 7 years, but last year Jen lost her job. Her pregnancy made gaining new employment difficult. Unemployed, her public health insurance was canceled. The gynecologist required $2,000 before providing pregnancy care. Immigration officials told her she should go home. We admitted her to the hospital. Jen left with a $4,000 hospital bill.

When does a migrant become "Canadian enough" to be granted access to maternal care? Jen could not access any antenatal care. Her obstetrical emergency could have been prevented, preventing an expensive hospital bill and harm to her and her unborn child.

Many pregnant women attending our CCRIHC clinics report similar experiences. In 2017, at shelters for both newly arrived undocumented refugee claimants and government-assisted refugees with health coverage, women initially hid their pregnancies from our medical staff. They avoided attending health clinics for both pregnancy and other needs, confiding later they feared deportation if their pregnancy was discovered.

In our clinic, where free healthcare is provided to all immigrants and refugees without health insurance, the majority of attendees (66%) have been female; 19% of all patients sought maternity care. We found that 80% of pregnant women who have come to our clinic had deficiencies in prior antenatal care ranging from having lacked adequate provider contact, pelvic examination, screening for diabetes, or counseling about the use of folic acid. Mean gestational age at presentation is 23 weeks. Patients who present near term are delivered by midwives and obstetricians chosen according to the mother's risk factors.

Policy Failure, Social Responsibility, and Access to Healthcare in Receiving Nations

Every refugee's journey is treacherous. Over 1,200 new migrations begin every hour, with the refugees fending for themselves, crossing the sea, the desert, through no fault of their own. How well is the world doing to create access to much-needed healthcare on their journeys and in receiving countries? What is our responsibility to this staggering apocalyptic refugee crisis?

Policy-driven access barriers to essential health services for forced migrants and refugees have persisted in wealthier receiving nations with advanced public health plans.[23] As numbers grow and rising levels of medical needs appear, fear, xenophobic attacks, the erection of walls and fences, and restrictions to healthcare for asylum seekers take hold. Unwelcoming efforts often drive refugees into the hands of smugglers and traffickers.

In North America, yesterday's pioneers were refugees and immigrants who built the foundations of today's strongest economies. Yet in today's world migration crisis, their descendants have replaced altruism with harsh national populace policies, including travel bans, exclusion, protectionism, fear, and rejection. The United States imposed severe immigration restrictions in 2016, but it is not alone. Many European nations have laid down their own nationalist-driven unwelcome mats. In 1956 the world opened its arms to Hungarian refugees; today Hungary erects fences to keep refugees out.

In response to actions taken by the United States, Canada's prime minister sent out a welcoming tweet to the world's refugees on January 28, 2017:

> To those fleeing persecution, terror & war,
> Canadians will welcome you, regardless of your faith.
> Diversity is our strength.

Nearly 50,000 people claimed asylum in Canada in 2017, including 20,600 who crossed the US border, mostly in Quebec.[34] Originally fleeing unsafe nations, they took Canada's welcome at face value, crossing a dangerous frozen northern border on foot or hidden in trucks. Yet Canadian government policy subsequently accepted only 63% of these refugee claims.[35] In 2017–18 only 7% of refugee claims by Haitians have been accepted. Access to public healthcare was delayed for months for many we treated. Uninsured pregnant mothers went without antenatal care. Children with asthma found it harder to breathe. Rejected refugee claimants became medically uninsured undocumented immigrants.

Government policy obstructing healthcare access for forced migration populations in Western nations is being used for immigration enforcement purposes. This is a direct challenge to the moral foundations of medical care and the social responsibility of physicians to access equity.

In 2002 the Medical Professionalism Project authors were moved to emphasize this threat to physician altruism, social responsibility, and health care equity in the *Charter on Medical Professionalism in a New Millennium*.[36] The charter asserts that changes to healthcare delivery systems in countries throughout the industrialized world threaten the foundations of medical professionalism:

> The conditions of medical practice are tempting physicians to abandon their commitment to the primacy of patient welfare . . . the objective of all healthcare systems is the availability of uniform, equitable access. Physicians must individually and collectively strive to eliminate discrimination barriers to equitable healthcare access whether based on race, gender, socioeconomic status, ethnicity, religion, or any other social category. Altruism contributes to the trust that is central to the physician–patient relationship. Market forces, societal pressures, and administrative exigencies must not compromise this principle.[36(pp243-246)]

This is becoming harder to do. The macro level of policymaking where corporate pressures trump ethical healthcare values cannot be trusted to make medically and socially responsible healthcare access decisions. It is too disconnected from the reality of the micro level, where endless lived realities of being undocumented and medically uninsured meet disease, disability, and death head on. Being in the room with a migrant 3-year-old refugee girl struggling to breathe for want of a $10 asthma inhaler is as compellingly and shamefully grotesque an argument as can be made for affirmative social responsibility action.

Withholding basic healthcare access through an immigration-health policy matrix is not prudent for Western nations to take. Pushing healthcare costs down the line, letting diseases worsen, and harming an essential human labor force is arguably counterproductive and expensive. Public health and public safety research demonstrates the risks to societies of leaving infectious diseases untreated, persons unimmunized, and patients with serious mental health problems unmanaged. In 2003, with severe acute respiratory syndrome (SARS) and again in 2014 with the Ebola virus, asylum seekers without access to health insurance were arriving at our center from endemic geographies but were unable to afford community clinics and hospital screening.

Arguably, physicians hold their medical skills in trust for the society they serve—all its residents. When physicians are neutral on healthcare denial and inequity, they have chosen to side with those who create unjust policies. Threats to their careers, jobs, and remuneration can ensue for taking a stand. Sadly, medical ethics are not enforceable when governments are complicit in access and social responsibility violations through their policies.

The current stance of European countries makes a farce of the UN conventions that they have all ratified, which include guaranteeing the right to health care for undocumented migrants. All member states should detach health care from immigration control and take the necessary measures to ensure that access to health care for undocumented migrants is uniformly implemented by national and local authorities.[37]

Conclusion

In this chapter, we examined systemic barriers to healthcare for refugees and undocumented immigrants based on our experience at the CCRIHC. Although we focused on the Canadian healthcare system, our experiences can be generalized elsewhere. A 2012 review showed that only 5 of 27 European states were fully meeting their internationally agreed-to responsibilities for access to healthcare set down in United Nations and European Union agreements for undocumented migrants, including recently failed refugee claimants.[20] While we recognize some of the information may be out of date, in all cases government policies were responsible for restricting access.

Migration is a major issue facing the world today; the plight of refugees and undocumented immigrants is only expected to get worse.

> Today, as yesterday, a nation is judged by its attitude towards refugees.
> —Elie Wiesel, Nobel Laureate and human rights leader

References

1. Caulford P, Vali Y. Providing health care to medically uninsured immigrants and refugees. *Can Med Assoc J*. 2006;174(9):1253–1254. doi:10.1503/cmaj.051206
2. United Nations. *New York Declaration for Refugees and Migrants. Resolution A/71/L.1*. New York; 2016.

3. United Nations. *International Migration Report 2017*. New York; 2017.
4. International Organization for Migration (IOM). *Migration Terms*. https://www.iom.int/key-migration-terms.
5. United Nations High Commission for Refugees. *Global Trends: Forced Displacement in 2016*. 2017. www.unhcr.org/statistics. Accessed March 15, 2018.
6. United Nations High Commission for Refugees. *Figures at a Glance*. 2017. unhcr.org. Accessed March 15, 2018.
7. United Nations High Commission for Refugees. *UNHCR Global Trends: Forced Displacement in 2014*. 2015. www.unhcr.org.
8. United Nations. *Population Facts*. Department of Economic and Social Affairs, Population Division. www.unpopulation.org.
9. de Leon Siantz ML. Feminization of migration: a global health challenge. *Glob Adv Health Med*. 2013;2(5):12–14. doi:10.7453/gahmj.2013.065
10. Adanu RMK, Johnson TRB. Migration and women's health. *Int J Gynaecol* 2009;106(2):179–181. doi:10.1016/j.ijgo.2009.03.036
11. United Nations Office of Drugs and Crime. *Global Report on Trafficking in Persons*; 2014.
12. Jewkes R. Intimate partner violence: causes and prevention. *Lancet*. 2002;359(9315):1423–1429. doi:10.1016/S0140-6736(02)08357-5
13. Blitz B, d'Angelo A, Kofman E, Montagna N. Health challenges in refugee reception: dateline Europe 2016. *Int J Environ Res Public Health*. 2017;14(12):1484. doi:10.3390/ijerph14121484
14. Keygnaert I, Dialmy A, Manço A, et al. Sexual violence and sub-Saharan migrants in Morocco: a community-based participatory assessment using respondent driven sampling. *Glob Health*. 2014;10(1):32. doi:10.1186/1744-8603-10-32
15. Puri L. Op-ed: Empowering women and girl migrants and refugees. September 2016. http://www.unwomen.org/en/news/stories/2016/9/op-ed-empowering-women-and-girl-migrants-and-refugees.
16. Piwowarczyk L, Fernandez P, Sharma A. Seeking asylum: challenges faced by the LGB Community. *J Immigr Minor Health*. 2017;19(3):723–732.doi:10.1007/s10903-016-0363-9
17. Equal Rights Coalition. Statement on Situation in Chechnya, April 26, 2017. http://international.gc.ca/world-monde/issues_development-enjeux_developpement/human_rights-droits_homme/eqr-ced.aspx?lang=eng.
18. Chávez KR. Identifying the needs of LGBTQ immigrants and refugees in southern Arizona. *J Homosex*. 2011;58(2):189–218.doi:10.1080/00918369.2011.540175
19. Newbold KB, McKeary M. Journey to health: (re) contextualizing the health of Canada's refugee population. *J Refug Stud*, published March 3, 2018. doi:10.1093/jrs/fey009
20. Cuadra CB. Right of access to health care for undocumented migrants in EU: a comparative study of national policies. *Eur J Public Health*. 2012;22(2):267–271. doi:10.1093/eurpub/ckr049

21. Moris D, Kousoulis A. Refugee crisis in Greece: healthcare and integration as current challenges. *Perspect Public Health*. 2017;137(6):309–310. doi:10.1177/1757913917726019
22. World Health Organization. *Migration and Health: Key Issues*. Office for Europe euro.who.int. Accessed March 15, 2018.
23. Graetz V, Rechel B, Groot W, Norredam M, Pavlova M. Utilization of health care services by migrants in Europe—a systematic literature review. *Br Med Bull*. 2017;121(1):5–18. doi:10.1093/bmb/ldw057
24. Mahon A, Merry L, Lu O, Gagnon AJ. Postpartum pain in the community among migrant and non-migrant women in Canada. *J Immigr Minor Health*. 2017;19(2):407–414. doi:10.1007/s10903-016-0364-8
25. McKeary M, Newbold B. Barriers to care: the challenges for Canadian refugees and their health care providers. *J Refug Stud*. 2010;23(4):523–545. doi:10.1093/jrs/feq038
26. Campbell RM, Klei AG, Hodges BD, Fisman D, Kitto S. A comparison of health access between permanent residents, undocumented immigrants and refugee claimants in Toronto, Canada. *J Immigr Minor Health*. 2014;16(1):165–176. doi:10.1007/s10903-012-9740-1
27. Kalich A, Heinemann L, Ghahari S. A scoping review of immigrant experience of health care access barriers in Canada. *J Immigr Minor Health*. 2016;18(3):697–709. doi:10.1007/s10903-015-0237-6
28. Ahmed S, Shommu NS, Rumana N, Barron GRS, Wicklum S, Turin TC. Barriers to access of primary healthcare by immigrant populations in Canada: a literature review. *J Immigr Minor Health*. 2016;18(6):1522–1540. doi:10.1007/s10903-015-0276-z
29. Gagnon AJ, Dougherty G, Wahoush O, et al. International migration to Canada: the post-birth health of mothers and infants by immigration class. *Soc Sci Med*. 2013;76:197–207. doi:10.1016/j.socscimed.2012.11.001
30. Guilfoyle J, Kelly L, St Pierre-Hansen N. Prejudice in medicine: our role in creating health care disparities. *Can Fam Physician*. 2008;54(11):1511–1513, 1518–1520.
31. Hynie M, Ardern CI, Robertson A. Emergency room visits by uninsured child and adult residents in Ontario, Canada: what diagnoses, severity and visit disposition reveal about the impact of being uninsured. *J Immigr Minor Health*. 2016;18(5):948–956. doi:10.1007/s10903-016-0351-0
32. Wilson-Mitchell K, Rummens J. Perinatal outcomes of uninsured immigrant, refugee and migrant mothers and newborns living in Toronto, Canada. *Int J Environ Res Public Health*. 2013;10(6):2198–2213. doi:10.3390/ijerph10062198
33. Shah RR, Ray JG, Taback N, Meffe F, Glazier RH. Adverse pregnancy outcomes among foreign-born Canadians. *J Obstet Gynaecol Can* 2011;33(3):207–215.
34. Siegfried K. *The Refugee Brief-22 March 2018*. United Nations High Commission for Refugees; 2018.

35. Immigration and Refugee Board of Canada. Refugee Protection Claims by Country of Alleged Persecution-2017. www.irb-cisr.gc.ca. Accessed March 15, 2018.
36. ABIM Foundation. American Board of Internal Medicine, ACP-ASIM Foundation. American College of Physicians-American Society of Internal Medicine, European Federation of Internal Medicine. Medical professionalism in the new millennium: a physician charter. *Ann Intern Med.* 2002;136(3):243–246.
37. Access to health care for undocumented migrants in Europe. *Lancet.* 2007;370(9605):2070. doi:10.1016/S0140-6736(07)61872-8

4 RURAL WOMEN

PLACE, COMMUNITY, AND ACCESSING HEALTHCARE

Christy Simpson and Fiona McDonald

Introduction

The provision of health services to rural and remote residents and the ethical questions that arise from this are underanalyzed.[1-3] In this chapter we focus on rural women, a group that is reported to face a "double disadvantage," due to their gender and rural place of residence, when making decisions about healthcare and/or accessing health services.[4(p2)] We argue that gendered and place constructions of "good" rural women and the roles "good" women should play in rural communities intersect with the values of place and community that, in earlier work, we have argued may characterize rural health ethics and may influence health decision making.[1] This nexus is important to understand as these factors may impact rural women, communities, and the ways in which we design and deliver health services. It may also reinforce gender and place stereotypes that can have positive and negative implications for rural women and rural communities more generally.

First, we critically examine stereotypes of what constitutes a "good" rural woman and how this connects with views of rural life as being either idyllic or deficient (the deficit perspective). We then provide an overview of the values of place and community in rural health ethics. Bringing these concepts together, we then examine how these intersecting conceptualizations of rural women, rural life, and the values of place and community may impact rural women's decision making about accessing health services. We employ Penchansky and Thomas's[5] taxonomy of access to analyze access-related issues. We have chosen this taxonomy as traditional analyses of access-related issues focus predominantly on cost and availability of services and overlook other important and relevant issues that impact rural women's access to or choices about accessing health services.

An understanding of the broader context in which rural women may make decisions is important as "behaviors that can look irrational to health professionals often have readily understandable origins in the complex sociospatial structures that constitute women's lives."[6(p875)] When we provide health services to rural women, do we think about how attached they may be to their place and/or community and how difficult it might be for them emotionally, psychologically, and financially to receive care outside of their familiar place? Do we consider how difficult it might be for rural women to access health services when they may be responsible for providing care to children in an area where childcare may be difficult or impossible to access? Do we think about the expense of accessing health services associated with travel, accommodation, and other costs? Or do we make assumptions that subsidies (if they are available) are sufficient, when a subsidy does not pretend to cover the complete costs and we know that some rural residents are poor? Do we consider how stereotypes of the "good" rural woman may influence the ways in which women access health services and the ways in which we design those services? And, even more fundamentally, do we question the stereotypes of the "good" rural woman? Or do we simply accept without question that all rural women conform to these stereotypes? It is our contention that a more nuanced understanding of the ways in which rural women may navigate decisions to access health services may be beneficial at both the individual and health systems levels.

The "Good" Rural Woman

There has been research that indicates an association of rurality with certain traits of character. For example, rural residents are stereotypically seen as being hard-working, self-reliant, virtuous, and stoic, as taking great pride in their independence, and as being "exemplars of traditional values."[7(p1),8-11] Given this, it is no surprise that rural residents have reported defining health in terms of one's ability to work and be independent[8,11] and as being more comfortable with and accepting of death.[12] Further, rural residents are reported and theorized to be more aware of community and social networks, to value them more highly, and to acknowledge responsibilities to other members of that community.[1,9,11] These characteristics of rural residents feed into the gendered concept of the "good" rural woman who is expected to confirm to these place norms.

One of the traditional values[7] is a perspective on gender roles and relationships.[13-17] The "good" rural woman is one who assumes a traditional gender role: she cares for her children, her partner, her extended family, and the community, often sacrificing her own needs.[13-17] She does what is needed to keep things going on the domestic, professional or work, and community fronts, often balancing multiple different demands and being proud of her ability to do so.[16] A rural woman is "level headed, practical, sensible and loyal."[14(p412)]

It is also expected that rural women will undertake the (bulk of the) caring work, which includes emotional work; this reflects broader social expectations of what constitutes a "good" woman.[17] Others note that this caring focus in the rural context is broader than caring for immediate family and includes the maintenance of relationships that are necessary to make communities function.[17] A need for a well-functioning community is recognized as being of particular importance in rural contexts as there are fewer people and "neighbours are not just nice, they are necessary."[9(p6),1,18] A "good" rural woman then may be expected to care for community as well as family.

This description of the "good" rural woman is of course heteronormative and assumes that a woman will have children, and both of these assumptions can and should be contested. However, they both feed into the conceptualization of the "good" rural woman. Not all rural women are accepting of this stereotype; they suggest that they can be "good" rural women in other ways, but they also may acknowledge that this pervasive stereotype is a reality within which they must navigate.[15]

Notwithstanding this, this familiar stereotype of the "good" rural woman is still limited, as other factors specific to perspectives about rural life also contribute to the conceptualization of a "good" rural woman. As Thien and Hanlon note,[19(p157)] "what are the implications, for example, when caring behaviours are not only dictated by gender, but subsumed within place-based expectations of 'independence', 'resilience' and 'self-reliance' in diverse, non-urban places?"

"Good" Rural Women: The Rural Idyll and the Rural Deficit

The "good" rural woman construct is further mediated through stereotypes about the nature of rural life. There are two predominant framings of rural life: the rural idyll and the rural deficit.[1,7,17,20,21] The rural idyll paints rural life as idyllic, focused on close community bonds, quiet healthier lives, connection to land or landscape, and a genuine society in which traditional values are upheld; for example, people take responsibility for each other's welfare. Indeed, some rural women report choosing rural communities because of the desire to live in a strong, close-knit community.[22,23]

In contrast, the deficit model emphasizes everything that rural societies lack and their geographic isolation. In the health context, for example, the poorer health outcomes of rural residents are emphasized, as is the lack of access to services, issues around difficulties in recruiting and retaining health professionals, and the challenges associated with rural health practice. Elsewhere we have argued that these framings should be contested, but they persist because they have elements that reflect the lived realities of rural life.[1] In this chapter, we engage with these framings and the ways in which they may mediate access to health services for (some) rural women.

As Little and Austin note, "The rural idyll has traditionally included very conventional images and expectations of women's place in rural society; at the heart of the family, the centre of the community. There can be no doubt that the woman of the rural idyll is the wife and mother, not the high-flying professional, the single childless business entrepreneur."[24(p106)] In this, we can see how both place-based and gender norms come together to maintain traditional gendered roles for rural women that prioritize mothering and caring.[24] The narrative of the rural idyll also reinforces the importance of social connectedness and social caring in rural communities. As caring is traditionally "women's work," this positions rural women as carers for community as well as family.[24,25] This is mirrored in the deficit perspective of rural living where the emphasis is on the gaps in service provision and the expectations that women, as carers, will fill these gaps as much as possible to ensure community functioning.[1,15,16]

Research is showing there are different ways in which rural women have been engaging with the idyll/deficit and "good" rural women narratives.[16,24,26] The limited research shows that rural women recognize these narratives and acknowledge, to some extent, that they influence, and potentially limit, the way in which they live their lives. Some women appear to accept limitations as part of a tradeoff for them and their children to live an "idyllic" rural life.[24,27] However, other women acknowledge that while they feel pride in fulfilling their role as a "good" rural woman they also worry that this role will subsume other parts of their identity and therefore they will lose their individual sense of self.[16] This illustrates the complexity of women's responses to these stereotypes around place, community, and gender and that these responses are not homogenous. So, if women are making choices to live a rural life and to work within, or outside, these narratives of the "good" rural woman, we then need to be attentive to the values that may inform those choices and to how these values may impact decision making.

The Values of Place and Community

Rural communities, in general, are smaller and more intimate such that relationships and social connectedness take on a greater importance to support individual and community functioning. The ways in which the stereotype of the "good" rural woman is constructed draws upon some values we argued are particularly relevant to rural health ethics,[1] notably the values of community and place.

We developed the values of place and community by using insights from feminist epistemology and feminist standpoint theory.[1] In our view, the benefit of using these theories is that they highlight the perspectives of those who are in nondominant or disadvantaged groups, which for us includes rural women, who may be doubly disadvantaged by gender and place.[4] Epistemology is the systematic investigation of knowledge and beliefs. Feminist epistemology encourages the examination of gendered and other perspectives (discussed above) about constructions of knowledge. Within the field of feminist epistemology, we drew on standpoint theory, which is based on the concept that who we are and what we value is shaped by where we come from. Where we come from refers to the values, beliefs, and norms associated with a place, community, and time.

The value of place has four components that may be differentially weighted, depending on the individual: (a) geography; (b) emotional connections to land, a feature of the landscape, or location; (c) a sense of belonging to a place; and (d) a sense of identity associated with that place.[1] In other words, the value of place is about the value people accord to their relationship with a place. The attachment that some rural women have to "their" land—the land they or they and their family farm—and to the rural environment within which they live are important factors in why these women continue to live in these settings and make the option of moving away or moving into an urban setting unappealing or challenging.[15] Other women who live in rural areas, even if they are not involved in farming, also express attachment to place. Rural settings are seen as desirable places to live, emphasizing the ability to be closer to nature or more natural surroundings and as a better place to raise children.[27]

The value of community is about the sense of obligation that people may have to those in their community.[1] In other words, the value of community is about the value people place on their relationship with their community or communities. We theorize that the value of community has two components, namely solidarity and reciprocity.[1] Solidarity captures the sense that "everyone is in this together," emphasizing the need to work with each other. Reciprocity focuses more on the nature of doing something for others, who then may have a perceived obligation to provide assistance in the future as a fellow community member. Rural women who hold the value of community may enact this via either solidarity or reciprocity or both. For example, if a rural woman feels she has obligations to her community, she may feel reluctant to leave this community, even for needed healthcare, recognizing that her absence may impact others and feeling guilty about adding to their burdens. Or, she may not want to be "ill" and choose to return to her community sooner than recommended in order to reduce this burden on others to take care of her and her family. A strong community can also be a source of emotional, financial, and practical support for women and their families during health crises because that community values solidarity and/or reciprocity. An older rural woman receiving treatment for breast cancer who was a participant in a study undertaken by Sawin[28(p7)] describes her experience as "I pretty much used up the neighbourhood, but I always had somebody to take me [to her treatment, which was just under 100 km away, over a mountain range]." Sawin[28(p8)] also noted, "Communities were aware of the financial strain that cancer treatment put on the participants and their families. One woman's church gathered up $1,100 to pay for the gasoline needed for transportation to cancer treatment."

From psychology, we understand that some may experience so strong an attachment to place and/or community that there may be psychological consequences or distress accruing from disassociation with that place/community.[29-32] Drawing from epistemology we have argued that attachment to place/community can also, for some, be significant in the construction of their identity.[1] If we accept that, for some, their identity is tied up with their attachment to or the way in which they value place and/or community, then health professionals and the health system, in our view, have a moral obligation to be respectful, attentive, and responsive to the ways in which (access to) health services can impact a person's decision making and sense of self.

We acknowledge that not every rural woman will hold the value of place and/or community, but some will—and some may hold the value or values quite strongly. If some do hold these values, in our view, this requires that these values, along with the needs of rural women, are engaged with by those providing or designing health services.

Jane, a 38-year-old, presents at her family doctor's office. She has been diagnosed with breast cancer and needs to decide whether to undergo a mastectomy versus breast-conserving surgery (lumpectomy) and radiation therapy. Mastectomy can be done at the local hospital, which is 30 minutes away by road. Breast-conserving surgery and radiation therapy requires travel to a larger hospital that is much further away for a six-week period. The recommendation from the specialists is that she is a good candidate for lumpectomy and radiation therapy.

But what other factors may be important to, and potentially influence, Jane's decision?

Jane has two children under the age of five. She and her partner run a small dairy farm. They have no family in the area. There are no formal daycare services for children in the immediate area. The area is in drought and it is difficult for them to raise the money to purchase water and feed for the cows, let alone hire someone to care for the farm or the children. Neither she nor her partner knows anyone in the town where the larger health facility is located. There is no healthcare travel subsidy available in this region. However, Jane is aware that the community has undertaken fundraising in the past to help cover the costs of going away for treatment. Jane and her partner had initially moved to the area as they were able to purchase land relatively cheaply. Now Jane cannot imagine living anywhere else and loves the view of the stars over the river. Jane does a lot of volunteer activities in the community and is well liked and respected.

What would you decide if you were in Jane's position or recommend if you were her family doctor?

The "Good" Rural Woman: Access to Health Services

Bringing together the insights from rural health ethics (and the values of place and community) and from the ways the stereotypes about the "good" rural woman and rural life are constructed and negotiated, we examine a critical issue for all rural residents: access to health services. In this section we unpack the concept of access and how it relates to rural women's decision making about healthcare, using Penchansky and Thomas's[5] taxonomy. Penchansky and Thomas[5] define access as the degree of fit between the patient and the healthcare system, arguing that the concept of access to health services has five dimensions: availability; affordability; accessibility; acceptability; and accommodation.

Availability refers to the sufficiency of the supply of health professionals, health facilities, and health services, with reference to the health needs of a population or group.[5] This is very commonly discussed in the rural health and rural health ethics literature.[1,33–38] It is a well-recognized fact that internationally most countries experience distribution issues, with many health professionals clustered in urban regions and fewer choosing to practice in rural areas.[39–44] This means that many rural residents may not be able to access health professionals in their community as regularly, or that they may need to travel. Similarly, there are fewer hospitals in rural areas, and they often offer a more limited range of services; for example, they may not offer obstetrics and gynecology.[1,33]

Most rural residents will face availability constraints. However, rural women may experience availability issues differently than rural men. This may be attributed to a number of factors. The neoliberalist approach to health services focuses on centralizing services in regional areas, limiting service provision in the name of efficiency and an increasing expectation that communities (e.g., volunteers) or families will fill in some of the "gaps" left by this process.[1] Women also experience different patterns around their need to access health services (e.g., higher utilization by women in reproductive years, much higher rates of domestic violence).[45] These specialized services are often the type that are most affected by neoliberalist reforms and are less likely to be available locally.

Also, rural women often are the ones seeking care for any children or older family members or community members for whom they have responsibility or have assumed responsibility—the gendered face of the value of community. Accordingly, any "gaps" between what health services are needed by rural women themselves and/or those they care for require them to navigate between what is available locally and what one must travel for, and their day-to-day responsibilities in work, household, and community as mediated by the "good" rural woman stereotype.[22]

Affordability, as defined by Penchansky and Thomas,[5] draws attention to the costs of health services, health insurance, and ability to pay. Affordability is discussed in the rural health ethics literature, but as that literature primarily comes from the United States, the discussion focuses on the issue of rural residents of that country not being able to afford health insurance and so not being able to afford to access health services.[8,33,46] This is a significant problem in the United States, especially given the changes to Obamacare, and has the potential to unduly affect rural women, who have higher poverty rates than rural men (see the section on accessibility to healthcare). It is less of a concern in countries such as Canada, Australia, and New Zealand, where universal health systems cover the direct costs of medically necessary services. The indirect costs of travel for rural women and their impact on accessibility are discussed in the next section.

This dimension also addresses patients' perspectives on the value of a health service in comparison to its overall cost.[5] Rural women's perspectives on the value of health services may be mediated through the values of place and community and the stereotypes of the "good" rural woman and rural life. The "cost" of healthcare should not be narrowly construed to be about just financial cost (although this is of course significant) but should also appreciate the social costs that may arise from making decisions about accessing health services. These social costs are intangible but may be highly important influences on rural women's decision making, in addition to family considerations. For example, if a rural woman has a network of friends or acquaintances who value community, those people may be willing to offer support with the understanding that this is just what community members do to support each other or that the rural woman in question will "pay this back" and reciprocate by providing support in similar circumstances at some point in the future. However, this ability to reciprocate in the future may be influenced by the nature of the illness or injury (e.g., if it is a long-term illness or requires many trips to town for care). Some rural women may defer asking for support at one point in an illness in anticipation that they will need further support later, not wanting to "overdraw their account." Others with a life-limiting illness may recognize that they will not be able to reciprocate in the future and underestimate the previous contributions they have made to community functioning. While in many cases community members may offer support, despite the internal questioning of women as to whether they are "owed" it, if a community is under stress (e.g., drought, bush fires), the ability of the community and of other rural women to lend assistance for healthcare needs may be diminished. A rural woman may choose to not share or reveal her or her family's health needs so as not to add to the collective burden faced by the community. While the rural idyll and the value of community suggests that a caring community will take care of its own, we need to be cautious about assuming that all rural communities and all rural women are caring in these ways and/or are able to care in all circumstances. Awareness of the limits of what can be truly reciprocated under times of stress (and more generally) in a community and by individual rural women, and the "cost" to them of accessing health services in terms of community functioning, needs to be taken into account as part of the overall picture of what access to healthcare means in rural settings.

Accessibility is also very commonly discussed in the rural health and rural health ethics literature[1,8,9,33] as this dimension focuses on how far and under what conditions a patient needs to travel to access health services and the costs both direct (e.g., gas, accommodation, food) and indirect (e.g., absence from work, childcare) of that travel.[5]

On average, rural residents are in a lower socioeconomic bracket than their urban counterparts; to put it bluntly, levels of poverty are higher per capita in rural areas than in urban ones.[6,8,47] Within this context, rural women are even more impacted by poverty: "Rural poverty affects women disproportionately, because of the gendered nature of paid work, childcare, and transportation."[6(p872)] Other factors affecting poverty rates for rural women may include longevity, marriage breakup, and an inequitable distribution of family income.[26]

As already discussed, rural residents often have to travel for some, if not all, health services. In some places (e.g., some Australian states), a travel subsidy may be provided for rural residents who must travel and stay in urban areas for medically necessary treatment that cannot be provided reasonably proximate to their community.[48] Despite this, it is a *subsidy* for accommodation and transport only. It does not cover all costs of travel or accommodation, nor does it cover food and other indirect costs arising from that travel. These nonsubsidized costs may place additional strains on low-income rural residents, who may have to choose between accessing health services and balancing their budgets. This may result in delays in accessing treatment or even a decision to not access this treatment, or the patient may fall more deeply into debt when unable to pay other pressing expenses. This point was highlighted by a Christmas fundraising appeal for the Australian Salvation Army in 2017–2018. The appeal focused on the true story of a family living in a remote rural area whose daughter was seriously injured falling out of a tree. The father was a shift worker who had to lose shifts because of his daughter's injury, as well as the costs to the family, who needed to travel to access the necessary health services.[49] The print advertising read, "Living in a remote rural area always has its challenges, but after the floods two years back, then the drought, now this [her daughter's injury] . . . we'd be lucky to keep the electricity on, let alone buy presents . . . Christmas was a luxury we simply couldn't afford."[50] This appeal highlights the precarious position of rural families who incur additional costs associated with injuries or illness and whose incomes are insufficient or uncertain, and thus they struggle to cope with these additional, unplanned costs.

Due to greater poverty rates, more rural women will be affected proportionately by what is or is not covered by subsidies. There are other, even less direct costs that may be experienced by rural women. If women have children, there may be childcare-related costs, or the costs of bringing the children with them when these women are having treatment. If rural women and/or their partners are self-employed or undertake casual work, there also may be issues with taking significant or any time off work, especially if that woman is a single mother or if she or the family have a single income. When a family is on the edge of poverty, even the loss of a single shift can create financial hardship. Additionally, not all universal health systems provide or subsidize items like medications or assistive devices, which places additional financial burdens on women and their families.

Accessibility may also have a disproportionate impact on rural women if traditional gender roles are at play; the assumption may be that their "work" is less important than male work, and therefore women are expected to both organize and undertake any travel for health services.[2] It is also the case that rural women who assume traditional gender roles (i.e., the "good" rural woman) may not be the ones who make financial decisions or who have control of the household budget.[21] This may mean that further negotiating about access to health services that require a budgetary outlay will occur outside of the healthcare consultation and could potentially add to the stress that women feel about accessing health services. And if, as was discussed earlier, there is a tradition of stoicism within the rural community and/or household, this may create some additional difficulties in having such discussions with one's partner, even though there may be a gendered acceptance that it is more acceptable for women to be affected by illness and/or be in charge of accessing health services for themselves and their family. These negotiations may be invisible to referring local health professionals, who may not want to know too many details of their neighbors' family structures and private lives, who may not have the time to inquire into family dynamics, or who may not even consider these issues, instead focusing solely on clinical ones.

An additional dynamic to consider could be intimate partner violence (IPV). Research has shown that rural women may be more likely to be affected by IPV.[28,51–53] IPV makes negotiations about travel to and costs associated with accessing health services even more fraught, as Sawin[28(6)] noted: "For the women who were in abusive relationships, the role of partner-as-driver put him into an increased position of power and control. One woman described trying not to rock the boat because, 'I was dependent on him. In every way. Because he was the one taking me to [urban medical center] all the time.'" This equally applies to discussions about the cost of travel and obtaining treatment.

Acceptability, as another dimension of access, focuses on the relationship between patients' attitudes toward their health providers and vice versa.[5] This may be on an individual level between a patient and a provider; it can also be considered more generally in terms of the attitudes and perspectives of, for example, urban physicians and other health professionals in providing care for rural women (and vice versa). While this dimension is most often explored in terms of religion, age, sex, ethnicity, and socioeconomic status, we are focusing primarily here on acceptability with respect to rurality and gender. How this might arise in terms of acceptability is that some rural women may only have access to health professionals locally who may not have a good understanding of, or empathy toward, rural women's health issues. Hence rural women have to choose between receiving health services from this health professional or the "costs" of travel to receive health services from either a female health professional, if this is desired, or to another health professional who may be more understanding of their needs. Rural women who accept or do not contest in whole or in part the expectations related to the "good" rural woman may respond differently to health professionals who assume that this is the role that they inhabit, rather than those who inquire about how a rural woman sees herself and her role vis-à-vis accessing health services for herself, her partner, and/or her children.

Some rural residents have reported feeling that they have been treated differently by health professionals based on negative stereotypes about rural residents being uneducated, ignorant "hicks".[7,19,54] Inappropriate assumptions and/or a lack of information about what it means to live in a rural area can impact how healthcare is delivered as well as how this care is perceived by rural residents and their willingness to access it. If rural women are stigmatized when receiving health services based on their rural residence and any negative stereotyping of rural women overall, they may face a "double disadvantage" of stigma that may impact their decision making as to accessing health services. Both stigma and bonds to family, place, and community may explain why some rural women (and men) choose, if possible, to receive services locally, even if service quality may be lesser, or may refuse treatment that would take them away from their community for an extended period.[1]

Based on the assumption that it is the woman's role to care, a possible consequence of the "good" rural woman stereotype is that rural women may bear the brunt of criticism for why they did not get their male partner to see a doctor or nurse sooner. While this may also be experienced by urban women, it seems plausible that rural women may have this happen more frequently. This may be especially so if rural women are perceived by health professionals to be in more traditional gender- and place-related roles. Also, there is evidence that suggests rural men are particularly resistant to seeking health services in a timely way.[55,56]

Rural women (and men) may further experience a sense of dislocation if they are required to travel for an appointment or to receive health services. They may not be familiar with the city to which they have been referred, and it can be stressful navigating busier roads, finding parking, and going into unfamiliar health facilities; they may feel "out of place" and alienated. This may be so even for people who do not hold the value of place. If they do hold the value, then they may experience the sense of disorientation and exile from home more acutely. Some health professionals recognize the additional stresses this type of travel places on persons from rural areas and provide support to help make it more familiar (e.g., patient information brochures on where to park, clear directions about where to go in the health facility), recognizing that some of the stress associated with unfamiliarity may decrease as familiarity with the city increases. However, some patients need to travel out of their home community for a sustained period to a place that is "foreign" and lacks the familiar markers of home (e.g., a particular view of a geographic feature). This loss of the facets of place that give one a sense of self and are linked to who one is and what one values can be particularly distressing for some people.[1] This dislocation can create psychological distress and may influence whether one wants to leave one's community because of these attachments to place, community, and people. A person may be reluctant to "travel into the city" due to this. These stressors may have a greater impact on rural women as they may be required to travel more often and may be required to reassure and support their children, partner, and/or other community members whom they care for who are feeling this sense of "displacement."

Accommodation, as another dimension of access, refers to the ways in which health services are organized and how well or able patients are to accommodate, and perceive the appropriateness of, this organization.[5] While

Penchansky and Thomas[5] focus on the ability of the patient to accommodate to the system, we have argued that a patient-centered system should accommodate (within reason) to the needs of patients, especially those who must travel long distances.[1,57] The rural health and rural health ethics literature discusses several facets of accommodation in the organization and delivery of health services.[1,9,13] Scheduling systems for appointments do not necessarily take into account how far some patients may need to travel, the implications if health professionals cancel at the last minute, and whether such travel is truly needed (especially if it is a short appointment or if the check-in with the patient could be accomplished in another fashion). As well, when there are structural factors that affect whether a patient can make an appointment (e.g., the "wet," snowstorms) that may be very place-dependent and only affect some patients who require a specialized health service, it is unclear whether this type of "barrier" to access is considered or addressed when an appointment needs to be rescheduled. More recent discussions about access for rural and remote patients to health services have focused on the possibilities of telehealth, telemedicine, and e-health to reduce the need for travel to access some specialized health services.[3,43,58–61] These types of changes to both scheduling and/or alternative methods for delivering appropriate health services could be beneficial for all rural patients.

At the same time, we should consider whether there are any differences in perceived appropriateness and accommodation by, in this case, rural women if these approaches to health service delivery are used. It is possible that online service delivery may reduce some concerns about privacy and confidentiality of health information, especially in respect of more intimate women's health needs. For particular health conditions, telemedicine, telehealth, and e-health may have the potential to mitigate the need for rural women to travel to access health services. This may be beneficial as those women who feel tied to their place and/or community do not have to leave it as frequently and incur the associated costs. However, research has suggested that engagement with online health activities does vary by rurality and gender, and that the impact of technological, health, and e-health literacy does affect the uptake and use of this form of healthcare.[58,62,63] Accordingly, a "one size fits all" approach to telehealth or e-health may not be appropriate in order to effect the best possible health outcomes. Further research is needed to examine how rural women from a variety of different rural contexts perceive alternate modes of health service provision.

Conclusion

We started this chapter by examining the decision making of rural women when accessing health services, as these women are a group that is reported to face a "double disadvantage" due to their gender and rural place of residence.[4(p2)] We agree with Dolan and Thein[64(p39)] that rural life can be experienced as "a specific space of power and oppression that is co-implicated with processes of gendering identity." We have argued in this chapter that gendered and place constructions of "good" rural women and the roles "good" women should play in rural communities intersect with the values of place and community that may characterize rural health ethics and may influence health decision making. This nexus is important to understand as it may impact women, communities, and the ways in which we should design and deliver health services. It also may reinforce gender and place stereotypes, such as the rural deficit and rural idyll, all of which can have positive and negative implications for rural women and rural communities more generally. One of the most problematic aspects of the "good" rural women stereotype, as reinforced by the rural idyll/deficit stereotypes with their emphasis on caring communities, is the assumption that rural women will "naturally" be carers for not only their family but also their communities. In and of itself the value that some people place on communities as sites of mutual support and assistance is highly positive. However, what is less positive is if there is a perception that one gender should predominantly assume the role of holding that community together in terms of the provision of informal community caring. It is also highly problematic if policy is made to remove and centralize some forms of health and other social supports from communities, assuming that the community (i.e., "good" rural women) will fill the void left by the removal of services hitherto provided by the state. In this context we agree with Bondi that this "has the potential to oppress both carers and cared for,"[65(p250)] although we have primarily focused in this chapter on the "carers."

We deliberately chose to use a broad taxonomy of access to health services as some of these broader dimensions have significant impacts upon rural women but are largely unexplored in the ethics literature. In examining the different dimensions of access and analyzing their application to rural women we have illustrated the complex interplay between the stereotypes of the "good" rural women, the rural idyll/deficit, and the values of place and community. While accessibility and, in the United States, affordability have been acknowledged as key issues mediating the ability of all rural residents to access health services, the gendered analysis in this chapter of all dimensions of access to health services illustrates the subtleties of how some rural women may negotiate decisions about, for example, travel to access specialized health services and highlights issues such as the indirect "costs" of seeking to access health services.

Ultimately, if we truly intend to improve women's health, understanding how rural women make health decisions and the factors that may influence their decision making is important. One of the issues with gender- and place-based stereotypes is the assumption that all rural women will behave the same way. While stereotypes can be powerful in influencing behaviors, some rural women will embrace, some will resist, and some will selectively engage with these stereotypes as they develop their identity, so we cannot assume that all rural women will act in the same ways. We also cannot assume that rural women will hold the values of place and/or community, and those who hold those values may do so strongly or weakly. It is important that we critically examine the implications that these stereotypes and values may have for rural women, rural communities, health professionals, and health systems to ensure that the implications of these issues on decision making and the health of rural women are fully appreciated.

Acknowledgment

We thank the editors for their thoughtful feedback on this chapter.

Notes

1. We acknowledge that there can be multiple communities within one geographic area. For example, a rural community can have a geographic location, but within that community there may be an agrarian community, a mining community, an Indigenous community, women's communities, and so on. We also acknowledge that values associated with these communities can overlap, and for some there will not be a binary distinction between place and people.
2. We recognize this will also apply to urban women; however, some urban women may have lesser gendered expectations, and travel may be simpler and less time-consuming, proportionally speaking.
3. Of course, for these types of innovations in healthcare to succeed, there is a need for infrastructure that ensures reliable mobile and internet coverage in rural settings that is of a sufficient quality that it will not interfere with any clinical assessments and discussions. This needs to be a national priority for countries where these approaches are being considered and/or implemented.

References

1. Simpson C, McDonald F. *Rethinking Rural Health Ethics*. Basel: Springer International; 2017.
2. Nelson W, Lushkov G, Pomerantz A, Weeks W. Rural health care ethics: is there a literature? *Am J Bioethics*. 2006;6(2):44–50.
3. Nelson W, Greene M, West A. Rural healthcare ethics: no longer the forgotten quarter. *Camb Q Healthc Ethics*. 2010;19:510–517.
4. Chapman P, Lloyd S. *Women and Access in Rural Areas: What Makes the Difference? What Difference Does It Make?* Aldershot, UK: Avebury; 1996.
5. Penchansky R, Thomas J. The concept of access: definition and relation to consumer satisfaction. *Med Care*. 1981;19(2):127–140.
6. Sutherns R, Bourgeault IL. Accessing maternity care in rural Canada: there's more to the story than distance to a doctor. *Health Care Women Int*. 2008;29:863–883.
7. FrameWorks Institute. How to talk about rural issues. http://www.frameworksinstitute.org/assets/files/PDF_Rural/How_to_Talk_Rural.pdf. Published 2008. Accessed January 31, 2018.
8. Nelson W. The challenges of rural health care. In: Klugman C. Dalinis P, eds. *Ethical Issues in Rural Health Care*. Baltimore, MD: Johns Hopkins University Press; 2008:34–59.
9. Pesut B, Bottorff JL, Robinson CA. Be known, be available, be mutual: a qualitative ethical analysis of social values in rural palliative care. *BMC Med Ethics*. 2011;12(19):1–11.
10. Hull M, Fennell K, Vallury K, Jones M, Dollman, J. A comparison of barriers to mental health support-seeking among farming and non-farming adults in rural South Australia. *Aust J Rural Health*. 2017;25(6):347–353.
11. Gessert C, Waring S, Bailey-Davis L, Conway P, Roberts M, VanWormer J. Rural definition of health: a systematic literature review. *BMC Public Health*. 2015;15(387):1–14.
12. Gessert C. Rural-urban differences in end-of-life care: reflections on social contracts. In: Klugman C, Dalinis P, eds. *Ethical Issues in Rural Health Care*. Baltimore, MD: John Hopkins Press; 2008:15–33.
13. Pugh R, Cheers B. *Rural Social Work: An International Perspective*. Bristol, UK: Policy Press; 2010.
14. Little J. "Riding the rural love train": heterosexuality and the rural community. *Sociol Ruralis*. 2003;43(4):401–417.
15. Tickamyer A, Henderson D. Rural women: new roles for the new century? In: Brown D, Swanson L, eds. *Challenges for Rural America in the Twenty-First Century*. University Park, PA: The Pennsylvania State University Press; 2003:109–117.

16. Heather B, Skillen DL, Cross J, Vladicka T. Being a good woman: the gendered impacts of restructuring in rural Alberta. In: Leipert BD, Leach B, Thurston W, eds. *Rural Women's Health*. Toronto: University of Toronto Press; 2012:253–268.
17. Thien D. Well beings: placing emotion in rural, gender, and health research. In: Leipert BD, Leach B, Thurston W, eds. *Rural Women's Health*. Toronto: University of Toronto Press; 2012:423–440.
18. Bourke L. Rural communities. In: Lockie S, Bourke L, eds. *Rurality Bites*. Melbourne: Pluto Press; 2001:118–120.
19. Thien D, Hanlon N. Unfolding dialogues about gender, care and "the North": an introduction. *Gend Place Cult*. 2009;16(2):155–162.
20. Seebach M. Small towns have a rosy image. *Am Demogr*. 1992;14(10):19.
21. Sutherns R. So close yet so far: rurality as a determinant of women's health. *Can Womens Stud*. 2005;24(4):117–122.
22. Bourgeault I, Sutherns R. Gender, health, care and place: living in rural and remote communities. In: Kuhlmann E, Annandale E, eds. *The Palgrave Handbook of Gender and Healthcare*. 2nd ed. Basingstoke, UK: Palgrave McMillan; 2012:287–302.
23. Leipert BD, Reutter L. Women's health in northern British Columbia: the role of geography and gender. *Can J Rural Med*. 2005;10(4):241–254.
24. Little J, Austin P. Women and the rural idyll. *J Rural Stud*. 1996;12(2):101–112.
25. Bondi L. Counselling in rural Scotland: care, proximity and trust. *Gend Place Cult*. 2009;16(2):163–179.
26. Bourgeault I, Sutherns R, Haworth-Brockman M, Dallaire C, Neis B. Between a rock and a hard place: access, quality and satisfaction with care among women living in rural and remote communities in Canada. In: Jacobs Kronenfeld J, ed. *Access, Quality and Satisfaction with Care (Research in the Sociology of Health Care, Volume 24)*. Bingley, UK: Emerald Group Publishing Limited; 2007:175–202.
27. Struthers C, Bokemeier J. Myths and realities of raising children and creating family life in a rural county. *J Fam Issues*. 2000;21(1):17–46.
28. Sawin E. "My husband would not help me, so I was driving over there": older rural women experiencing breast cancer with a non-supportive intimate partner. *Rural Remote Health*. 2010;10(4):1536.
29. McMillan D, Chavis D. Sense of community: a definition and theory. *J Community Psychol*. 1986;14:6–23.
30. Perkins D, Long D. Neighborhood sense of community and social capital: a multi-level analysis. In: Fisher A, Sonn C, Bishop B, eds. *Psychological Sense of Community: Research, Applications, and Implications*. New York: Plenum; 2002:291–318.
31. Pretty G, Chipuer H, Bramston P. Sense of place amongst adolescents and adults in two rural Australian towns: the discriminating features of place attachment, sense of community and place dependence in relation to place identity. *J Environ Psychol*. 2003;23:273–287.

32. Scannell L. Gifford R. Defining place attachment: a tripartite organizing framework. *J Environ Psychol.* 2010;30:1–10.
33. Bushy A. A landscape view of life and health care in rural settings. In: Nelson W, ed. *Handbook for Rural Health Care Ethics: A Practical Guide for Professionals.* Hanover, NH: Dartmouth; 2009:15–41.
34. McDonald F, Simpson C. Challenges for rural communities in recruiting and retaining physicians: a fictional tale helps examine the issues. *Can Fam Physician.* 2013;59(9):915–917.
35. Simpson C, McDonald F. "Any body is better than nobody?" Ethical questions around recruiting and/or retaining health professionals in rural areas. *Rural Remote Health.* 2011;11:1867.
36. Humphreys J, Wakerman J, Pashen D, et al. *Retention Strategies and Incentives for Health Workers in Rural and Remote Areas: What Works?* Canberra, ACT: Australian Primary Health Care Research Institute; 2010.
37. Wakerman J, Humphreys J. Sustainable primary health care services in rural and remote areas: innovation and evidence. *Aust J Rural Health.* 2011;19(3):118–124.
38. Wakerman J, Humphreys J. Sustainable workforce and sustainable health systems for rural and remote Australia. *Med J Australia.* 2012;1(Suppl 3):14–17.
39. Institute of Medicine Committee on the Future of Rural Health Care. *Quality Through Collaboration: The Future of Rural Health Care.* Washington DC: National Academies Press; 2005.
40. OECD. *OECD Reviews of Health Care Quality: Australia 2015: Raising Standards.* Paris: OECD Publishing; 2015.
41. Queensland Health. Queensland remote and rural services framework. https://publications.qld.gov.au/storage/f/2014-06-06T00%3A38%3A43.498Z/rural-remote-service-framework.pdf. Published June 6, 2014. Accessed November 1, 2017.
42. Romanow R. *Building on Values: The Future of Health Care in Canada. Final Report.* Ottawa: Commission on the Future of Health Care in Canada; 2002.
43. Rural Health Services Review Committee. *Rural Health Services Review: Final Report.* Edmonton: Government of Alberta; 2015.
44. World Health Organization. *Increasing Access to Health Workers in Remote and Rural Areas Through Improved Retention: Global Policy Recommendations.* Geneva: WHO; 2010.
45. Roy K, Chaudhuri A. Gender differences in healthcare utilization in later life. In: Kuhlmann E, Annandale E, eds. *The Palgrave Handbook of Gender and Healthcare.* 2nd ed. Basingstoke, UK: Palgrave McMillan; 2012:256–272.
46. Purtilo R, Sorrell J. The ethical dilemmas of a rural physician. *Hastings Cent Rep.* 1986;16(4):24–28.
47. Bushy A. Health issues of women in rural United States: an overview. In: Leipert B, Leach B, Thurston W, eds. *Rural Women's Health.* Toronto: University of Toronto Press; 2012:80–97.

48. Queensland Government. Travel assistance: patient subsidy scheme. https://www.qld.gov.au/health/services/travel/subsidies. Published 2017. Accessed November 22, 2017.
49. Salvation Army Christmas Appeal (television ad). "Telling the kids there'd be no Christmas was heartbreaking". Also available on: https://salvos.org.au/christmas/give-back-this-christmas/donate-to-the-christmas-appeal/. Published 2017. Accessed November 29, 2017.
50. Salvation Army Christmas Appeal (print ad). *"Telling the kids there'd be no Christmas was heartbreaking"*. Published 2017. Copy on file with author (received November 29, 2017, Brisbane, AU).
51. Dillon G, Hussain R, Loxton D. Intimate partner violence in the young cohort of the Australian longitudinal study on women's health: urban/rural comparison and demographic associations. *Adv Mental Health*. 2015;13(1):18–29.
52. Peek-Asa C, Wallis A, Harland K, Beyer K, Dickey P, Saftlas A. Rural disparity in domestic violence prevalence and access to resources. *Res J Womens Health*. 2011;20(11):1743–1749.
53. Edwards KM. Intimate partner violence and the rural-urban-suburban divide: myth or reality? A critical review of the literature. *Trauma Violence Abuse*. 2015;16(3):359–373.
54. Kelly S. Bioethics and rural health: theorizing place, space and subjects. *Soc Sci Med*. 2003;56(11):2277–2288.
55. Men's Health and Wellbeing WA Sector Report. *A quiet crisis: male health in rural, remote and regional Western Australia*. Men's Health and Wellbeing WA; https://www.menshealthwa.org.au/a-quiet-crisi-male-health-in-rural-remote-and-regional-western-australia/. Published December 2016. Accessed January 31, 2018.
56. Roy P. Help seeking among male farmers: connecting masculinities and male health. *Sociol Ruralis*. 2014;54(4):460–476.
57. Bell A, McDonald F, Hobson T. The ethical imperative to move to a seven-day care model. *J Bioethic Inq*. 2016;13(2):251–260.
58. Goldner M, Hale TM, Cotton SR, Stern MJ, Drentea P. The intersection of gender and place in online health activities. *J Health Commun*. 2013;18:1235–1255.
59. World Health Organization. *Telemedicine: Opportunities and Developments in Member States*. Geneva: WHO; 2010.
60. Institute of Medicine. *The Role of Telehealth in an Evolving Health Care Environment: Workshop Summary*. Washington DC: National Academies Press; 2012.
61. Standing Council on Health. *National Strategic Framework for Rural and Remote Health*. Canberra: Department of Health; 2011.
62. Neter E, Brainin E. eHealth literacy: extending the digital divide to the realm of health information. *J Med Internet Res*. 2012;14(1):e19.

63. Kontos E, Blake KD, Wen-Ying SC, Prestin A. Predictors of eHealth usage: insights on the digital divide from the Health Information National Trends Survey 2012. *J Med Internet Res*. 2014;16(7):e172.
64. Dolan H, Thien D. Relations of care: a framework for placing women and health in rural communities. *Can J Public Health*. 2008;99:S38–S42.
65. Bondi L. On the relational dynamics of caring: a psychotherapeutic approach to emotional and power dimensions of women's care work. *Gen Place Cult*. 2008;15(3):249–265.

NEW AND EMERGING THEMES

5 DRIVERS AND DILEMMAS OF FEMALE GENITAL COSMETIC SURGERY

Dorothy Shaw and Nicole Todd

Introduction: "Size" of the Problem

Women are the primary consumers of cosmetic surgery. Female genital cosmetic surgery (FGCS) is a surgical procedure that women request for reasons that are not medically indicated. Although frequently presented as enhancing women's autonomy, FGCS raises complex ethical issues that have been underdescribed in the bioethics literature and in medical training. There are significant concerns about patient safety and whether practitioners are operating in an ethical manner. Further, there is a gap in the feminist ethics literature about FGCS, indicating the need for more conceptual and normative research. This chapter explores medicoethical considerations related to these procedures.

Requests for FGCS demonstrated a striking 44% increase over a single year.[1] Yet, there are no current data to suggest that the overall size, shape, and health of the external genitals are changing with time, suggesting that sociocultural drivers are at play.[2] FGCS includes many procedures undertaken at the request of the woman, the vast majority of which are for reasons that are not medically indicated and where long-term effects are unknown. Some terms used to describe surgical or laser procedures that purportedly enhance appearance or sexual satisfaction include "vaginal rejuvenation," "revirgination," "designer vaginoplasty," and "G-spot amplification." Such procedures are not only relatively new but also poorly understood and are not part of the training of gynecologists or plastic surgeons during residency. These procedures also include labiaplasty, clitoral hood size reduction, perineoplasty, vaginoplasty, and hymenoplasty, some of which are not medically recognized and are considered marketing terms.[3] Female genital surgical procedures following female genital mutilation/cutting will be discussed separately. These procedures include defibulation, which may be considered medically indicated, and re-infibulation, which is controversial.

FGCS, labiaplasty in particular, has been hotly debated over the last decade or so, with a key driver identified as the ethical principle of autonomy and self-determination. The increasing requests for such procedures, performed alone or in combination, are occurring in a context of lack of knowledge of normal anatomic variation and sexual response, creating significant ethical concerns regarding informed consent, autonomy, and beneficence, as well as conflict of interest. Many of these procedures are being performed in a private-pay environment as they are not medically indicated. Informed consent is deficient, as there is publication bias within the literature with incomplete reporting of the risks, complications, and side effects. The limited amount of peer-reviewed evidence regarding FGCS outcomes does not include long-term follow-up; thus, there are no long-term outcomes available. This is concerning as it impacts the ability to provide full and appropriate informed consent. As such, professional organizations responsible for women's health have issued guidelines or policies calling for avoidance or a cautionary approach. This uncertainty emphasizes the need for an ethical discussion framework to assist us as health professionals to provide the best care for our patients. Cain and colleagues integrate this framework in discussing the macro-ethical and micro-ethical issues of FGCS.[4]

This chapter will explore the normal physiologic development of female genitalia as it pertains to knowledge of what is "normal," expression of autonomy regarding changing societal norms, and the ethical responsibility of the physician to provide accurate information about FGCS, including potential harms and benefits.

Normal Female Genital Development

The labia majora, labia minora, and clitoral hood have a variety of appearances that fit within normal. The labia minora are composed of erectile-like connective tissue, dense blood supply, and nerve endings.[5,6] This underlying structure contributes to the female sexual response.[6] Unlike Tanner staging of breasts and pubic hair, the initiation and completion of genital development is not known. The prepubescent vulva may present with very small labia minora. While the precise development of the external genitalia is not completely known, adolescence is a time of genital growth. Labial growth during puberty may incite concern within the young woman, given prepubescent appearance and lack of discussion regarding normal development. It is unclear whether the labia grow symmetrically at the same velocity, or when development is complete.[7] Accompanying the physical changes, cognitive changes abound. Adolescence is a time of decreased self-esteem, starting at 11 years in Caucasian girls, followed by regaining of self-esteem in high school.[8] The development and relationship of genital self-image and self-esteem is not known in childhood and early adolescence. Thirty percent of women requesting labiaplasty first noted dissatisfaction between 11 and 15 years, 15% between 16 and 20 years, and 21% in their 20s and 30s.[9] In this study, girls as young as 10 years voiced genital dissatisfaction. Given that development is ongoing, and the potential nadir in self-esteem in adolescence, offering FGCS is problematic from an ethical perspective, with many considerations, including professional ethics, generally overriding the normal evolving autonomy of the adolescent. The focus on an educational physical exam (description of normal anatomy, variance in normal appearance, contribution to sexual function) and addressing contributors to low self-esteem are more consistent with non-maleficence.

In reproductive-age women, a wide variety of genital appearances are present. The external genitals change with age, parity, and menopausal status. However, clear criteria defining abnormal labia minora do not exist.[10] Contributing to this is a lack of consistent measurement of labial width. In one study, the labia minora ranged from 7 to 50 mm in asymptomatic women.[11] While the authors were expecting small deviations around the mean, these measurements demonstrated the breadth of diversity in appearance. The external genitals may appear different in standing, lying, and frog-legged positions and during sexual arousal. Further, removal of genital hair can make the vulva more visible.

Reasons for Requests for FGCS

Ostrzenski summarized reasons for seeking FCGS into four categories: anatomic abnormality, functional symptoms, emotional and social disturbance, and aesthetic dissatisfaction.[12] Women may present with physical and psychological complaints. A prospective study by Crouch and colleagues demonstrated that 60% of women desired labiaplasty for improved appearance and 18% to reduce discomfort.[9] In one of the largest cohort studies, 87% of women cited aesthetic concerns and 26% to 64% physical discomfort as reasons for surgery.[13] However, in the women with physical symptoms, only 18% believed surgery would help.[9] While in this study 18% experienced physical symptoms, 18% experienced genital teasing from a partner and 9% from a peer, and 54% did not elaborate on the etiology of the heightened physical awareness.[9] Young adolescents may first complain of physical symptoms, followed by concerns from the mother.[3] Older adolescents have aesthetic concerns, as well as fear of a partner's perception.[3] Women may describe rubbing, chafing, sticking to underwear, and interference with menstrual hygiene products and sexual intercourse. However, over half (57.1%) of women interviewed after undergoing labiaplasty indicated that the postoperative appearance did not meet their expectations, including women who primarily had physical complaints.[14] This demonstrates the underlying concern with appearance. Women may worry about the opinions of peers and current and future sexual partners. This leads women with normal labia minora to pursue FCGS. In the prospective study by Crouch and colleagues, all women requesting labiaplasty had labia that measured within normal published limits.[9] One cross-sectional study (involving women aged 18 to 72 years) failed to demonstrate a difference among women's perceptions of their vulva.[15] This could indicate that genital self-image is stable in adulthood, lending support to the argument that FGCS should be deferred into adulthood.

Self-Image and the Drivers of Genital Self-Image

The media and its unrealistic representations are drivers associated with body dissatisfaction.[16] Women seek genital references from their mothers, peers, and the media. Sources within media include the internet, women's magazines, and pornography.[15] The majority of women (78.6%) who had undergone labiaplasty first heard about FGCS through television and other media.[14] Younger age is associated with use of pornography and friends as a source of information.[15] Adolescents are also more likely to seek sexual information from online sources.[15] In one study, 28.6% of women acknowledged that media representations are unrealistic.[14] Interestingly, 71.4% of women in that study compared their labia to those on the "before" photographs on cosmetic websites and considered themselves worse.[14]

There is a trend in popular media toward the hairless, flat, prepubescent vulva.[15] Complete removal of hair is more commonly done in younger age groups (18 to 44 years).[15,17] Approximately 83.8% of women in one cross-sectional study acknowledged pubic hair removal, including 61% who have removed all their pubic hair at least once.[17] Motivations for this grooming include a perception of improved appearance of the vagina in 31.5% and perceived partner preference in 21.1%.[17] Removal of all pubic hair is associated with younger age, bisexual orientation, sexual activity, receipt of oral sex, and higher scores on genital self-image.[18]

Online pornography also depicts a less varied range of labia minora size.[19] Viewing modified images is not a benign act, as it adversely impacts a woman's self-image. Moran and Lee demonstrated that if women are primed by modified images, they are more likely to view these post-labiaplasty vulvas as normal.[20] Further in this study, all participants rated the postoperative labiaplasty vulvas as fitting with society's ideal. This increased access to genital images and cosmetic surgery could also contribute to increased requests, as it alters society's perspective of what is the norm.[2] Women perceive small, nonprotruding, symmetrical labia minora and a small clitoris as being representative of normal. Liao and Creighton, in their argument for caution around FCGS, note the lack of requests for female genital enlargement.[2] Further, women rated visual depictions of modified vulvas as more in keeping with society's ideal.[20]

The medical literature also fails to demonstrate accurate depictions. Only half of medical textbooks contained a vulva image, and the majority do not represent variety in the amount of labia minora protuberance.[19]

Beyond the media, there are both intrapersonal and interpersonal drivers in genital self-image.[21,22] Research is lacking in positive drivers of genital self-esteem. Genital self-image is higher in women who are sexually active, those who experience orgasm through oral sex or masturbation, and those who undergo gynecologic exams.[21,23] This could demonstrate that healthy sexuality is related to positive genital self-image, yet whether this relationship is correlation or causation has not been determined. Low genital self-image is presumed to be the underlying reason that women may seek these procedures, but the root causes of low genital self-image remain poorly characterized within the literature and poorly investigated by treating physicians. In their review, Swami and colleagues noted multiple studies supporting an association of body dissatisfaction with poor mental health, eating disorders, and low confidence in relationships.[16] There is a high proportion of body dysmorphic disorder in women pursuing FGCS.[24] Rates of self-harm and body image distortion are increased in similar populations requesting alteration of other sexual anatomy.[25] Harmful effects of cosmetic surgery in other body areas, such as breast augmentation, can be delayed for 10 years and result in a two- to three-fold increased risk of suicide and death from alcohol and substance use compared to women who did not undergo breast augmentation.

While there is a connection between low genital self-image and sexual dissatisfaction, there is a paucity of research demonstrating that FCGS improves both genital self-image and sexual satisfaction, suggesting resources should be directed at ensuring appropriate sexual health assessment and treatment. The role of perceived and experienced partner perceptions and genital teasing/shaming needs further exploration.

Erica is a 16-year-old who is referred to a gynecologist to discuss vulvar concerns. Her concerns began in grade 5 when she was changing and a friend made a comment about Erica's protruding labia minora. Initially Erica thought she would grow into them, but nothing has changed. She feels her labia minora stick out the sides of her thong underwear. Erica removes all of her pubic hair. She has difficulties with sports and has quit track and field, as she feels the labia rub together when she runs. She thinks about her labial appearance daily and hates how it looks. She was seen by a family physician, who told her that her labia were abnormal, and her mother agrees with this assessment. She has engaged in several relationships with males. She broke up with her last boyfriend as she was nervous about his opinion of her labia. She also experienced genital teasing from another non-romantic male. She is concerned about acne and denies other concerns with her weight and appearance. She struggles with social anxiety and has been seen by a counselor previously for depressive symptoms. Erica feels that her depression, social anxiety, and concerns about relationships would be solved with surgery on her labia minora. When asked about surgical expectations, she would like both labia minora "removed" so that they are not visible beyond the labia majora.

She was examined in standing and frog-leg position. Her left labia minora measured 4 cm and right minora 5 cm. Erica was told her appearance falls within normal limits. Counseling at the appointment focused on the range of normal genital appearance and that the appearance can change with age, and the paucity of research demonstrating improvement in symptoms with surgery. Risks of surgery were discussed. Options to improve discomfort were suggested, including avoidance of pubic hair removal; use of cotton, wide-gusset underwear; and use of lubricants prior to physical activity. Erica was advised to seek assessment and treatment of her mood and anxiety symptoms.

KEY DRIVERS

Low self-image
Depression, anxiety
Maternal perception of normal anatomy

Fears perception of future partners

ETHICAL PRINCIPLES

Respect, compassion, and dignity
Autonomy—evolving capacity of Erica (adolescent) to provide informed consent
Non-maleficence (do no harm)—evidence suggests labiaplasty for Erica may be harmful, and unclear if growth complete
Beneficence (do good)—no evidence that labiaplasty will be beneficial
Veracity (truth telling, transparency)—provide facts about normal anatomic variation, and risks, benefits, long-term outcomes of surgery

ETHICAL APPROACH TO MANAGEMENT

Reassure Erica, mother, and family physician that exam findings fall within normal variation of appearance.
Perineal hygiene to reduce discomfort
Referral for assessment and management of mental health

DILEMMA

Will Erica seek labiaplasty elsewhere?

Hymenoplasty—A Special Case?

Culture is also a driver for requests for hymenoplasty and virginity testing, which are typically more common in countries and cultures where women's rights and autonomy are compromised. Women in other cultures may also request hymenoplasty and vaginal tightening in the absence of vaginal trauma, presenting additional challenges. Knowledge about what constitutes virginity as opposed to chastity is usually lacking, as is an understanding of the nature of the hymen itself, which can place women at risk of violence and social isolation, or even death.[26] Studies have shown that a hymen can appear intact after vaginal intercourse and ruptured in women who have not had intercourse, as it varies in its structure, flexibility, and thickness.[27]

Physicians can feel pressured to support a woman whose life or well-being is threatened. Surgical options for hymenoplasty are described, but evidence is limited for their efficacy, and breakdown of the repair is one of the complications. Like other surgeries that are not medically indicated, they are not part of the postgraduate curriculum. Perhaps most significantly, the proof of virginity being sought is associated with bleeding at the time of first marital intercourse, yet this reportedly occurs no more than 50% of the time at first intercourse or after surgical repair, primarily due to the lack of vascularity in the hymen.[26,28] This creates unrealistic expectations from hymenoplasty that do not provide the desired outcome. Counseling is very important for women requesting hymenoplasty, with three-quarters of women in a study by van Moorst and colleagues deciding against surgery.[28]

Female Genital Mutilation

Given some similarities between FGCS and female genital mutilation (or cutting/circumcision [FGM/C]), it has been suggested that FGCS could qualify as type IIa (removal of the labia minora only) or type IV (all other harmful procedures to the female genitalia for non-medical purposes; e.g., pricking, piercing, incising, scraping, cauterization).[29] Both involve surgical procedures that are not medically indicated to change the appearance or to impact the function on physically healthy girls or women. FGCS is requested by women from early adolescence; younger patients are typically brought to a health provider by their mother. Mothers typically also bring their daughters for FGM/C, but less often to a surgical health professional. Since FGM/C is illegal in most high-prevalence countries, the cost for the procedure would be very high if they reached a willing surgical health professional. Cost comparisons are not available for FGCS and FGM/C.

In an Australian study by Simonis and colleagues, the incidence of FGCS in the age group 15 to 25 has matched that in the group aged 26 to 45, which is similar to findings in the United Kingdom and the United States.[30] The age at which FGM/C is performed varies, but it is mostly carried out on young girls from infancy to age 15. It is considered a violation of human rights of girls and women, a harmful traditional practice without consent of the girl or woman. FGM/C is illegal in 12 industrialized countries, including Canada, according to the Centre for Reproductive Rights.[31] Furthermore, the wording of the legislation could be interpreted to read that any female genital surgery on adolescents under age 18 that is not medically indicated is also illegal, as consent is not considered valid.[32]

The main differences, other than legality, involve the purpose and the lack of voluntary informed consent. In theory, FGCS is performed for women wishing to enhance their appearance and/or sexual satisfaction, whereas FGM is intended to control women's sexuality and chastity before marriage. Voluntary informed consent, with provisos mentioned elsewhere, is part of

FGCS, whereas this is rarely the case for FGM. Coercion, however, can occur in adolescents or young women in the context of their lives. For example, the situations of a younger adolescent whose mother indicates an abnormality of the labia in her daughter that must be "fixed" or a partner who tells the woman she is not normal and should have surgery hardly fulfill the requirement for voluntary informed consent, with a woman exercising her autonomy.

Reinfibulation

Reinfibulation may be requested after giving birth by a woman who has undergone the infibulation type of FGM (type III), which includes suturing the labia majora together, leaving a small opening. This woman will require defibulation or opening of the sutured tissue of the vulva in order to give birth vaginally. She may request to be resutured or reinfibulated, because to her that feels "normal."

In discussions during education sessions, postgraduate trainees have often queried why this request should not be honored, given the woman is now able to exercise her autonomy, whereas FGM is performed without consent. What is poorly understood by physicians in countries where women have migrated from countries with a high prevalence of FGM/C, is that in their countries of origin, reinfibulation is not an autonomous decision but the result of persuasion by a birth attendant, who typically stands to profit from the procedure, and to perpetuate cultural values.[33] In Canada and other countries, FGM/C is illegal, as discussed earlier in the chapter.[32] It would follow that reinfibulation is also illegal, given that it is not medically indicated and is meant to control a woman's sexuality.

A discussion with the woman and her partner should be undertaken during pregnancy so that she understands that reinfibulation is of no benefit to her and has implications for long-term complications. It also impacts sexual experience as well as the need to defibulate with any subsequent planned vaginal births. These discussions are not optimally timed for a trainee who is faced with repairing the vulva after birth and has never met the woman until she was in labor.

Ali is a 23-year-old who presents to your office for vaginal rejuvenation. Ali has never been sexually active. She has never undergone a gynecologic exam. She has normal menses, without concern. She is otherwise healthy and has received HPV vaccination. She is engaged and would like to ensure her vagina is "ready" for her partner. She has not looked at her vulvar anatomy. She has not engaged in self-touch. She was told by family members that her new husband would expect her to bleed at the time of first intercourse to prove she was a virgin. Ali is a competitive swimmer and is concerned that her use of tampons has made her vaginal opening "loose." She does not want to discuss the use of tampons with her female family members or future husband, as she was told not to use them.

On examination, her external genital anatomy is normal. With labial traction, the vaginal opening is visualized and the exam is normal. The variation in hymen appearance was emphasized as well as the infrequency of bleeding with first intercourse, and she is informed that the hymen may have been stretched by other activities. It was also discussed that vaginal rejuvenation is an advertising term and that there is a publication bias in aesthetic medicine whereby only positive results are published. Ali seems reassured by this discussion and will consider bringing her future husband in to discuss the matter further.

KEY DRIVERS
Cultural expectations regarding virginity/bleeding at first intercourse
Concerns regarding tampon use also widening vagina

ETHICAL PRINCIPLES
Respect, compassion, and dignity
Non-maleficence (do no harm)—no indication for surgery. Surgery does not ensure that bleeding will occur with first intercourse.
Beneficence (do good)—no evidence that surgery would address her concern
Veracity (truth telling, transparency)—provide facts about normal variation in hymen, bleeding at first intercourse, lack of research on aesthetic medicine

ETHICAL APPROACH TO MANAGEMENT
Reassure on variety of hymen appearances and vaginal tone related to tampon use.
Provide facts about normal anatomic variation and frequency of lack of bleeding at first intercourse.
Educate Ali and offer to educate her partner.

DILEMMA
Does cultural expectation place her at risk?

Statements from Professional Societies

The available guidelines on FGCS from professional associations, including the Society of Obstetricians and Gynaecologists of Canada (SOGC), the American College of Obstetrics and Gynecology (ACOG), the Royal Australian and New Zealand College of Obstetricians and Gynaecologists (RANZCOG), the Royal College of Obstetricians and Gynaecologists (RCOG), and the International Federation of Gynecology and Obstetrics (FIGO), all state that they cannot clearly support such surgery ethically.[3,33-38] All refer to the need for informed consent and the lack of clear evidence on which to base such consent. Further, there is consensus that terms commonly used to advertise these procedures are poorly understood and that the procedures are not medically indicated and are not part of the training of gynecologists or plastic surgeons during residency. The lack of knowledge of normal female anatomic variation and developmental changes during adolescence is highlighted by several organizations. Several of the groups raise concerns regarding conflict of interest and the veracity of web-based advertising. Labiaplasty is the exclusive focus of the recent ethical opinion paper of the RCOG, primarily due to the continuing increase in requests for the procedure.

Counseling, screening for body dysmorphic disorder, and referral as appropriate for all patients seeking FGCS, are recommended by SOGC, ACOG, and FIGO.[3,34,37] Several organizations recommend that the procedure not be offered to individuals under age 18. As noted, ACOG, RCOG, SOGC, RANZCOG, and FIGO have all issued statements on the need to exercise caution in providing FGCS.[3,34-38] The message is clear: there is inadequate evidence to support the beneficial claims of FCGS.

So where does that leave the clinician? Gynecologic exams that provide unbiased education on the normal appearance of the vulva should be routine. Genital image is higher in women who undergo gynecologic assessment.[21,23] Care in the use of language in genital description is key. In one study, women were told they had "labial hypertrophy," yet all measurements were less than 5 cm.[7] There is no pathology seen with "labial hypertrophy," as demonstrated in one pathology study that was stopped prematurely, given that all excised labia were histologically normal.[13]

Clinicians must not only include discussion of a variety of genital appearance but should specifically discuss the unattainable images appearing in the media and provide strategies for managing maladaptive behaviors.[39] This is in keeping with the principle of beneficence in promoting a healthy self-image. In a prospective study, there was no improvement in psychological symptoms with FGCS.[24] Mental health screening (for depression, anxiety, eating disorders, body dysmorphic disorder), providing teaching on normal genital appearance, and discussing the publication bias within aesthetic medicine should be included in all assessments of women requesting FCGS. In the adolescent population, young women, and their mothers, may be looking for confirmation of normal development. Shaving and regular use of pads can be irritating to the vulva. Women experiencing symptoms should be counseled about the use of emollients, avoidance of hair removal on the mons, and use of natural/cotton menstrual hygiene products and underwear.

Veracity is imperative in discussions of genital anatomy and the risks of surgery. Surgical risks include incisional dehiscence (7% to 13.3%), wound hematoma (4.7% to 40%), allodynia, paresthesia, infection, damage to adjacent structures, asymmetry, scarring, and impact on sexual function, including dyspareunia (23%).[12,13] In one study reoperation occurred in 7% of patients, and 4% of patients would opt not to have the procedure performed.[13] While most of the data describing surgical complications are of low quality, the risks cannot be ignored.

Non-maleficence should underpin the counseling of patients, given our responsibility to do no harm. These patients should be clearly counseled that surgery is for appearance alone, and improvements in self-image and sexual function cannot be expected.[40] A large cohort demonstrated that only 88% of women were satisfied with the resultant appearance.[13] Braun's review could not demonstrate an association between FCGS and improved sexual function.[41] Goodman and colleagues demonstrated initial improvement in arousal and satisfaction, but it returned to preoperative levels within 6 to 9 months.[24] Some claim that a potential increased risk for suicide, as seen in long-term follow-up of cosmetic breast surgery patients, is a reason to avoid FGCS. Others, however, suggest that it identifies a population at increased risk who require a more fulsome preoperative assessment with a surgical, medical, and psychosocial history as well as a possible model for suicide prevention.[42] Further research into the overlapping predictors is warranted, and its connection to FGCS must be explored.

Role of the Clinician: Dilemmas

As a medical community, we have not done enough to fully explore the indications, surgical techniques, and outcomes (psychological, physical) to offer our patients safe care. A 2015 review of 19 articles by Motakef and colleagues found seven different surgical techniques for labiaplasty in 1,949 patients.[43] Motakef and colleagues also proposed a classification system based on the distance of the lateral edge of the labia minora from the labia majora, not the vaginal introitus, but in the absence of postgraduate education based on evidence, best practice has yet to be established. Cosmetic surgery often occurs outside the public sector, where audit and publication are not required.[44] In one review of cosmetic gynecology, there were 72 peer-reviewed publications, compared to 1,100 articles from marketing literature.[12] The criteria for publishing within advertising does not require use of the rigorous scientific method and unbiased review by scientific peers. The peer-reviewed studies are also of poorer quality, as only two met level II for evidence-based medicine.[12] Another review indicated there are no published studies on failed techniques for labiaplasty, further demonstrating publication bias.[41] Improved methodologic rigor and use of validated assessment tools are needed. Further, long-term follow-up studies are required, both for nonsurgical and surgical approaches to genital dissatisfaction.

The limited peer-reviewed literature places clinicians in a difficult ethical situation. When it comes to anatomic cosmetic surgery, the vulva is different—it is so integral to the woman's sexual response, and appearance is not a de facto determinant of that complex response. Sexual response is in the realm of the gynecologist and the psychologist and is not part of the training of aesthetic surgeons, some of whom advertise widely regarding FGCS and its benefits in improving sexual satisfaction.

To ensure that a woman's right to education and information is met, much more is required in terms of an ethical approach than naively agreeing to a request on the basis of personal autonomy. Is this request coerced in any way? Aesthetic surgeons need to have skills in assessment for mental health, including depression, anxiety, body dysmorphic disorder, and sexual dysfunction. Gynecologists should seek additional training in these and should partner with aesthetic surgeons to produce high-quality, evidence-based medicine. Instead of creating divisions, these health professionals need to provide a safe, unified front to advocate for the best interests of women and adolescent girls.

The Ethical Dilemma of Declining Surgery

Clinicians must balance patient discontent with avoidance of surgical risk when there is no indication. Working through a formal ethical framework can be helpful in navigating this physician/patient divide.[4,45] When surgery occurs outside the confines of a therapeutic benefit, in the face of surgical risk, a well-informed patient may wish to access surgery through the principle of autonomy.[46] Since FGCS procedures are not medically indicated, FGCS is not part of the postgraduate training curriculum for either obstetrician/gynecologists or aesthetic surgeons. Yet the demand for and provision of these procedures continues to climb at a rapid and disturbing rate. For some cultures, hymenoplasty and reinfibulation are requests where a harm-reduction approach is argued by some to be ethical in approaching the issue of autonomy or life-threatening situations.[26,33] Our first and overriding ethical principle as physicians is that of non-maleficence—to do no harm. Although we are obligated to treat the patient with dignity and respect, we are not obligated to carry out procedures that are not medically indicated. A patient may wish to achieve a "normal" vulva, but as clinicians, we have no definition of this. The lack of established norms, standard of practice, and training programs is a very real concern.[40] There are studies in which labiaplasty is offered to symptomatic women where the labial width exceeds 5 cm or the asymmetry between labia exceeds 2 cm.[7,9] In a cross-sectional survey of physicians, 75% felt that abnormal labia span was beyond 5 cm.[10] While many women appear satisfied in the short term with their surgery, there is no long-term follow-up and the quality of the follow-up data is not robust overall.

If a clinician feels there is no anatomic concern, the patient is pushed into aesthetic medicine. Of those who were refused surgery within the public sector, 36% accepted a mental health referral and 40% pursued a second opinion.[9] Aesthetic medicine, as the patient's first consultation, or her option once declined from the public sector, needs to uphold the professional ethical tenets of veracity, integrity, stewardship, and transparency. Ethical principles dictate that the clinician must ensure there are no interfering psychological comorbidities, or coercion.[40] The clinician must ensure that he or she is free from bias, including disclosure of financial involvement in proprietary procedures. Advertisements for FGCS by health professionals should uphold these ethical standards. Proprietary naming of procedures and naming of techniques with positive bias (i.e., "rejuvenation") should be avoided as they interfere with informed consent, trustworthiness, and transparency.

Publications reporting the "satisfaction" of patients are a further threat to transparency if they do not include the regular use of validated questionnaires or assessment tools. For example, one review examined positive patient outcomes in nine papers; five of these did not describe data acquisition, and four used nonvalidated questionnaires.[44] However, the patient may believe these outcomes to be positive given the conclusions drawn by the authors. Follow-up of these studies is often short and incomplete.

Conclusion

The topic of FGCS is very timely given the rapidly increasing demand—for labiaplasty in particular. The drivers of FGCS include heightened awareness of genital anatomy, perceived anatomic abnormality, functional symptoms, emotional and social disturbance, and aesthetic dissatisfaction. The role of the media is problematic, given the lack of accurate knowledge and education on normal development of female external genitalia in both public and medical education systems.

The ethical principle of autonomy and self-determination is described as a driver of aesthetic surgery such as FGCS, though conflict of interest is difficult to avoid in a private-pay environment for these procedures that are not medically indicated. Advertising is also a driver and may promise results that have not been proven by appropriate levels of evidence in peer-reviewed literature.

The tension between the ethical principles of respect for autonomy and non-maleficence creates dilemmas for practitioners. Patients may argue that the surgical indication for pathology is moot: if we do not have a set norm, it is impossible to have an abnormal. RCOG defines a "medically indicated" procedure as one in which functional problems rather than genital appearance leads to the request, but the group goes on to state that the definition of direct clinical care relates to the prevention, diagnosis, or treatment of illness.[36] Agreeing as health professionals when procedures such as labiaplasty are medically indicated and merit payment through a public health system is also a dilemma, especially where access to gynecologic consultation and surgery for other gynecologic, medically indicated procedures may be compromised, bringing to the fore the utilitarian ethical principle. Until such agreement is reached using an appropriate ethical framework, the focus should be on broad education about normal anatomy, fully informed consent, screening for body dysmorphic disorder, and acquisition of good-quality evidence. Physicians should collaborate to ensure procedural justice is addressed. The risk to physicians, in denigration of the reputation of those who ethically decline to perform FGCS procedures that are not medically indicated, has not been explored to date, but sites such as RateMDs.com are being used by dissatisfied patients.[47]

The knowledge of adolescent developmental changes in anatomy and declining to perform genital cosmetic surgery until age 18 is relevant to the ethical principle of beneficence as well as utilitarianism. Clinicians need to protect vulnerable populations.[37] While adolescents may be able to understand and make a fully informed decision, this population is vulnerable. Given that adolescence is a time of physical, cognitive, and emotional development, FGCS cannot be ethically justified in this population. Similarly, sociocultural drivers for hymenoplasty and reinfibulation typically do not occur in a context where women have true autonomy; they are preferably addressed by education and provision of factual information. The debate as to the ethics of health personnel providing surgery that is not medically indicated in a woman of any age will continue until evidence or social norms change.

References

1. American Society for Aesthetic Plastic Surgery. 2013 Cosmetic Surgery National Data Bank Statistics. https://www.surgery.org/sites/default/files/Stats2013_4.pdf
2. Liao LM, Creighton SM. Female genital cosmetic surgery: a new dilemma for GPs. *Br J Gen Pract*. 2011;61(582):7–8.
3. Shaw D, Lefebvre G, Bouchard C, et al. Female genital cosmetic surgery. *J Obstet Gynaecol Can*. 2013;35(12):1108–1112.
4. Cain JM, Iglesia CB, Dickens B, Montgomery O. Body enhancement through female genital cosmetic surgery creates ethical and rights dilemmas. *Int J Gynaecol Obstet*. 2013;122(2):169–172.
5. Iglesia CB, Yurteri-Kaplan L, Alinsod R. Female genital cosmetic surgery: a review of techniques and outcomes. *Int Urogynecol J*. 2013;24(12):1997–2009.
6. Ginger VA, Cold CJ, Yang CC. Structure and innervation of the labia minora: more than minor skin folds. *Female Pelvic Med Reconstr Surg*. 2011;17(4):180–183.
7. Michala L, Koliantzaki S, Antsaklis A. Protruding labia minora: abnormal or just uncool? *J Psychosom Obstet Gynaecol*. 2011;32(3):154–156.
8. Biro FM, Striegel-Moore RH, Franko DL, Padgett J, Bean JA. Self-esteem in adolescent females. *J Adolesc Health*. 2006;39(4):501–507.
9. Crouch NS, Deans R, Michala L, Liao LM, Creighton SM. Clinical characteristics of well women seeking labial reduction surgery: a prospective study. *Br J Obstet Gynaecol*. 2011;118(12):1507–1510.
10. Lowenstein L, Salonia A, Shechter A, Porst H, Burri A, Reisman Y. Physicians' attitude toward female genital plastic surgery: a multinational survey. *J Sex Med*. 2014;11(1):33–39.
11. Lloyd J, Crouch NS, Minto CL, Liao LM, Creighton SM. Female genital appearance: "normality" unfolds. *Br J Obstet Gynaecol*. 2005;112(5):643–646.

12. Ostrzenski A. Cosmetic gynecology in the view of evidence-based medicine and ACOG recommendations: a review. *Arch Gynecol Obstet.* 2011;284(3):617–630.
13. Rouzier R L-SC, Paniel BJ, Haddad B. Hypertrophy of labia minora: experience with 163 reductions. *Am J Obstet Gynecol.* 2000;182:35–40.
14. Sharp G, Mattiske J, Vale KI. Motivations, expectations, and experiences of labiaplasty: a qualitative study. *Aesthet Surg J.* 2016;36(8):920–928.
15. Yurteri-Kaplan LA, Antosh DD, Sokol AI, et al. Interest in cosmetic vulvar surgery and perception of vulvar appearance. *Am J Obstet Gynecol.* 2012;207(5):428 e1–7.
16. Swami V, Taylor R, Carvalho C. Body dissatisfaction assessed by the Photographic Figure Rating Scale is associated with sociocultural, personality, and media influences. *Scand J Psychol.* 2011;52(1):57–63.
17. Rowen TS, Gaither TW, Awad MA, Osterberg EC, Shindel AW, Breyer BN. Pubic hair grooming prevalence and motivation among women in the United States. *JAMA Dermatol.* 2016;152(10):1106–1113.
18. Herbenick D, Schick V, Reece M, Sanders S, Fortenberry JD. Pubic hair removal among women in United States: prevalence, methods and characteristics. *J Sex Med.* 2010;7(1):3322–3330.
19. Howarth H, Sommer V, Jordan FM. Visual depictions of female genitalia differ depending on source. *Med Humanit.* 2010;36(2):75–79.
20. Moran C, Lee C. What's normal? Influencing women's perceptions of normal genitalia: an experiment involving exposure to modified and nonmodified images. *Br J Obstet Gynaecol.* 2014;121(6):761–766.
21. DeMaria AL, Hollub AV, Herbenick D. The Female Genital Self-Image Scale (FGSIS): validation among a sample of female college students. *J Sex Med.* 2012;9(3):708–718.
22. Swami V. Body appreciation, media influence, and weight status predict consideration of cosmetic surgery among female undergraduates. *Body Image.* 2009;6(4):315–317.
23. Herbenick D, Reece M. Development and validation of the female genital self-image scale. *J Sex Med.* 2010;7(5):1822–1830.
24. Goodman M, Fashler S, Miklos JR, Moore RD, Brotto LA. The sexual, psychological, and body image health of women undergoing elective vulvovaginal plastic/cosmetic procedures: a pilot study. *Am J Cosmetic Surg.* 2011;28(4):219–226.
25. Lipworth L, Nyrén O, Ye W, Fryzek JP, Tarone RE, McLaughlin JK. Excess mortality from suicide and other external causes of death among women with cosmetic breast implants. *Ann Plast Surg.* 2007;59(2):119–123.
26. Shaw D, Dickens BM. A new surgical technique for hymenoplasty: a solution, but for which problem? *Int J Gynaecol Obstet.* 2015;130(1):1–2.
27. Adams JA, Botash AS, Kellogg N. Differences in hymenal morphology between adolescent girls with and without a history of consensual sexual intercourse. *Arch Pediatr Adolesc Med.* 2004;158(3):280–285.

28. van Moorst BR, van Lunsen RHW, van Dijken DKE, Salvatore CM. Backgrounds of women applying for hymen reconstruction, the effects of counselling on myths and misunderstandings about virginity, and the results of hymen reconstruction. *Eur J Contracept Reprod Health Care.* 2012;17(2):93–105.
29. World Health Organization. *WHO Guidelines on the Management of Health Complications from Female Genital Mutilation.* 2016. Published by WHO Document Production Services, Geneva, Switzerland.
30. Simonis M, Manocha R, Ong JJ. Female genital cosmetic surgery: a cross-sectional survey exploring knowledge, attitude and practice of general practitioners. *BMJ Open.* 2016;6(9):e013010.
31. Center for Reproductive Rights. Female genital mutilation (FGM): legal prohibitions worldwide. 2009. https://www.reproductiverights.org/document/female-genital-mutilation-fgm-legal-prohibitions-worldwide.
32. Criminal Code RSC, 1985, c. C-46, s.268;1997, c. 16, s. 5. Assault . <http://canlii.ca/t/53gxz> retrieved on 2018-11-26
33. Serour GI. The issue of reinfibulation. *Int J Gynaecol Obstet.* 2010;109(2):93–96.
34. ACOG. Vaginal "rejuvenation" and cosmetic vaginal surgeries. ACOG Committee Opinion No. 378. *Obstet Gynecol.* 2007;110:737–738.
35. Royal Australian and New Zealand College of Obstetricians and Gynaecologists. Statement :Vaginal rejuvenation, laser and cosmetic procedures. 2008, amended 2016. https://www.ranzcog.edu.au/RANZCOG_SITE/media/RANZCOG-MEDIA/Women%27s%20Health/Statement%20and%20guidelines/Clinical%20-%20Gynaecology/Vaginal-rejuvenation,-laser-and-cosmetic-procedures-(C-Gyn-24)-Amended-July-2016.pdf?ext=.pdf
36. Royal College of Obstetricians and Gynaecologists. Ethical considerations in relation to female genital cosmetic surgery (FGCS). 2013.
37. FIGO Committee for the Ethical Aspects of Human Reproduction and Women's Health. Ethical considerations regarding requests and offering of cosmetic genital surgery. *Int J Gynecol Obstet.* 2014;128(1):85–86.
38. <Cosmetic Vaginal Procedures ACOG Clin Pract Guideline 2007.pdf>.
39. Noser A, Zeigler-Hill V. Investing in the ideal: does objectified body consciousness mediate the association between appearance contingent self-worth and appearance self-esteem in women? *Body Image.* 2014;11(2):119–125.
40. Goodman MP. Female cosmetic genital surgery. *Obstet Gynecol.* 2009;113(1):154–159.
41. Braun V. Female genital cosmetic surgery: a critical review of current knowledge and contemporary debates. *J Womens Health.* 2010;19(7):1393–1407.
42. Manoloudakis N, Labiris G, Karakitsou N, Kim JB, Sheena Y, Niakas D. Characteristics of women who have had cosmetic breast implants that could be associated with increased suicide risk: a systematic review, proposing a suicide prevention model. *Arch Plast Surg.* 2015;42(2):131–142.

43. Motakef S, Rodriguez-Feliz J, Chung MT, Ingargiola MJ, Wong VW, Patel A. Vaginal labiaplasty: current practices and a simplified classification system for labial protrusion. *Plast Reconstr Surg*. 2015;135(3):774–788.
44. Liao LM, Michala L, Creighton SM. Labial surgery for well women: a review of the literature. *Br J Obstet Gynecol*. 2010;117(1):20–25.
45. <BCWH-BCCH-Ethics-Framework-Dec-2016.pdf.pdf>.
46. Kelly B, Foster C. Should female genital cosmetic surgery and genital piercing be regarded ethically and legally as female genital mutilation? *Br J Obstet Gynecol*. 2012;119(4):389–392.
47. Todd, NJ. RateMD.com use by patients whose request for non-medically female genital cosmetic surgery was declined. Personal communication, November 2017.

6 ETHICAL ISSUES IN THE CARE AND SUPPORT OF WOMEN LIVING WITH HIV

Ruby Rajendra Shanker, Angela Underhill,
Valerie Nicholson, Logan Kennedy, Denise Jaworsky,
and Mona Loutfy

Introduction: A Brief History of Women and HIV

She is the leading lady in the AIDS epidemic. She was under the surface, hidden, but finally emerged, rushed forward with newfound breath, born into existence with twin shoves: first, feminism; next epidemiological fathomability and visibility.[1]

Women have overcome complex challenges throughout the history of the human immunodeficiency virus (HIV) epidemic and have been at the forefront of the response to HIV. Despite remarkable resilience, gender inequities continue to minimize the experiences of women living with HIV and have led to systemic and societal impediments to action. Even the initial surveillance case definition of the US Centers for Disease Control and Prevention (CDC) from 1987 to 1993 focused solely on the disease manifestations in men, despite the 18,000 US women who had already lost their lives to acquired immune deficiency syndrome (AIDS).[1] Unified voices of several women's interest groups in the US eventually led to expansion of the CDC surveillance case definition to include manifestations of HIV in women, including persistent or recurrent vaginal infections. Advocacy and research, often driven by affected women, has since paved the path for more visibility of women's health issues as they relate to HIV and/or AIDS. In practice, these efforts are still subject to the complex dynamics of oppressive social structures that compound gender inequity. Further, there has been insufficient acknowledgment and response within the HIV epidemic regarding the multiple roles that women have as mothers, grandmothers, daughters, caregivers, partners, breadwinners, peer leaders, advocates, and role models. Often, the competing social roles women fulfill in others' lives are prioritized above their personal needs, and they often put their own care last.

By the end of 2016, the World Health Organization (WHO) estimated there were 36.7 million people living with HIV globally; women made up 17.6 million of the 34.5 million adults.[2] Estimates of people newly acquiring HIV in 2016 were 1.8 million. When examined further, these numbers demonstrate that the rate of new infections among women has been steadily growing over the past two decades, even though there has been a decline in overall new HIV infections.[3] In Canada, women now represent nearly one-quarter of people living with HIV, and these numbers relay the staggering reality of how many women are estimated to be directly affected globally and in Canada.[3] What these numbers fail to account for, though, is the disproportionate number of women who may experience marginalization due to their gender identity, ethnicity, power imbalance in relationships, experiences of violence and abuse, substance use, poverty, and/or lack of access to safe and appropriate services. HIV affects or potentially affects all dimensions of women's sexual, reproductive, physical, and mental health through the lifespan, and the social, economic, and political insecurities that women face continue to gravely affect access to treatment, combination antiretroviral (ARV) therapy utilization, and quality of care received.[4,5]

With this chapter, we aim to explore some of the ethical issues that arise when providing clinical care and support to women living with HIV in a high-income country such as Canada. We note here that by virtue of historical injustices and socio-political structures, certain populations or geographic areas within resource-rich countries face detrimental health inequities. In the Canadian context, we particularly underscore the experiences of inequity faced by women who identify as Indigenous, who are refugees and newcomers, who lack health insurance, and who face many barriers and life challenges. To be authentic to this aim, it is imperative to uphold the principles of the Greater Involvement of People Living with HIV/AIDS (GIPA) and Meaningful Involvement of People Living with HIV (MIPA). These principles seek to recognize the contributions and expertise of people living with HIV and to create space for their involvement and active participation in shaping care, education, and research on the response to the HIV epidemic.[6-8] Accordingly, we honor the experiences of a woman living with HIV who, as a peer research associate, knowledge keeper, and front-line warrior, and through her Indigenous identity, lends crucial insight to the discourse. She speaks from her own experiences as well as those of the numerous women whose lives she has touched. Her experiences enrich the perspectives of an ethicist, a nurse, a doctoral student, and two physicians who together have three decades of experience working with women living with HIV.

Our discussion will follow a life-course analysis of women living with HIV from prepubescence and adolescence, youth and midlife, to older years. To orient this chapter, we will draw upon the four principles of biomedical ethics as described by Beauchamp and Childress (autonomy, beneficence, non-maleficence, and justice).[9] Further, the chapter will be guided by a feminist interpretation of each principle and commentary highlighting the experiences of women living with HIV. Our ethical interpretation will explore critical concepts of intersectionality and oppression that women are prone to experience due to social stigma across their lifespan.

HIV as a Feminist Ethics Issue

In the response to the HIV epidemic, women have consistently been described as more vulnerable than men, owing to a multitude of biologic, social, and systemic issues.[10-14] Such labeling has potentially occurred due to the increased biologic and socio-political susceptibility of women to HIV across the lifespan. In the initial response to HIV in North America, women represented a minority and were underrepresented among decision-making authorities, leading to service establishments where the comprehensive care needs of women ended up being sidelined.[15] In reviewing several studies, O'Brien and colleagues note that even within resource-rich settings where medical advances offer safer care, gaps exist in the availability of contraceptive counseling, pregnancy planning supports, cancer screening, aging and menopause support, as well as management of comorbidities.[16] These gaps are a result of the historical social injustices, stigma of contagion, discrimination, and violation of human rights that women with intersecting identities have had to, and continue to, experience. Taboos surrounding sexual health and well-being compound these stigmata and push care for women living with HIV to the liminal zones of considerations for resource allocation.

The four principles of biomedical ethics as described by Beauchamp and Childress have guided clinicians and healthcare workers in defining professional obligations toward caring for patients.[9,17] These principles are autonomy, beneficence, non-maleficence, and justice. In the context of care for women living with HIV, we shall further explore these principles through a feminist lens, while interpreting the principle of justice in light of interlocking and intersecting influences of power and oppression.

As outlined by Beauchamp and Childress, autonomy may be understood as respect for persons and their right to self-determination.[9] Applying a feminist lens, we interpret autonomy in its relational form, whereby the ability to self-determine derives from how one is situated within personal and social relationships.[18] This nuanced interpretation of autonomy is important if we are to acknowledge the multiple roles women embody and how these roles influence their healthcare decision making. Relational autonomy also recognizes identity—from where values and beliefs originate and guide decision making—as primarily belonging to and deriving from communities.

Beneficence is broadly understood as the moral obligation to act in a person's best interests, and furthering the important and legitimate interests as defined by the person.[9] It embodies the promotion of good for others, which is why within clinical practice, the principle of beneficence tends to be misconstrued as paternalistic protection for those who may be perceived as vulnerable, and can result in overriding the autonomous wishes of persons. Due to variable interpretations, the clash between autonomy and beneficence often sets the scene for ethical dilemmas within clinical practice. Where the clinician–patient relationship is already subject to power imbalances around knowledge and skills, applying beneficence within its paternalistic interpretation can contribute to silencing and erasure of the unique experiences of patients, particularly those who may experience this silencing and erasure in other realms of their lives. Additionally, from a public health and policy perspective, a liberty-limiting notion of beneficence may justify actions that position the greater good of others over that of the individual's right to privacy and confidentiality. Such an interpretation may only be justified where harm to others is of more immediate concern. A feminist reorientation toward the principle of beneficence stems from how women living with HIV define key values and goals that ought to guide their care. Clinicians ought to apply the principle of beneficence from an understanding of the values most closely held and expressed by the patient, not merely what may be considered clinically beneficial.

Non-maleficence goes hand in hand with beneficence and refers to the principle of "do no harm."[9] The conventional interpretation for non-maleficence within clinical practice involves proceeding through options with graduated degrees of invasiveness or risk. Yet, risk can have multiple connotations based on personal preferences, and decisions to weigh risks and benefits are guided by personal values and experiences. As we move toward underscoring key values as defined by women living with HIV, the principle of non-maleficence also means that risk or harm *as defined by them* must be taken into consideration. This is of utmost importance where social insecurities, life challenges, and cycles of violence and abuse underlie care considerations. An approach of harm reduction, and more recently the concept of trauma-informed care, includes feminist interpretations of non-maleficence, and in turn beneficence as well.[19]

The principle of justice may be thought of as how individuals ought to be treated where claims to freedom, opportunity, and resources converge. As per Aristotelian notions, justice is conceptualized as either horizontal or vertical.[20] Horizontal justice is the treatment of like cases alike, or that persons in equal need ought to be treated the same. Vertical justice involves proportionality, where persons in unequal need ought to be treated in proportion to the inequality in need.[20] Distinguishing the two concepts is paramount within healthcare. Where horizontal justice or "equality" means equal care to all without consideration of any special claims, vertical justice or "equity" refers to the provision of care to individuals that seeks to address systemic, historical, and socio-political injustices that contribute to gaps in healthcare.[21] The notion of equity also offers a foundation for embracing the related concept of social justice, which refers to how the rights of those who face socio-political inequities may be maximized, while critiquing the influence of power as privilege and oppression.[22]

Within the realization of power relations, individual social identities and structural inequities form interdependent and mutually constitutive relationships known as "intersectionality," as coined by the feminist legal scholar, critical race theorist, and civil rights advocate Kimberlé Williams Crenshaw.[23] According to Crenshaw, an individual's many identities intersect and provide a more complex realization of the privileges enjoyed and oppressions faced. Political theorist and feminist scholar Iris Marion Young further categorized these complex experiences of oppression as exploitation, marginalization, powerlessness, cultural domination, and violence.[24] Depending on the space and/or system, these identities may intersect and manifest in various ways, including systemic violence. In the context of care for women living with HIV, intersecting and interlocking oppressions ought to be considered closely and addressed within the clinician–patient relationship, as well as where public health policies apply.[25]

With these concepts now elucidated, we delve into the ethics and complex considerations of care and support across the lifespan for women living with HIV. To offer opportunities for ethical reflection, we present the narrative of a hypothetical woman living with HIV as she accesses healthcare at different stages of her life. Corresponding to each life stage (prepubescence and adolescence, youth and midlife, and older years), we offer scenarios that build upon the realities she encounters, followed by the ethical themes and considerations from the literature for clinical practice. Each scenario concludes with poignant commentary from one co-author, who offers her perspective on these scenarios as a woman living with HIV. We encourage readers to consider the multiplicity and complexity of women's lives and to appreciate how a simple scenario will never encapsulate everyone's experience.

Prepubescence and Adolescence

> Christina is a healthy 15-year-old young woman who is living with HIV. She acquired HIV perinatally. As a young girl she lost both of her biological parents to AIDS, and she is currently living with her adoptive parents. Christina has just begun high school and is finding the transition to young adulthood challenging as she faces the loss of her biological parents and reconciles her own reality as a woman living with HIV. To cope with these emotional complexities, she has lately taken to drinking alcohol. Christina also has a new boyfriend with whom she is hoping to become more intimate, but she is struggling with the idea of disclosing her status for the first time.

Young age, in addition to gender, disability, poverty, and periods of socioeconomic-cultural transitions can contribute to the disenfranchisement from HIV care of prepubescent and adolescent people living with HIV. Accordingly, two key populations deserve special focus for ethical considerations—those who acquire HIV perinatally or in childhood, and those who acquire HIV in adolescence.

Children or adolescents living with HIV face unique healthcare experiences, such as engagement in specialized pediatric HIV care to ensure optimal virologic suppression, as well as challenges associated with the clinical management of a chronic illness in children. There was a time in the not-so-distant past that pediatric HIV care offered much less promise of health than it does today. With the overall success of combination ARV therapy and specifically the increase in pediatric dosing guidelines, from a biomedical perspective pediatric HIV has become a manageable, chronic health condition. However, the clinical care of children and adolescents living with HIV is inextricably linked with the challenges associated with disclosure, family structure, and often complex social/familial situations. Persistent stigma and lack of understanding within schools and the community severely limit safe situations in which to disclose, and thus many children and adolescents living with HIV rarely disclose their diagnosis, thus restricting possible support from friends, relatives, or community organizations. Daily medication requirements can interfere with social engagement when the diagnosis must be kept a secret.[26]

Parents of children who have acquired HIV perinatally may have their own health issues to address and may be reluctant to access services due to fear that this would affect their children. Parents not wanting to address their own health concerns may unwittingly impart patterns of health avoidance behaviors to their children or may not access available support for their children. On the other hand, parents who have been supported and engaged regarding their own health are likely to pass on similar patterns of health-seeking behaviors to their children. The mental, social, and physical health of the parents, and/or the social stigma surrounding HIV, could also lead to children and adolescents living with HIV being forcibly extracted from mothers, orphaned, in foster care, or adopted, which in itself poses ethical issues.

For those who acquire HIV as children, adolescence can present unique challenges. It is important that confidence and self-esteem be nurtured to support them through navigating their relationships. However, empowering their sense of autonomy can be challenging for healthcare providers. If followed from a young age, healthcare providers may be able to provide education and counseling as appropriate for the developing adolescent, with an emphasis on information about transmission, risk reduction, and encouraging healthy sexuality. Adolescence is also an important time to instill autonomy related to treatment adherence, engagement in care, and supporting the development of life goals beyond the teen years. Encouraging sexual agency and normalizing sexual desires, intimacy, and satisfaction are important aspects of clinical care for youth living with HIV that should be included in discussions on how to negotiate risk and safety around HIV transmission through sexual intercourse.[27]

The focus of counseling on public health safety can often overshadow appropriate support toward understanding what risk and safety means within personal relationships. These conversations may be challenging enough for adult women living with HIV who, as per Hankins and colleagues, tend to go through a "sexual adjustment period" after an HIV diagnosis that may last from 1 month to 5 years.[28] Given this adjustment period for adults, additional care needs to be considered for children and youth. Children and adolescents living with HIV need to be offered more support around how to disclose their diagnosis within safe relationships. Contributing social determinants of health must be addressed where violence and criminalization may be present. Most importantly, these conversations between the adolescent living with HIV and the clinician should be open, in an environment that is safe and free from stigmatizing influences.

Commentary by a Woman Living with HIV: For children and youth, peer support is essential and can come in many forms. They may receive support from other children and youth, but guidance from an older individual living with HIV can provide them with a source of knowledge and also a sense of safety and security. I feel honored when a young person calls me to ask advice on healthy sexuality or when I am able to use my knowledge to provide them with reassurance. The trust that forms between older peers and youth often leads to a long-lasting nurturing relationship.

Youth and Midlife

> Christina is now 18 years old. She continues to struggle with her use of alcohol and is facing a very unstable time in her life. While she expresses feeling sad often, she finds that support from peers living with HIV offers her great strength and an important sense of community. She does not wish to stay with her adoptive parents anymore and seeks the natural transition to adulthood that comes with independent living. With the potential of being unstably housed, there are some concerns around her safety and the potential for experiencing violence on the streets.

Ethical considerations in caring for youth living with HIV must begin with a close examination of intersecting social determinants of health and how poverty, education, and employment can impact their lives. The complex social locations of many young and middle-aged women living with HIV creates a disproportionate burden of poverty within the community, thus limiting access to education opportunities and employment, and resources overall. Impairment of cognitive or adaptive functions in instances of in utero drug or alcohol exposure, HIV-progressive encephalopathy in infancy, and/or growing up in a suboptimal social environment may impart greater vulnerabilities.[26] Some may also be newcomers on account of migration for kinship, for better employment and educational opportunities, or due to fleeing from war and persecution. They may experience challenges of adjusting to a new culture, language, or social expectations as compared to their country of origin. Where a young woman living with HIV's identity intersects with belonging to a marginalized or oppressed community, there may be stark experiences that may contribute to psychological stressors.[29] Housing insecurities compound how youth living with HIV navigate healthcare, as some may be in care of Child and Family Services (CFS) and may experience a sudden loss of support/housing when discharged at 18 or 19 years of age. Many may also be struggling to understand their gender identity and sexual orientation and/or to have their gender and/or sexual identity accepted.

As youth reach the age of 18 or 19, they experience the social service phenomenon termed "aging out." During this transition, their access to both clinical and CFS-funded support services can change dramatically, even overnight. Youth make the switch from pediatric to adult HIV care in their late teens or early twenties. Although many pediatric clinics are now allowing for an overlap period to allow for successful continuity of care, loss to follow-up and poor engagement in care during and/or post-care transitions has been found to persist, with poor clinical outcomes being more notable in young women after the care transition.[30] To support optimal transition, literature supports a gradual process beginning in the early teens, maintaining relationships with longstanding pediatric providers, offering choices in the transition process, and most of all ensuring it is a coordinated, person-centered process.

For young women newly diagnosed with HIV, there may be several issues that crop up in the treatment cascade. Stigma and misconceptions around HIV are still prevalent among healthcare providers, resulting in disjointed access to ancillary healthcare services. HIV care centers and HIV specialists may not be readily accessible due to physical distance or due to institutional policies that do not fully consider the gender-specific needs of young women. Additionally, youth living with HIV may have to shoulder the burden of disclosing their status and avoiding transmission to sexual partners without adequate support or guidance.[26] Disclosing one's status may put youth living with HIV at acute risk of violence and death.

Mental health and substance use are important issues to reflect upon when caring for youth living with HIV. Poverty and multiple overlapping traumas are some of the many psychological stressors that can exacerbate mood and anxiety disorders. In the context of substance use, healthcare providers must discard their biases and focus on providing care and support rather than attributing blame. For youth who use substances, adopting a harm reduction approach respects their autonomy and fosters a clinical care space that can build trust.

Commentary by a Woman Living with HIV: We need to acknowledge that youth transitioning from pediatric to adult care must be considered long-term survivors. Many of them have been living with HIV their entire lives. When they enter adult care, they are often treated as someone who needs basic education on HIV, and this failure to recognize their expertise is insulting and can damage the therapeutic relationship. Many youth, particularly those from racialized communities, are missing connections with their culture and their land. Culture is a strong medicine. For youth impacted by substance use, trauma, and mental health challenges, reclaiming identity and drawing strength from culture may help them to navigate their own healthcare and help prepare them to take ARV medications.

> Christina has matured into an energetic 24-year-old. She currently participates in providing education and counseling as a peer supporter toward empowering other youth living with HIV. She has been doing well in a nurturing relationship. Christina and her partner have been thinking about getting pregnant.

Pregnancy planning can simultaneously be a joyous and complex experience for women living with HIV. Due to stigmatizing attitudes about parenting from healthcare providers, many women living with HIV may face challenges when speaking to their healthcare provider about pregnancy options. Historically, fertility clinics have not provided assisted reproduction for women living with HIV.[31,32] Although healthcare providers may now be more accepting, unfortunate experiences with the healthcare system may lead some women living with HIV to feel as though they may not have a right to pregnancy and parenting.[33] Some may be fearful to disclose their HIV status in the context of pregnancy planning. Additionally, unintended pregnancies among women living with HIV may in part be due to fear of disclosing a desire for pregnancy at the risk of being judged by healthcare providers. In some cases, women learn of their positive HIV status during their pregnancy, a discovery that may contribute to additional stress and the fear of being judged when medical surveillance around the mother's health behaviors is already heightened. Also, finding out one may be pregnant at the same time a new diagnosis of HIV is made could be an emotionally overwhelming situation for women and their partners.

Healthcare providers need to normalize conversations about reproduction with their patients who are living with HIV. By routinely asking patients living with HIV about their intentions and desires to have children, they open up conversations about minimizing the risk of vertical and horizontal transmission (if applicable) and they ultimately make space for patients to raise any reproduction questions/concerns at later times. People change their minds about having children as their life circumstances change, so it is important to ask these questions over the lifespan. With medical advances and accessibility, women living with HIV now have a variety of options for family planning, and all possible options should be presented to support the autonomy of women living with HIV. It is vital to share with women living with HIV that when ARVs are taken as soon as possible preconception or in pregnancy, they can help someone achieve undetectable viral loads and reduce the risk of transmission to a fetus to virtually zero. The effects of HIV and ARVs in pregnancy are still being investigated; as such, any fears related to medication use in pregnancy should be discussed. As a result of these ongoing investigations, and the higher incidence of some adverse birth outcomes such as small for gestational age, increased medical follow-up is recommended in pregnancies among women living with HIV. Women living with HIV should fully understand this and be encouraged to ask questions and voice concerns. Beyond these concerns, healthcare providers should be aware of the healthcare services and institutions in their area and direct their patients accordingly; ideally, women living with HIV should be cared for by an experienced team to ensure optimal, stigma-free prenatal care.

Pregnant women living with HIV may consider opting for a midwife to provide care. However, it should be noted that in Canada midwifery may not be available for people living with HIV or may not be covered under public health insurance.[33] Options for assisted reproduction exist for those women living with HIV who may also be experiencing infertility; however, the associated costs may be inequitably prohibitive, depending on the jurisdiction where they live. These issues around exercising choice and access raise important questions about justice.

It is equally important to offer adequate support and guidance to women living with HIV and their partners who become pregnant but consider terminating their pregnancy for a multitude of reasons that may have nothing to do with HIV: perhaps they have something happening in their lives, or they simply do not want to be a parent. Regardless of the reason, women's choices must be respected and healthcare providers must empower women living with HIV to make informed and autonomous choices.[34] Throughout the pregnancy journey, healthcare professionals must provide holistic support to women, addressing their physical, emotional, and spiritual needs.

They must explore women's fears and uncertainties, some of which may be exacerbated by experiences of stigma.

Commentary by a Woman Living with HIV: Many healthcare providers focus on what is happening to the mother's body but do not spend enough time educating mothers about what this all means for their babies. They are not told about the implications of maternal medications or warned about all of the tests that will need to be done on the baby. This can be very scary, especially for women who fear that their child will be apprehended.

Christina has recently given birth following a healthy pregnancy. Although expressing deep joy, she says she feels like a "lot has been going on." Christina is hoping to receive some guidance around self-care and newborn care during this visit. She has been having some difficulty adhering to her medication regimen, as opposed to when she was pregnant, and may be experiencing postpartum depression. She mentions feeling fearful as she received a call from Child Services last week, after they received an anonymous tip about substance use, even though she has been sober for 3 years.

With the arrival of a new baby, women living with HIV are prone to experience the stresses of caring for an infant like anyone else. However, there may be additional considerations or triggers that may contribute to their experiences. Support from the partner or family may be crucial in addressing some anxieties around self-care and care of the newborn, but healthcare providers must recognize that these supports are not available to all women. An important ethical theme to consider is medication adherence for implications on autonomy. During pregnancy, women living with HIV might be motivated to follow their medication regimen to protect their developing baby from HIV transmission and the risk of other infections. Following birth, competing priorities in addition to cultural or familial pressures that compound stress while caring for the newborn can impact her self-care.

Infant feeding can also be wrought with complex considerations. In Canada, new mothers living with HIV are currently recommended to exclusively formula feed.[35] This can contribute to confusion, particularly for those who have immigrated from resource-limited settings where they may have been counseled to breastfeed as a means to counter the more likely dangers of malnutrition. To best support women and families, a comprehensive and supportive discussion about infant feeding should take place during pregnancy. While the Canadian recommendation to formula feed should be clearly communicated, clinicians should also be prepared to support families regardless of their decision. With formula feeding, clinicians should ensure that families with less financial means have access to formula either through a provincially subsidized program or other compassionate grounds. Alternative options for bonding ought to be discussed. In the rare instance where breastfeeding remains the preference of families, the care team needs to work together to meet the needs of that family with the goal to uphold the woman's right to make autonomous decisions.

Child welfare agencies have had an unfortunately tumultuous history of discrimination toward mothers with HIV.[36,37] Stigma and paternalistic attitudes, and moral judgments on what parenting ought to embody, have resulted in children being taken away from mothers with HIV. This history is part of colonial oppressive attitudes that have also been responsible for separating women with Indigenous identities from their children, often with no course to reconciliation.[38] In Canada, this history includes the "Sixties Scoop," which refers to the mass removal of Indigenous children from their families into the child welfare system, and builds on the destructive legacy of residential schooling.[39,40] Yet injustice within the child welfare system is an ongoing reality for many Indigenous women in North America. Colonial attitudes about what it means to be a parent often disregard the diversity of cultural beliefs regarding childcare. Further, the fear of being surveilled can weigh heavily on mothers with HIV, especially where there may have been a history of mental illness or substance use. The intersecting stigmas of HIV and substance use can have a profound impact on mothers living with HIV.

In Canada, one of the first calls many women living with HIV receive after their doctors determine pregnancy is from Public Health, asking them if they have disclosed their status to their partner(s). This is an example of how the gender-based discriminatory nature of laws and policies places a huge burden on pregnant women living with HIV who are trying to navigate many complexities in their lives. Further, HIV criminalization laws can have a detrimental effect on women living with HIV who are pregnant or who have recently given birth. There are a few notable cases, particularly one where a woman living with HIV was convicted for not disclosing her HIV status to her healthcare providers during delivery, where disclosure could have mitigated the risk of HIV transmission to the baby.[41] The baby tested positive for HIV soon after birth and the mother was charged with failure to provide necessities of life; she received a 6-month conditional sentence followed by 3 years of probation.[41] This case provides pause for reflection on the social forces that may contribute to pregnant women not being able to disclose their HIV status, or feeling as if it would be unsafe to do so. The association of criminal penalties with disclosing status can be discouraging to women living with HIV who plan to start a family.[42,43]

Intertwined here are narratives of pregnant women living with HIV who experience many barriers and challenges; who have had prior encounters with the criminal justice system; who are sex workers or part of sex trade; and who may also encounter challenges with mental illness and substance use and have likely experienced stigma in healthcare systems due to these experiences. An attitude of compassion and patience ought to underlie healthcare providers' approaches toward optimizing agency and autonomy for pregnant women living with HIV, rather than paternalism that only serves to perpetuate stigma.

Commentary by a Woman Living with HIV: Women often find themselves under constant surveillance, and criminalization laws vary by jurisdiction and are difficult to interpret. Women are often so fearful of judgment and criminalization that this becomes a barrier to seeking care. They worry that if they go to the doctor too often, this will be seen as a sign that they are not well enough to be a mother. They worry that their baby will be taken away. This constant fear can transform a joyful time into a traumatic experience.

Christina's daughter is now 10 years old. They have moved from a region with universal government-funded ARVs to one where the medication are covered only for people receiving disability assistance. Due to medication costs Christina must apply for disability assistance, which precludes her from full-time work. She is concerned about food security and supporting her family on her partner's limited income.

Discourses within care for people living with HIV do not adequately address the multiple roles that women might have in their personal lives. Caregiving responsibilities tend to traditionally fall upon women, and these stresses may contribute to an inability to adhere to medications while caring for others. Further, not being able to work can create food insecurity and lead to experiencing poverty, which bodes poorly for the woman's health in general and can impact medication absorption.

As mothers with growing children, women living with HIV may experience a different facet of the fear of surveillance. Trust may be difficult to build with teachers or healthcare providers who may interact with her children often, as the fear of being separated may always loom. Women who were previously comfortable disclosing their HIV status may no longer be able to for fear that their children may be impacted by HIV stigma, and this can lead to feelings of isolation. Here, healthcare providers may find it necessary to offer safe opportunities to women living with HIV to be able to express their worries and to link them with supportive social services that ease their burden for caregiving, without casting aspersions. Words and actions must be aligned with building trust, optimizing agency, and addressing the inequities women living with HIV face due to their identities and life circumstances.

Commentary by a Woman Living with HIV: Although stigma exists in healthcare settings, it can be even more pervasive in education settings. Teachers may be uninformed about HIV, and their fears can lead to discrimination within the classroom. In these cases, it is not surprising that women living with HIV do not feel they can develop trusting relationships with teachers. Safe spaces for children impacted by HIV are crucial, and programs such as dedicated camps for children and youth affected by HIV can provide peer support for children and also offer parents time to focus on their own self-care.

The Older Years

> Now in her 50s, Christina is recovering in the hospital from a sudden cardiac event. She has also been diagnosed with diabetes while in the hospital. She has been employed part time as an office assistant but is not eligible for benefits. Christina expresses that some healthcare providers in the hospital may be biased toward her because of her HIV status. She has been worried about the effects of aging and HIV on her memory and wishes to receive support with advance care planning.

Women living with HIV may face further stigma and discrimination as they age.[44] Historically, cardiovascular conditions and metabolic disorders affecting endocrine function (e.g., diabetes and thyroid disease) have been inadequately addressed in the care of women as they age, and living with HIV may unfortunately obfuscate attention to these comorbidities. Although many HIV providers are beginning to offer comprehensive comorbidity assessment and management, uptake of this practice is variable. Aging ought to be considered as an important lifespan theme, and not only in relation to physiologic shifts in women like menopause.

HIV can have long-term effects on cognition, vascular health, and neuromuscular activity.[45,46] With longstanding ARV regimens, as women living with HIV age, they may come to experience long-term side effects that may compound symptoms of menopause like reduced bone density. Some ARV side effects may also include premature ovarian failure and early menopause.[45] Sexual agency, pleasure, and satisfaction may be affected as well, and many aging women living with HIV may feel discouraged or embarrassed to raise these concerns with their primary healthcare providers.[27] Developing other comorbid conditions may lead to an increased frequency of having to access acute care services. In these encounters, communications with new healthcare providers may reveal discrimination in healthcare settings that may be less knowledgeable in caring for women living with HIV.

Through the spectrum of aging, we acknowledge that discussions around goals of care and advance care planning as initiated by healthcare providers are inconsistent and deserve greater attention.[47] With women living with HIV, these discussions take on equal, if not more, importance to offer opportunities for reflection around personal values and beliefs that will guide treatment decision making and personal care, including where one may choose to live when unable to care for oneself. Women living with HIV should be offered the same range of advance care planning options as everyone else. However, assisted living and other care facilities may be inexperienced in providing services to women living with HIV, and efforts are needed to destigmatize HIV in these settings. As noted throughout this chapter, providing education around options at every stage of life elevates relational autonomy for women living with HIV, supporting them to consider the trajectory of their care in the future in relation to their key values, meaningful relationships, and life priorities.

Commentary by a Woman Living with HIV: As I age, I worry that as my health conditions accumulate I may become a burden on my children. I worry that if I develop memory issues I may forget to take my ARVs. I want to stay healthy and I do not want to end up in a care facility. If I do need a care facility in the future, I fear stigma and discrimination if the staff are not adequately trained to support people living with HIV. We are just starting to understand the impact of HIV on aging, and there are so many uncertainties. Despite how far we have come in the 13 years that I have been living with HIV, my biggest fear is dying of AIDS.

Emerging Issues of Recent Times and Policy Implications

First and foremost, policy that impacts women living with HIV must be driven by women living with HIV. Women living with HIV must be given the opportunity to hold leadership roles and influence policy. Their involvement must be meaningful and not simply tokenistic. They ought to be acknowledged as service providers and experts rather than always seen as patients or clients.

A group of researchers, clinicians, and women living with HIV in Canada (of whom we are a part) have come together to develop and carry out research regarding issues of top priority to women living with HIV.[48,49] This has led to the Canadian HIV Women's Sexual and Reproductive Health Cohort Study (CHIWOS).[48] This study was developed to longitudinally investigate the concept of Women-Centered HIV Care (WCHC) and its impact on overall and HIV health outcomes; quality of life; preventive cancer screening; mental health; sexual health, functioning, and satisfaction; and reproductive health outcomes of women living with HIV. Given the distinct ways that women with HIV are situated with respect to structural inequities, social roles, biologic needs, and healthcare complexities, it is crucial to address women with HIV's specific health needs. Recently, WHO released a consolidated guideline on the sexual and reproductive health and rights of women living with HIV.[50] This guideline calls for women-centered care, although to date it remains unexplored in practice. As such, we have come together to develop and investigate the impact of WCHC as a model of care in addressing these inequities. Toward developing a WCHC model, the group has conducted a literature review, 11 focus groups with women living with HIV, and quantitative analyses.[16,51]

Through the literature review and focus groups, the definition of WCHC that emerged refers to "care that supports women living with HIV to achieve the best health and wellbeing as defined by them."[48] Further, this model of care recognizes, respects, and addresses diverse health and social concerns as connected. Driven by diverse experiences, it takes into consideration the different needs of women. This care model has been gaining operational prominence as it is aware of trauma and violence; is person-centered; delivers competent HIV, women's healthcare, and mental health care; and links patients to peer support and leadership opportunities. Further efforts are aimed at testing the flexibility of the model for delivery, grounding in anti-oppression practices, and recognition of social determinants of health.

Conclusion

This chapter presents only a brief overview of some of the complex issues and considerations when providing care for women living with HIV, from a feminist ethical perspective. There are many challenges that must be considered and service gaps to address when providing care for women living with HIV. It is beyond the scope of this chapter to discuss these in detail, but the following list provides a starting point for discussion:

- Care delivery ought to reflect the multiple needs of women throughout their lives and be founded upon women-centered care models that are informed by feminist and trauma perspectives.
- Holistic interdisciplinary clinics are needed that support women's physical and mental health and provide opportunities for peer support and leadership.
- There is a need to bridge the service gaps that exist when youth make the transition from pediatric to adult care and services.
- There are significant geographic discrepancies in service access, and additional efforts are needed to support women living with HIV outside of urban areas.
- Care and medications ought to be universally accessible and affordable.
- Research and programing must prioritize women-specific issues rather than simply adapting lessons from male-dominated studies.

We end with words from the experiences of our co-author who is a woman living with HIV: "When I started working as a peer researcher at my medical clinic, they could not see me as anything other than a patient. It took delicate navigation and reflection on both my own journey and the journey of the clinic staff throughout the history of HIV to break this false dichotomy. Tears welled up in my eyes the day they hung a sign bearing my name and provided me with my physician's office to use for my research, because for once, I truly felt valued."

References

1. Dworkin SL. Who is epidemiologically fathomable in the HIV/AIDS epidemic? Gender, sexuality, and intersectionality in public health. *Culture Health Sexuality.* 2005;7(6):615–623.
2. World Health Organization's International HIV data. http://www.who.int/hiv/data/epi_core_2016.png?ua=1. Published 2016. Accessed March 22, 2018.
3. Public Health Agency of Canada (PHAC). Summary: Estimates of HIV incidence, prevalence and proportion undiagnosed in Canada. https://www.canada.ca/content/dam/canada/health-canada/migration/healthy-canadians/publications/diseases-conditions-maladies-affections/

hiv-aids-estimates-2014-vih-sida-estimations/alt/hiv-aids-estimates-2014-vih-sida-estimations-eng.pdf. Published 2014. Accessed March 22, 2018.
4. Gupta GR, Parkhurst JO, Ogden JA, Aggleton P, Mahal A. Structural approaches to HIV prevention. *Lancet.* 2008;372(9640):764–775. doi: 10.1016/S0140-6736(08)60887-9 PMID: 18687460.
5. Auerbach JD, Parkhurst JO, Caceres CF. Addressing social drivers of HIV/AIDS for the long-term response: conceptual and methodological considerations. *Global Public Health.* 2011;6(Suppl 3):S293–309. doi:10.1080/17441692.2011.594451 PMID: 21745027.
6. The Denver Principles. http://data.unaids.org/pub/externaldocument/2007/gipa1983denverprinciples_en.pdf Published 1983. Accessed March 22, 2018.
7. Greater Involvement of People Living with HIV (GIPA): UNAIDS Policy Brief. http://data.unaids.org/pub/briefingnote/2007/jc1299_policy_brief_gipa.pdf. Published March 2007. Accessed September 23, 2017.
8. Meaningful Involvement of People Living with HIV (MIPA): UNAIDS resource. https://www.aidsunited.org/resources/meaningful-involvement-of-people-with-hivaids-mipa. Accessed March 22, 2018.
9. Beauchamp TL, Childress JF. *Principles of Biomedical Ethics.* New York, NY: Oxford University Press; 2012.
10. Exner TM, Dworkin SL, Hoffman S, Ehrhardt AA. Beyond the male condom: the evolution of gender-specific HIV interventions for women. *Ann Rev Sex Res.* 2003;14(1):114–136.
11. Exner TM, Seal DW, Ehrhardt AA. A review of HIV interventions for at-risk women. *AIDS Behav.* 1997;1(2):93–124.
12. Gupta GR. Gender, sexuality, and HIV/AIDS: the what, the why, and the how. *SIECUS Rep.* 2001;29(5):6.
13. Reid PT. Women, ethnicity, and AIDS: what's love got to do with it? *Sex Roles.* 2000;42(7-8):709–722.
14. Simoni JM, Walters KL, Nero DK. Safer sex among HIV+ women: the role of relationships. *Sex Roles.* 2000;42(7):691–708.
15. Steiner RJ, Finocchario-Kessler S, Dariotis JK. Engaging HIV care providers in conversations with their reproductive-age patients about fertility desires and intentions: a historical review of the HIV epidemic in the United States. *Am J Public Health.* 2013;103(8):1357–1366.
16. O'Brien N, Greene S, Carter A, et al. Envisioning women-centered HIV care: perspectives from women living with HIV in Canada. *Womens Health Issues.* 2017;27(6):721–730.
17. World Medical Association's Declaration of Geneva. https://www.wma.net/policies-post/wma-declaration-of-geneva/. Published September 1948. Updated October 2017. Accessed March 22, 2018.
18. Sherwin S. A relational approach to autonomy in health care. In: *Readings in Health Care Ethics.* 2000:69–87.

19. Huckshorn KE, LeBel JL. Trauma-informed care. In: Yeager K, Cutler D, Svendsen D, Sills GM, eds. *Modern Community Mental Health Work: An Interdisciplinary Approach*. New York, NY: Oxford University Press, 2013:62–83.
20. Culyer AJ, Wagstaff A. Equity and equality in health and health care. *J Health Econ*. 1993;12(4):431–457.
21. Bambas A, Casas JA. Assessing equity in health: conceptual criteria. *Equity and Health: Views from the Pan American Sanitary Bureau*. 2001:12–21.
22. Powers M, Faden RR. *Social Justice: The Moral Foundations of Public Health and Health Policy*. New York, NY: Oxford University Press; 2006.
23. Crenshaw K. Mapping the margins: intersectionality, identity politics, and violence against women of color. *Stanford Law Rev*. 1991:43(6):1241–1299.
24. Young IM. *Justice and the Politics of Difference*. Princeton, NJ: Princeton University Press; 2011.
25. Carter A, Greene S, Nicholson V, et al. CHIWOS Research Team. "It's a very isolating world": the journey to HIV care for women living with HIV in British Columbia, Canada. *Gender Place Culture*. 2016;23(7):941–954.
26. Alimenti A, Sauvé L, Pick N. Transition of HIV-infected adolescents to adult care in British Columbia. http://www.bcwomens.ca/Professional-Resources-site/Documents/revised%20Aug%202015%20Transition%20policy%20BC%20from%20Sept%202013%20%20AA%20LS%20NP.doc. Accessed March 22, 2018.
27. Carter A, Greene S, Money D, et al. The problematization of sexuality among women living with HIV and a new feminist approach for understanding and enhancing women's sexual lives. *Sex Roles*. 2017;77(3):1–22.
28. Hankins C, Gendron S, Tran T, Lamping D, Lapointe N. Sexuality in Montreal women living with HIV. *AIDS Care*. 1997;9(3):261–272.
29. Woodgate RL, Zurba M, Tennent P, Cochrane C, Payne M, Mignone J. A qualitative study on the intersectional social determinants for indigenous people who become infected with HIV in their youth. *Int J Equity Health*. 2017;16(1):132.
30. Kakkar F, Van der Linden D, Valois S, et al. Health outcomes and the transition experience of HIV-infected adolescents after transfer to adult care in Québec, Canada. *BMC Pediatr*. 2016;16(1):109.
31. Yudin MH, Shapiro HM, Loutfy MR. Access to infertility services in Canada for HIV-positive individuals and couples: a cross-sectional study. *Reprod Health*. 2010;7(1):7.
32. Gruskin S, Ferguson L, O'Malley J. Ensuring sexual and reproductive health for people living with HIV: an overview of key human rights, policy and health systems issues. *Reprod Health Matters*. 2007;15(29):4–26.
33. Margolese S. You can have a healthy pregnancy if you are HIV positive. Canadian AIDS Treatment Information Exchange resources. http://www.catie.ca/en/practical-guides/pregnancy. Accessed March 22, 2018.
34. Marlatt GA, Larimer ME, Witkiewitz K, eds. *Harm Reduction: Pragmatic Strategies for Managing High-Risk Behaviors*. New York, NY: Guilford Press; 2011.

35. World Health Organization. *Guidelines on HIV and Infant Feeding 2010: Principles and Recommendations for Infant Feeding in the Context of HIV and a Summary of Evidence.*
36. Greene S, Tucker R, Rourke SB, et al. "Under my umbrella": the housing experiences of HIV-positive parents who live with and care for their children in Ontario. *Arch Womens Mental Health*. 2010;13(3):223–232.
37. Greene S, Ion A, Elston D, Kwaramba G, Smith S, Loutfy M. Othering with HIV: resisting and reconstructing experiences of health and social surveillance. In: Hogeveen B, Minaker JC, eds. *Criminalized Mothers, Criminalizing Motherhood*. Ontario: Demeter Press; 2015:231–263.
38. McKenzie HA, Varcoe C, Browne AJ, Day L. Disrupting the continuities among residential schools, the Sixties Scoop, and child welfare: an analysis of colonial and neocolonial discourses. *Int Indig Policy J*. 2016;7(2). doi:10.18584/iipj.2016.7.2.4
39. Sinclair R. Identity lost and found: lessons from the sixties scoop. *First Peoples Child Family Rev*. 2007;3(1):65–82.
40. Woodgate RL, Zurba M, Tennent P, Cochrane C, Payne M, Mignone J. "People try and label me as someone I'm not": the social ecology of Indigenous people living with HIV, stigma, and discrimination in Manitoba, Canada. *Soc Sci Med*. 2017;194:17–24.
41. Priest L. Mother convicted of hiding HIV status for son's birth. *Globe and Mail*. https://www.theglobeandmail.com/news/national/mother-convicted-of-hiding-hiv-status-for-sons-birth/article1101486/. Published August 2006. Accessed March 22, 2018.
42. Loutfy MR, Margolese S, Money DM, Gysler M, Hamilton S, Yudin MH. Canadian HIV pregnancy planning guidelines. *Int J Gynecol Obstet*. 2012;119(1):89–99.
43. Emlet CA. "You're awfully old to have this disease": experiences of stigma and ageism in adults 50 years and older living with HIV/AIDS. *Gerontologist*. 2006;46(6):781–790.
44. Deeks SG, Lewin SR, Havlir DV. The end of AIDS: HIV infection as a chronic disease. *Lancet*. 2013;382(9903):1525–1533.
45. Brew BJ. Has HIV-associated neurocognitive disorders now transformed into vascular cognitive impairment? *AIDS*. 2016;30(15):2379–2380.
46. Rodriguez-Penney AT, Iudicello JE, Riggs PK, et al. The HIV Neurobehavioral Research Program (HNRP) Group SP. Co-morbidities in persons infected with HIV: increased burden with older age and negative effects on health-related quality of life. *AIDS Patient Care STDs*. 2013;27(1):5–16.
47. Heyland DK, Barwich D, Pichora D, et al. ACCEPT (Advance Care Planning Evaluation in Elderly Patients) Study Team. Failure to engage hospitalized elderly patients and their families in advance care planning. *JAMA Intern Med*. 2013;173(9):778–787.

48. Loutfy M, de Pokomandy A, Kennedy VL, et al. Cohort profile: the Canadian HIV Women's Sexual and Reproductive Health Cohort Study (CHIWOS). *PLoS One*. 2017;12(9):e0184708.
49. Loutfy M, Greene S, Kennedy VL, et al. Establishing the Canadian HIV Women's Sexual and Reproductive Health Cohort Study (CHIWOS): operationalizing community-based research in a large national quantitative study. *BMC Med Res Methodol*. 2016;16(1):101.
50. World Health Organization's consolidated guideline on sexual and reproductive health and rights of women living with HIV. http://www.who.int/reproductivehealth/publications/gender_rights/Ex-Summ-srhr-women-hiv/en/. Published 2017. Accessed March 22, 2018.
51. Carter AJ, Bourgeois S, O'Brien N, et al. Women-specific HIV/AIDS services: identifying and defining the components of holistic service delivery for women living with HIV/AIDS. *J Int AIDS Soc*. 2013;16:17433.

7 ETHICAL ISSUES IN HEALTHCARE FOR WOMEN IN THE CONTEXT OF VIOLENCE

Rochelle Einboden and Colleen Varcoe

Introduction

Interpersonal violence is rooted in inequity and power differentials and is contiguous with structural inequities. Interpersonal violence thus most commonly is committed against those who are positioned to be most vulnerable in society. Violence against women, the focus of this chapter, is rooted in gender inequity, and women who are further disadvantaged by poverty, racism, heterosexism, and stigma related to mental health problems or (dis)abilities experience even higher levels of violence.

This chapter examines the ethical issues involved in providing healthcare to women in the context of violence against women, including intimate partner violence and sexual assault. It begins by defining violence against women. It then traces the roots of violence against women to the social contexts within which it occurs, making explicit the interconnectedness of interpersonal and structural forms of violence against women. The ethical analysis begins with a discussion of the issue of violence against women through a traditional bioethical lens. Insights, limitations, and consequences of applying principles such as beneficence, non-maleficence, respect for persons, and justice to support ethical deliberations around responses to violence against women are considered. Next, a critical feminist perspective is offered to deepen the analysis by drawing attention to relational ethics. Such an analysis includes attention to context, the power relations within which women live and within which healthcare is provided, and the structural conditions of women's lives. This ethical orientation supports an analysis of women's roles as mothers and consequently takes into account the complex ethical issues that must be considered given that children are exposed to violence. This analysis includes but is not limited to directly seeing or hearing (witnessing) violence perpetrated against their mothers, and that child maltreatment overlaps with violence against women.

Healthcare responses to violence are shifting, guided by this critical social understanding of violence and ethical perspectives. Policies and practices that are informed by these perspectives are culturally safe and trauma- and violence-informed and consider that any person may have a history of, or currently be experiencing, violence, as well as the complexity of ethical issues related to disclosure. Because those who are positioned to be most vulnerable in society experience the most violence, they are also least likely to be able to access supports. Thus, an ethical response needs to include policies and practices that support individual women and families, as well as their care providers, with an appreciation for the social context of women's lives, roles, and relationships.

What Is Violence Against Women?

The United Nations (UN) defines violence against women as "any act of gender-based violence that results in, or is likely to result in, physical, sexual or psychological harm or suffering to women, including threats of such acts, coercion or arbitrary deprivation of liberty, whether occurring in public or in private life."[1] A variety of terms are used to describe the issue of violence against women in their private lives, including *intimate partner violence, domestic violence,* and *family violence.* In this chapter we will use the term *violence against women* because the other terms are not gender-specific and this term extends across public and private domains. Regardless of gender, anyone can be either a victim or perpetrator of violence; however, the term *violence against women* emphasizes the gendered nature of violence that women and girls experience.

Women, and people who do not conform to the gender binary male/female, have different experiences of violence than men. A disproportionate amount of violence against women is perpetrated by men. Further, unlike men's experience of violence, women are much more likely to experience violence in the context of family and intimate relationships.[2] UN Women estimates that

35 per cent of women worldwide have experienced either physical and/or sexual intimate partner violence or non-partner sexual violence. However, some national studies show that up to 70 per cent of women have experienced physical and/or sexual violence in their lifetime from an intimate partner.[3(p2)]

This distinct pattern of gender-based violence against women by men from within the family is significant because it points to both the insidious nature and complexity of the violence women experience. Just because this violence is perpetrated by known abusers does not make it any less severe or dangerous to the health and well-being of women. In fact, violence has direct and indirect consequences for women's health, details of which will be discussed in more detail later in the chapter.

Roots of Violence Against Women

As a social phenomenon, violence against women represents, generates, and sustains a hierarchical social ordering, where women are positioned with lower social status than men. Thus, "[t]here is increasing international consensus that the abuse of women and girls, regardless of where it occurs, should be considered as 'gender-based violence', as it largely stems from women's subordinate status in society with regards to men."[2(p11)] Social ordering starts early in our lives and requires violence. Violence perpetrated against particular women functions indirectly to promote compliance with the social order, through the nonspecific *threat* of violence for all women. For example, sexual assaults directed at specific groups of women may be interpreted by women in general in various ways (e.g., "It happens to 'other' women" or "that could be me"). These interpretations are integrated into other social norms and steer understandings such as where women might expect to be safe from assault and what public behaviors are considered acceptable.

While intersecting situational and interpersonal factors contribute to particular incidents of violence, social structures and norms that dictate and differentiate the roles of men and women, including how they should be or behave, create the foundation and justification for violence against women.[2(p25)] These gender roles are socially constructed yet legitimized by discourses of nature, which make the political and cultural relations that support them invisible and difficult to critique. Oppressive gender roles are a structural form of social violence. Following Galtung, Farmer and colleagues argue that social "arrangements are structural because they are embedded in the political and economic organization of our social world; they are violent because they cause injury to people (typically, not those [people] responsible for perpetuating such inequalities)."[4(p. e499)] The violence that can be attributed to these structures is indirect and systematic, generated diffusely from everywhere and everyone within the social order.[4]

Structural violence informs "the study of the social machinery of oppression. Oppression is a result of many conditions, not the least of which reside in consciousness."[5(p307)] For instance, consider the dominant positioning of men as head of the family with authority for decision making and finances, while women typically are positioned with domestic responsibilities such as childrearing and sustenance work. Consider also how women's roles within the home isolate them and limit their social networks and mobility. Normative social roles are oppressive because they constitute women with limited power in relation to men.[i] How we understand women and the feminine within society is relevant to violence against women. Gender roles are structurally violent because they constitute social relations that put women in harm's way. Generally speaking, healthcare providers are not supported to understand social relations and the resulting structural violence. They are poorly supported to intervene at the social level and focus instead in a limited way on how to support women to navigate violence to maintain their own safety.

Gendered patterns of violence highlight how violence against women is rooted in dominant oppressive social values and beliefs. These oppressive values in relation to gender create conditions for violence against women. For instance, research across multiple societies consistently shows how challenges to dominant gender roles and norms trigger violence against women.[6] Challenges include:

> not obeying the husband, talking back, not having food ready on time, failing to care adequately for the children or home, questioning him about money or girlfriends, going somewhere without his permission, refusing him sex, or expressing suspicions of infidelity.[2(p25)]

Normative performances of gender roles for men and women also create conditions for violence against women. While masculinity is characterized as dominant, aggressive, independent, and competitive, femininity is characterized as nurturing, passive, dependent, and altruistic. These characteristics, along with the relegation of women to domestic roles, have been naturalized through biologic essentialisms and anchored to women's reproductive capacity. Yet, tracing the production of these gendered roles historically reveals socio-political influences instead of biologic ones.[7,8]

In ancient Western society, women's roles in production and reproduction were respected as essential to life. However, women were associated with nature and thus subordinate to men's civilizing cultural pursuits in politics and arts.[9] During the shift to capital economic systems, production, and the accumulation of surplus, women's roles in production and reproduction (production of a labor force) were revalued, thus improving women's social status.[8] However, this improvement was short-lived because with industrialization, the rise of the factory separated the sites of production from reproduction, creating a divide between public and private labor.[8] At the same time, capitalism reframed the economic unit from the community to the family and introduced the idea of private property; thus, kin alliances became the mechanism of property accumulation and transfer.[10] When women's domestic and reproductive labor was not allocated monetary value within the capitalist economy, patriarchy was institutionalized and intensified.[8] This shift eroded respect for women's contributions, exploited women's reproductive labor, and redefined women and children as family property.[8,9]

The movement of women into public labor has occurred over time, with a notable acceleration during World War II. At the end of the war, middle-class women's participation in paid work was thwarted by governments, who initiated a resurgence of normative gender roles to allow jobs to become available for returning soldiers. Thus, in the 1950s, women were sent back into the home to enact their domestic duties with renewed discourses of authority over the governance of children and the home (e.g., the "domestic goddess").[10] While given a domain of authority, women's power was still limited and subordinate.

This brief historical account details some of the political mechanisms within which normative gender roles are enacted, although within dominant contemporary discourse they are framed as emerging from biology alone. Analysis of violence against women as an ethical issue requires an understanding of the gendered nature of the violence and the underpinning political relations.

Violence Against Women Through a Traditional Bioethics Lens

Violence against women is an ethical issue. Traditional bioethical perspectives and principles offer some ethical guidance to health practice and policy in response to violence against women. In this section, principles of beneficence, non-maleficence, respect for persons, and justice will be considered. Despite the magnitude of the problem, healthcare practices and policies respond to violence against women in individualistic ways, for example by offering counseling services or forensic evidence collection. These responses aim to support women who have experienced violence to cope with their experiences. Beneficence and non-maleficence require that healthcare practices respond to violence against women in ways that benefit individual women as much as possible and minimize the potential for further harm, as well as respect women's autonomy, confidentiality, safety, and dignity.

While traditional bioethical principles offer some helpful guidance across healthcare practice to support health professionals to consider practices and policies that address violence against women, these ethical principles tend to be framed by deontological understandings and oriented toward individuals. A focus on individuals is at times useful to consider the approaches in one-on-one interactions with women who have experienced violence, yet they are limited and often consider the problem as if it were an individual's problem that could be addressed at an individual level. These types of responses often leave women facing unrealistic expectations to address the violence, such as requirements to leave an abusive situation. A gendered analysis of violence against women that considers the socio-political context encourages responses that create conditions for safety within the community and society. Further, healthcare professionals need to be cognizant about how narrow individualistic understandings about violence against women may lead to responses that inadvertently extend the violence women experience rather than address it.

The Need to Go Beyond Traditional Bioethical Perspectives

Hegemonic understandings of violence set up conditions for violence within the social mechanisms that address it. For example, that individual women could be responsible for the violence they experience is a central hegemonic belief that orients responses toward educating women and girls about how to behave to prevent or respond to defend themselves against violence situations. The hegemony of women's responsibility for the violence perpetrated against them removes from view the roots of violence, such as the ways women and children are constituted within proprietary family relations and how these constitutions lead to objectifications of women's bodies, the conditions that incite men to perpetrate violence against women. When the hegemonic belief that women are responsible for the violence they experience is challenged, another type of response can arise, such as a response that considers what education and socialization men and boys require to support them to avoid perpetrating violence. Further considerations of structural violence have implications for the development of responses within healthcare practices and policies, as well as legal and social responses.

Within legal responses to violence, the onus is on the victims to provide tangible (and often visible) evidence of the violent incident that identifies the perpetrator. Healthcare practices have evolved to support victims in fulfilling these prescribed legal responsibilities. Thus, in relation to responses to extreme physical and sexual assault, standardized forensic practices are improving the quality of evidence collected and used in police investigations and legal proceedings. Aided by technologies such as DNA testing and advanced imaging, forensic science is oriented to address violence through retributive forms of justice. While this medical-legal orientation has a role to play within healthcare responses to violence, these practices are only one aspect of the care that is required. From an ethical perspective, it should also be considered how, while offering some benefit to individual victims of interpersonal violence, these investigations entrench hegemonic understandings that define the problem as that of an individual perpetrator. The dominant nature of these practices is problematic because they entrench individualized understandings of violence against women. Further, they fail to resist an emphasis on individual responses *in lieu of social ones*.

Applied at the individual level, beneficence, non-maleficence, and respect for persons not only miss the social context that supports violence but contribute to legitimizing the violence within the structure of the legal system. Relational ethics require that individual responses be balanced with complementary social responses. These socially oriented responses are needed to disrupt the dominant hegemonies that set the conditions for violence against women and that place the responsibility to address this violence on the victims. A social perspective opens a dialogue about how we might begin to address violence against women differently. Acting relationally requires considering (a) how interpersonal violence and structural forms of violence are interconnected, (b) how these intertwined forms of violence operate in current policies, practices, and responses to violence against women, and (c) the need for alternative approaches that go beyond addressing individual acts of violence to address the conditions that perpetuate and sustain patterns of violence. To practice ethically is to ensure that our healthcare policies and practices do not cause further distress or harm, for individuals *and* for women across society.

Violence Against Women Through a Relational Ethics Lens

A relational perspective has expanded how we understand the traditional bioethical principle of justice. As we have discussed, legal and healthcare practices are primarily oriented toward justice at an individual level. However, the shift to a social justice framework is gaining momentum even within mainstream discourses. Social justice considers the structural issues, how injustices are systematically built into society and the implications for certain cohorts of the population. Violence against women is an ethical issue; the injustices experienced by girls and women are further intensified as they intersect with multiple forms of inequity, such as inequities based on racism, classism, ableism, heterosexism, and ageism.

As a mechanism that maintains social inequity, violence against women is a key issue for social justice. "Violence against women is the most pervasive yet under-recognized human rights violation in the world."[2(p9)] Violence against women occurs in a variety of social locations, from family homes to combat zones. Threats of or actual violence in any form enforces relations of power between individuals or groups of people. An obvious and extreme example of how violence operates as a technique of domination is in the strategic and pervasive use of sexual violence in warfare. Violence and its threat produce fear that can make bodies act and obey. It enforces a particular form of social order that limits women's access to certain spaces (e.g., public, corporate). A less obvious example is in the responses of universities to sexual assaults. A typical response is to warn women to protect themselves by limiting where they go, when, and with whom. The responsibility shifts onto women to prevent assaults and to change their movement and presence (e.g., "She was walking alone at night," "Why doesn't she leave him?").

Domination is evident in the limits placed on women's participation in social life, by violence and its threat. This includes influencing where to live and with whom; when, where, and how to travel; and whether to attend work, school, or other activities central to social life. Thus, violence against women can be seen as a technique of power and an integral mechanism of maintaining social hierarchy. Inequity requires violence, and responding to violence is a matter of social justice.[11] However, within dominant social discourse, violence is individualized and constituted as an issue of out-of-control male aggression or out-of-control sexual desire rather than domination. In this framing, the function of violence against women in establishing and maintaining social relations, and hence a means of social ordering, is obscured.[12] Yet, threats of violence against women are so common they often go unchallenged. "Despite the high costs of violence against women, social institutions in almost every society in the world legitimize, obscure and deny abuse."[2(p9)] The legitimization of abuse is evident by requiring women to shoulder the responsibility for the violence perpetrated against them. As we have discussed, an ethical analysis of violence against women from a relational perspective considers social justice and thus requires that men be consistently charged with a responsibility for addressing and not perpetrating violence, rather than women being charged with the responsibility to avoid it. Reconsidering healthcare policies and practice from this perspective highlights instead of obscures relations of domination. This perspective also emphasizes how violence maintains the social order, opening a place for discussion for ethical approaches that disrupt gender inequity.

Interpersonal Violence, Inequity, and Power Differentials

While a gendered analysis offers some key insights into the dynamics of violence against women, alone it is insufficient to capture the experience of most women. Gender is only one of many categories of difference used to position persons within the social order. Of the oppressive power relations underpinning violence, subjugation based on gender is one of various means of social ordering. Women who experience multiple forms of marginalization are much more likely to experience interpersonal violence.[13] And, while all women are influenced by oppressive gendered constructions, they experience these differently depending on other categorizations of difference in relation to their social position. For instance, despite pressure to focus on domestic life after World War II, many women from low socioeconomic situations continued to work in public labor as a matter of necessity. The opportunity to engage solely in domestic work was and continues to be an option available primarily to middle- and upper-class women. Further, the exclusion of many women from performing normative gender roles has inconsistent effects, and women who occupy low socioeconomic social positions experience more, not less, intense gender-based violence.[2]

Women who experience discrimination related to race, class, sexuality, or ability are disadvantaged further because violence converges on women who occupy marginalized social positions.[14] Intersecting forms of discrimination and marginalization set up social conditions that make more overt forms of violence possible. While "[a]ny woman ... has reason to fear rape,"[15(p62)] women who are marginalized experience associated material deprivations, setting social conditions and opportunities that make it more likely for them to be raped compared with the likelihood of rape for any woman. For example, a woman who is homeless is more likely to be raped than one who lives in a safe home. Yet, in dominant discourses marginalization is not usually considered violent, because material deprivations associated with marginalization are normalized as unfortunate but largely within the control of the individual woman. Dominant social discourse constitutes only spectacular and extreme forms of violence (e.g., death and obvious physical violence) as violence, with the broader dynamics of social positioning as incidental to, rather than integral to, how violence operates and flows. Yet, eruptions of spectacular forms of interpersonal violence are predicated by structural forms of violence. For example, in Canada, the disproportionate violence against Indigenous women in comparison to the general population repeatedly has been shown to be related to the underlying structural violence directed against Indigenous people.[16-20] After years of activism by Indigenous people, important attention has been drawn to the most spectacular forms of violence against Indigenous women, for example through the National Inquiry into Missing and Murdered Indigenous Women and Girls.[21] However, this violence is supported by and continuous with the pervasive experiences of structural violence (from poverty to institutional racism in healthcare, social services, and justice systems) experienced by many Indigenous people. For example, many Indigenous women are put at risk on the Highway of Tears (a stretch of highway in British Columbia along which many Indigenous women have disappeared or been killed) in part because, as a consequence of policy-induced poverty, they cannot afford private transportation and public transportation is not affordable or available. In healthcare, the attention of clinicians is directed to the spectacular through textbooks (e.g., by emphasizing dramatic physical injuries), policies (e.g., by advocating screening aimed at disclosure), and narrow understandings about the roots of violence (e.g., ones that apportion blame to victims for contributing through their behaviors).

While those who are positioned to be most vulnerable in society experience the most violence, conditions that allow for violence are set by the positioning of some groups as dominant in relation to others. Violence and its threat disrupt the image of society as safe, and as such are disturbing at a social level.[22] In order to contain the threat of violence, it is often constituted as something that happens outside of the dominant social group; for example, to "other" women by "other" men, or to "certain" women by "certain" men, defined variously by race, ethnicity, class, and ability (particularly related to mental health). This distancing preserves an illusion of safety for some, while concentrating the focus on the most spectacular and obvious forms of violence, allowing the conditions from which they arise to go unnoticed and undisturbed.[22] Violence is constituted as if it were the problem of, and originating from, individuals within marginalized groups. Thus, making explicit the connections between interpersonal and structural violence helps to resist simplistic and marginalizing understandings of violence against women. Making these connections explicit encourages discussion of the social conditions for violence, beyond those related to individual women, including accountability for social inclusion and equity.

Healthcare Policies and Practices in Response to Violence

Over the past several decades, increasingly the problem of violence against women has been taken seriously in healthcare settings. In this section, healthcare practices and policies are discussed. Universal screening, a key response to violence against women, is considered using a relational and ethical lens. Trauma- and violence-informed healthcare policies and culturally safe practices are discussed in the context to responding to violence against women in meaningful ways. Best practices such as "case finding" and developing a relational approach to violence against women are introduced to support a broad understanding of how these responses might support women in the context of their family relations and caregiving roles.

Screening and the Ethics of Disclosure

In North American healthcare contexts, efforts have focused largely on implementing universal screening by healthcare providers across a variety of healthcare settings, including emergency departments and maternal and primary care settings. A universal approach to screening mandates that all persons seeking care are asked whether they have a history of, or are currently experiencing, violence. Screening as an approach to responding to violence against women in healthcare is consistent with an understanding of violence as an individual problem. The logic to screening is that (a) a high proportion of people will have such experiences, (b) a disclosure of such experience is required to provide appropriate care, and (c) following disclosure, effective care will be provided. However, screening reinforces a focus on spectacular forms of violence (as the most obvious and extreme signs are most likely to be recognized) decontextualized from wider social conditions. Importantly, the focus on the individual woman as "victim" can obscure the effects on others, such the woman's children, friends, and other family members. The focus on spectacular forms of violence against women within practice and policy responses operates paradoxically because it effaces women's agency and constitutes them within discourses of passivity and victimisation.[23] Practices that constitute women as victims have implications for interpersonal violence, especially within the relationship with perpetrators, where such practices can increase the danger to women (e.g., advice to leave a partner in the absence of safety planning and adequate resources to foster safety).

Further, research has consistently shown that screening is not effective. While screening can result in clinicians increasing their recognition of such histories, it has not been shown to increase referrals to services or to improve outcomes.[24-26] Randomized controlled trials have shown that screening women and providing passive referrals (information cards or printouts) does not lead to improvements in life quality or mental health or a reduction in violence. Systematic reviews have routinely concluded there is insufficient evidence to recommend screening in healthcare.[27,28] Subsequently, the World Health Organization (WHO) and the Canadian Task Force on Preventive Health Care do not recommend screening.[29]

Responses to violence against women that focus on eliciting disclosures and substantiating abuse are limited. From a critical and relational ethics perspective, pinning practice to disclosure is one of the ways that the roots of violence are obscured and denied. Again, this is because these practices address violence at the level of the individual and after it has happened. It orients us away from the social problem of subordination of women and children, and away from considering the need for social responses. In this way, these practices perpetuate rather than interrupt violence.

Other ethical concerns in relation to disclosure include the need to consider affective responses to violence. Exposure to violence is disturbing because it highlights our embodied vulnerability.[22,30] Containing this anxiety is a priority and, as we have discussed, those in dominant social positions require mechanisms to create distance between themselves and the violence through "othering" both victims and perpetrators. Proximity to violence, especially proximity to violations of the body experienced in spectacular cases of abuse, intensifies anxiety and provokes what Julia Kristeva describes as abjection, contradictory but simultaneous experiences of fascination and repulsion.[31] This experience of fascination and repulsion is intensified by visual practices such as photography and other forms of imaging.[11,32] Abjection is a helpful concept to consider the ethics of contemporary responses to violence against women critically, because it suggests that these practices are vulnerable to voyeurism. Further, medico-legal responses require visual documentation of violence (e.g., photographs of injuries and video-recorded colposcopy are "gold standard" practices for physical/sexual assault). Considering how commonly violence against women occurs and how rare it is to be able to visualize its imprint on women's bodies, a critique of the visual medico-legal practices of evidence collection is needed. Rather than supporting justice for women, concentrating attention on physical evidence works paradoxically: it reproduces and incites violence by requiring its presentation in increasingly spectacular forms to justify a response.[33] This concentration simultaneously obscures and dismisses the invisible forms of violence, including mental, emotional, and financial abuse, that make up the majority of daily harms toward women. A relational ethical perspective that considers these complexities and appreciates the lure of the spectacular suggests that to practice ethically, revisiting contemporary practices and policies that require disclosure, physical assessment, and photographic documentation is needed.

In practical ways, pinning effective care to disclosure assumes that disclosure (a) will lead to beneficial responses and (b) is necessary for good care. However, disclosure does not always lead to responses that are beneficial for the person disclosing. First, when violence is historical, there may be nothing that can be done, or that the person would like done. Second, even when violence is ongoing, healthcare providers do not always know how to respond, nor do they have the resources to do so. Rather than focus on screening to identify individual "victims," the current emphasis is on building on the notion of trauma-informed practice. This approach to practice has been shown to be effective in mental health and substance use care settings[34] to create organizational cultures and approaches to practice that are safe for all patients and staff, particularly for those who have histories and ongoing experiences of interpersonal violence, regardless of disclosure. Drawing on a relational understanding of ethics, this approach has the potential to attend to those affected beyond the particular woman and to base practice on a broad contextual understanding of violence.

Trauma- and Violence-Informed Policies and Practices

Building on trauma-informed practice as developed within substance use and mental health contexts, current efforts are directed toward making all healthcare practice settings trauma- and violence-informed.[35,36] Such an approach takes into account that *any person may have a history of or currently be experiencing violence*. Taking this "universal precautions" approach means that healthcare providers are supported through policy and training to provide the emotionally safest possible care to all persons. This means that individuals do not have to disclose should they judge it not safe to do so. The onus for safety is on the health care organization and providers, not on the individual patient.

This approach is underpinned by an *understanding of the effects of violence*. Thus, healthcare providers are tasked with understanding how experiences of violence affect individuals physiologically (e.g., the relationship between violence experiences, chronic pain, substance use, and mental health) and socially (e.g., by interfering with trust and increasing wariness). Healthcare providers use such knowledge to create physically and emotionally safe care environments—for example, by expressing understanding of the health effects of violence and avoiding practices that can trigger unwanted memories or emotional responses. This requires supportive policies—for example, staffing levels adequate to provide such care, and the ability to afford privacy.

This approach is also underpinned by a relational understanding of autonomy. Healthcare providers who understand that violence is always an abuse of power explicitly seek to *foster opportunities for choice and collaboration with patients*, but they also understand that people make decisions "in relation" to others and the circumstances of their lives.[37] For example, women who are living with abusive partners make judgments about those relationships taking into account their level of danger, the potential impacts of their decisions on their children and others, and other aspects of their life circumstances.

This relational understanding considers individuals within their broader social circumstances and draws attention to the continuities between interpersonal and structural forms of violence. This understanding supports healthcare providers to consider the complexity of people's lives. So, for example, a provider ought not to urge a woman to leave an abusive partner without attending to the risks involved—for example, will difficulty finding safe housing and the related risks worsen the woman's danger? This in turn requires policies that support such attention—for example, safe discharge policies, referral pathways, outreach services, and so on. Practitioners who are supported to be trauma- and violence-informed on a routine basis are thus well prepared to engage in case finding and responding effectively to disclosures.

Best Practice Includes Case Finding

The WHO recommends that healthcare providers learn the signs and health presentations that are commonly associated with violence, such as mental health issues, chronic pain, and substance use.[38] Knowing the common issues associated with violence, and how violence manifests, positions providers to effectively inquire with individuals. Given the high association of violence and trauma with mental health issues and substance use, routine inquiry in mental health and substance use settings is recommended. Similarly, given the association between substance use and chronic pain, providers can reasonably inquire about a history of or ongoing violence when patients present with chronic pain. Case finding that begins with an individual's clinical presentation connects the person's concerns with inquiry and can contribute to the development of trust. That is, inquiring by saying that "people with chronic pain often have histories of experiencing violence" conveys recognition of the person's concern and is a very different opening than a screening question disconnected from the person's presentation.

Culturally Safe Practices and Policy

Trauma- and violence-informed practices must be emotionally and physically safe, which necessarily implies efforts toward cultural safety. Given the continuities between structural violence, including systemic racism, and interpersonal violence, attention to racism and other forms of discrimination is integral to trauma- and violence-informed practice. Cultural safety was initially developed to counter Indigenous-specific racism and discrimination and, given the disproportionate levels of violence against Indigenous women, is essential to such practice in Canada. Cultural safety, like trauma- and violence-informed care, puts the onus for safety on the healthcare organization and providers. Providers are tasked with understanding the impacts of history, including colonization, and the ongoing effects of racism and discrimination, and providing care based on such understanding.

Responses to Disclosure That Are Safe, Supportive, and Not Stigmatizing

A trauma- and violence-informed approach and cultural safety emphasize that the onus is on healthcare providers to respond in ways that communicate that it is safe to discuss violence with them. The WHO recommendations for responding to disclosures of violence are captured in the acronym LIVES: Listen, Inquire about needs and concerns, Validate, Enhance safety, and Support.[39] This suggests that responding safely to disclosures is not specialized; rather, empathetic, ethical practice is required. In order to engage in an empathetic and ethical way, a useful practice for care providers is reflexivity about assumptions about violence against women. This reflexive approach can be used following principles of cultural safety, while considering the context of gender (e.g., Where do I place responsibility for violence? What messages in my social context encourage me to see some groups as more "prone" to violence than others?). Examining assumptions about women and violence against women within its social and political complexity supports new understandings and practices. Specifically, recognizing how the social context supports violence against women, and what opportunities within the political context might disrupt the context, offers opportunities for change.

Best Practice Includes Considerations for the Social Circumstances and Family Members

Women's positions as stewards of the family have significant implications for them, and the effects of violence ripple out over family members for whom they care. The violence women experience is experienced also by others—children, elderly parents, or any individuals who rely on the woman for their needs. Further, because many women have little support in their caregiving roles, their vulnerability to violence spreads across all of those who rely on them. When violence interferes with the woman's ability to care for and protect those in her charge, she is at risk of being dispositioned from her responsibilities. In this way, the violence she experiences strikes twice. From an ethical perspective, responses need to consider how to protect the woman who is experiencing violence in the first instance, and to create space that enables her to continue caregiving responsibilities as she desires. From a relational ethics perspective, threatening removal of children extends the violence the woman experiences; thus, alternative approaches and resources for mothers and other caregivers are needed. Given the recent trend to consider the exposure of children to violence against their mothers as an issue of child protection, ethical considerations are crucially important.

Conclusion

This chapter has presented a gendered analysis of violence against women supported by a relational ethics. A gendered analysis illustrates how violence against women is an ethical issue related to social inequity and highlights how various other social positions (e.g., race, class, sexuality, age, or ability) may intensify or buffer the violence women experience. Such analysis encourages consideration of how the roots of violence against women are anchored deeply within society, and thus contemporary individualistic responses are not able to make meaningful differences for women collectively. From a relational perspective, responses that resist the dominant but narrow individualistic discourses and resist the focus on spectacular forms of violence are needed to avoid reproducing and perpetuating violence against women. This perspective highlights the need for ethical healthcare policy and practices to draw on social and relational perspectives to ensure that violence is addressed meaningfully (rather than being reproduced or further entrenched). Attending to ethical approaches calls for policies and practices that respond to the complexity of ethical issues related to disclosure, including case finding instead of routine screening, culturally safe and trauma- and violence-informed care, and consideration of the context of women's lives and relationships, especially their caregiving relationships.

Note

[i] Some Indigenous matriarchal societies represent an exception to this social construction.

References

1. United Nations General Assembly. *48/104 Declaration on the Elimination of Violence Against Women (Article 1).* 1994. www.un.org/documents/ga/res/48/a48r104.htm. Accessed December 5, 2018.
2. Ellsberg M, Heise L. *Researching Violence Against Women: A Practical Guide for Researchers and Activists.* Washington, DC, United States: World Health Organization, PATH; 2005. http://www.who.int/reproductivehealth/publications/violence/9241546476/en/. Accessed December 5, 2018.
3. UN Women. *In Brief: Ending Violence Against Women and Girls.* New York, NY: United Nations; n.d. http://www2.unwomen.org/~/media/headquarters/attachments/sections/library/publications/2013/12/un%20women%20evaw-thembrief_us-web-rev9%20pdf.pdf?v=2&d=20161013T141205. Accessed December 5, 2018.

4. Farmer PE, Nizeye B, Stulac S, Keshavjee S. Structural violence and clinical medicine. *PLoS Med*. 2006;3(10):e449. doi:10.1371/journal.pmed.0030449
5. Farmer P. An anthropology of structural violence. *Curr Anthropol*. 2004;45(3):305–325. doi:10.1086/382250
6. Heise LL. Violence against women: an integrated, ecological framework. *Violence Against Women*. 1998;4(3):262–290. doi:10.1177/1077801298004003002
7. Chodorow N. *The Reproduction of Mothering: Psychoanalysis and the Sociology of Gender: With a New Preface*. Berkeley, CA: University of California Press; 1999.
8. Zaretsky E. *Capitalism, the Family & Personal Life*. London: Pluto Press; 1976.
9. O'Neill J. *The Missing Child in Liberal Theory: Towards a Covenant Theory of Family, Community, Welfare, and the Civic State*. Toronto, ON: University of Toronto Press; 1994.
10. Donzelot J. *The Policing of Families*. New York, NY: Pantheon Books; 1979.
11. Einboden R. *Nowhere to Stand: A Critical Discourse Analysis of Nurses' Responses to Child Neglect and Abuse*. Doctoral dissertation, 2017. http://hdl.handle.net/2123/18349. Accessed December 5, 2018.
12. Nic Giolla Easpaig B, Fryer D. Dismantling dominant sexual violence research without using the master's tools. *GLIP Rev*. 2011;7(2):168–175.
13. Stockman JK, Hayashi H, Campbell JC. Intimate partner violence and its health impact on disproportionately affected populations, including minorities and impoverished groups. *J Womens Health*. 2015;24(1):62–79. doi:10.1089/jwh.2014.4879
14. Sokoloff NJ, Dupont I. Domestic violence at the intersections of race, class, and gender: challenges and contributions to understanding violence against marginalized women in diverse communities. *Violence Against Women*. 2005;11(1):38–64. doi:10.1177/1077801204271476
15. Young IM. *Justice and the Politics of Difference*. Princeton, NJ: Princeton University Press; 1990.
16. Varcoe C, Dick S. Intersecting risks of violence and HIV for rural and Aboriginal women in a neocolonial Canadian context. *J Aborig Health*. 2008;4:42–52. doi: https://doi.org/10.18357/ijih41200812314
17. Pedersen JS, Malcoe LH, Pulkingham J. Explaining aboriginal/non-aboriginal inequalities in postseparation violence against Canadian women: application of a structural violence approach. *Violence Against Women*. 2013;19(8):1034–1058. doi:10.1177/1077801213499245
18. Daoud N, Urquia ML, O'Campo P, et al. Prevalence of abuse and violence before, during, and after pregnancy in a national sample of Canadian women. *Am J Public Health*. 2012;102(10):1893–1901. doi: 10.2105/AJPH.2012.300843
19. Daoud N, Smylie J, Urquia M, Allan B, O'Campo P. The contribution of socioeconomic position to the excesses of violence and intimate partner violence among aboriginal versus non-Aboriginal Women in Canada. *Can J Public Health*. 2013;104(4):e278–e83. doi: http://dx.doi.org/10.17269/cjph.104.3724

20. Brownridge DA. Understanding the elevated risk of partner violence against Aboriginal women: a comparison of two nationally representative surveys of Canada. *J Fam Violence*. 2008;23(5):353–367. doi: https://doi.org/10.1007/s10896-008-9160-0
21. National Inquiry into Missing and Murdered Indigenous Women and Girls. *Interim Report: Our Women and Girls Are Sacred*. Her Majesty the Queen in Right of Canada; 2017. http://www.mmiwg-ffada.ca/files/ni-mmiwg-interim-report-en.pdf. Accessed December 5, 2018.
22. Žižek S. *Violence: Six Sideways Reflections*. London: Profile Books Ltd.; 2009.
23. Valentine K, Breckenridge J. Responses to family and domestic violence: supporting women? *Griffith Law Rev*. 2016;25(1):30–44. doi:10.1080/10383441.2016.1204684
24. MacMillan H, Wathen C, Jamieson E, et al. Screening for intimate partner violence in health care settings: a randomized trial. *JAMA*. 2009;302(5):493–501. doi: 10.1001/jama.2009.1089
25. Koziol-McLain J, Garrett N, Fanslow J, et al. A randomized controlled trial of a brief emergency department intimate partner violence screening intervention. *Ann Emerg Med*. 2010;56(4):413–423. doi: 10.1016/j.annemergmed.2010.05.001
26. Klevens J, Kee R, Trick W, et al. Effect of screening for partner violence on women's quality of life. *JAMA*. 2012;308(7):681–689. doi: 10.1001/jama.2012.6434
27. Ramsay J, Richardson J, Carter YH, Davidson LL, Feder G. Should health professionals screen women for domestic violence? Systematic review. *BMJ*. 2002;325(7359):314–318. doi: https://doi.org/10.1136/bmj.325.7359.314
28. O'Doherty L, Hegarty K, Ramsay J, Davidson LL, Feder G, Taft A. Screening women for intimate partner violence in healthcare settings. *Cochrane Database Syst Rev*. 2015(7):CD007007
29. Wathen CN, MacGregor JCD, MacMillan HL. *Research Brief: Identifying and Responding to Intimate Partner Violence Against Women*. London, ON: PreVAiL Research Network; 2016. http://prevail.wp.fims.uwo.ca/wp-content/uploads/sites/10/2018/01/PreVAiL-CE-IPV-Research-Brief-2016.pdf. Accessed December 5, 2018.
30. Shildrick M. *Embodying the Monster: Encounters with the Vulnerable Self*. Thousand Oaks, CA: SAGE; 2002.
31. Kristeva J. *Powers of Horror: An Essay on Abjection*. New York: Columbia University Press; 1982.
32. Sontag S. *Regarding the Pain of Others*. New York: Picador; 2003.
33. Zalewski M, Runyan AS. "Unthinking" sexual violence in a neoliberal era of spectacular terror. *Crit Stud Terror*. 2015;8(3):439–455. doi:10.1080/17539153.2015.1094253
34. Domino M, Morrissey JP, Nadlicki-Patterson T, Chung S. Service costs for women with co-occurring disorders and trauma. *J Subst Abuse Treat*. 2005;28(2):135–143. doi: 10.1016/j.jsat.2004.08.011

35. Varcoe C, Wathen CN, Ford-Gilboe M, Smye V, Browne AJ. *VEGA Briefing Note on Trauma- and Violence-Informed Care*. 2016. http://newvega.fims.uwo.ca/wp-content/uploads/sites/3/2016/10/VEGA-TVIC-Briefing-Note-2016.pdf. Accessed December 5, 2018.
36. Ponic P, Varcoe C, Smutylo T. Trauma- (and Violence-) Informed Approaches to Supporting Victims of Violence: Policy and Practice Considerations. Department of Justice, *Victims of Crime Research Digest*; 2016. https://www.justice.gc.ca/eng/rp-pr/cj-jp/victim/rd9-rr9/p2.html. Accessed December 5, 2018.
37. Sherwin S, Feminist Health Care Ethics Research Network. *The Politics of Women's Health: Exploring Agency and Autonomy*. Philadelphia, PA: Temple University Press; 1998.
38. World Health Organization. *Health Care for Women Subjected to Intimate Partner Violence or Sexual Violence: A Clinical Handbook*. Geneva: World Health Organization; 2014. https://www.who.int/reproductivehealth/publications/violence/vaw-clinical-handbook/en/. Accessed December 5, 2018.
39. World Health Organization. *Responding to Intimate Partner Violence and Sexual Violence Against Women: WHO Clinical and Policy Guidelines*. Geneva: World Health Organization; 2013. https://www.who.int/reproductivehealth/publications/violence/9789241548595/en/. Accessed December 5, 2018.

8 SEX WORK, ETHICS, AND HEALTHCARE

Victoria Bungay and Lauren Casey

Introduction

Historically, healthcare for women engaged in commercial sex work—defined as adult consensual commercial exchange of sexual services for money or other resources—has been overly informed by a narrow set of assumptions and stereotypes concerning the nature of sex work, reasons for entry, and the associated health "risks."[1,2] The emphasis on these narrow misconceptions has resulted in the range of female sex workers' healthcare needs being largely ignored while many rather basic questions remain unanswered, including how sex work is shaped by gender, income, and education.[2] Beginning in the 1980s and throughout the 1990s, for instance, researchers began to identify primary health risks they associated with sex work, including substance misuse, trauma/violence, and exposure to the human immunodeficiency virus (HIV) and other sexually transmitted infections (STIs).[3] With the rise of intervention-oriented research, sex workers were redefined as health risks within public health circles and as victims of sexual violence and childhood trauma within some feminist and social welfare circles. These depictions of sex work led to similarly crude health interventions, which many, especially sex work advocates, argued were aimed at social control. These crude interventions included unethical practices ranging from mandatory drug or disease testing[4] to moral condemnation[5] and outright refusal of treatment.[6,7] Some have additionally observed that these discriminatory practices are racialized and classed and thus magnified when the sex worker comes from a racial minority, is an immigrant, is transgendered, is using illicit substances, or is living in poverty.[7–10]

Perhaps one of the most recognized health concerns many health scholars argue are unique to sex workers is exposure to HIV and other STIs. Many studies situating sex work and HIV, however, have emerged from lower-income nations in Africa[11] and India,[12] where the spread of HIV is rampant and associated with inequities in essential determinants of health, including poverty and gender-based violence.

In Canada, sex work has been blamed for being a major contributor to these illnesses.[3,13] However, recent evidence illustrates that sex work accounts for limited HIV infections in Canada and many other industrialized nations and that rates of infection among some female sex workers may be well below the national average.[14-16] Additionally, HIV research among sex workers in Canada has tended to emphasize women working in street-level marketplaces where high rates of poverty, violence, housing instability, cocaine injection, heroin injection, and crack cocaine use occur.[17,18] The emphasis on sex work and HIV obscures the vulnerable and chaotic nature of women's lives in these situations and perpetuates assumptions about sex workers as disease vectors. The conflation of sex work and risk for infection also contributes directly to a disproportionate amount of attention and resources directed toward infectious disease prevention and management and inadequate healthcare and health policies to address the broader determinants of health that ultimately determine their vulnerability to infection and overall health outcomes.

Use of drugs and alcohol is an additional health concern emphasized in some scholarship concerned with health and healthcare among sex workers. Much of the research literature suggests either that sex workers use substances to cope with having to "prostitute" themselves or that they were using substances prior to entering the sex industry and turned to sex work in order to support their addiction.[19,20] The image created by these studies is of an inseparable link between sex work and substance use, usually explained through a history of victimization.[21] However, the co-trajectories of substance misuse and sex work are much more complex than the literature indicates and, as such, depend on a number of other dynamics, such as the structural conditions underlying sex work and substance use and significant contextual factors of race, gender, and class. For example, other research indicates that only a minority of persons in the sex industry report substance dependence; like other Canadians, they likely use substances for a variety of reasons, including recreational purposes[21] and the inability to receive effective health services to address mental health and/or chronic pain issues.[7]

Physical violence and trauma are health concerns several scholars argue are unique to sex workers, often positioning sex work as inherently violent.[17,22-25]

Others have illustrated, however, that the interrelationships between violence and sex work are embedded in the broader social relations of gender-based violence and intersecting forms of racism, classism, and heterosexism. Violence, for example, comes in all forms, including harassment from the police, the community, and/or clients.[26-28] One recent study suggested that transgender sex workers experience the most violence, such as episodes of gay bashing, violent attacks, and verbal and physical harassment from male pedestrians.[29] Violence typically occurs on the street; however, fear of being "found out," losing their children, or being assaulted by clients or members of the community have been identified by sex workers of all genders working in off-street establishments.[27,29-31] Moreover, it is well established that the socio-structural conditions of limited occupational health and safety regulations governing working conditions and client behaviors are significant contributors to violence against sex workers versus being engaged in sex work per se.[27,30,31]

Due to their stigmatization and discrimination, sex workers have become scapegoats caught in the fire of competing discourses, and this has significant consequence for ethical healthcare programs and practices. Weitzer, for example, argues that there is a growing moral panic over prostitution, fueled by the claims about drug addiction, the spread of HIV, and violence experienced by sex workers, furthering the agendas of abolitionists.[31] Accordingly, minimal attention has been paid to occupational health and safety to promote sex workers' health.[27] The media largely favor the abolitionist position in their portrayal of the sex industry, in part because it resonates with dominant moral values concerning women's sexuality and moral order.[3] Thus, the public understanding of the sex industry overplays portrayals of sex workers as female victims or villains, depending on whether one identifies more strongly with the criminological or victim-of-abuse rhetoric.[3] Stigmas about the sex industry contain notions of causality that do not take into account broader social processes and thus give rise to the impression that participation in sex work is a cause of an array of social ills and health risks.[32-37]

There are at least two types of stigmas that are especially relevant to the study of health and healthcare among sex workers. The first is disease- and illness-associated stigma (individuals are stigmatized because they have contracted an illness or disease or have been diagnosed with a health-related disorder that is associated with a particular set of negative attributes), and the second is group-associated stigma (discrimination based on such personal attributes as race, ethnicity, sex, gender, sexual orientation, and occupation).[34] Group-associated stigma translates into poor health outcomes due to stigmatized persons' inability to access social resources, causing many to see themselves from the negative perception of the community. This, in turn, results in lower self-esteem, demoralization, poor perceived quality of life, fear of being judged negatively, social withdrawal, and low expectations and few demands on services such as healthcare, law enforcement, and employment rights and benefits.[3,29,32-39] In turn, stigmatized persons may experience depression or other mental health problems, diminished social support networks, unstable housing, stress, and engaging in behaviors that could further compromise their health or the health of others (e.g., illicit substance use, smoking, unsafe sex, alcohol consumption).[9,26,28,40-44] The literature also suggests that individuals use various managing, coping, and resistance strategies to try to counteract the negative impacts of stigma, although these have been less well investigated.[32,43,55]

In this chapter we examine female sex workers' experiences of stigma and discrimination within the context of their health and engagement with the healthcare system. We specifically discuss how stigma and discrimination and ideologies of deviance underpin healthcare service programming and clinical encounters among this population. These issues are further nuanced in an analysis that illustrates the consequential and significant ethical concerns for clinicians and health service programming and the devastating effects for women's health, their rights to healthcare, and their opportunities to be active agents in decisions affecting their care.

Methods

Our findings are based on a subset of data from a larger project carried out between 2012 and 2016 examining the interrelationships between working conditions and the health and safety of people engaged in the indoor sex industry. The data drew from in-depth interviews with 51 women (including 8 who identified as trans persons) ranging 20 to 60 years of age who had been involved in sex work between 1 and 30 years. Many women had worked both in the street marketplace and indoor settings, including escort agencies, massage parlors, and their homes. Interviews began with asking women for a general description of their working conditions and consisted of probes to examine specific concerns relating to their health and safety, including their experiences with healthcare. A multi-method recruitment strategy situated within our western Canadian city locale was used. Our purposeful sampling strategies included posting online banner advertisements and posters in physical and web-based locations derived from ethnographic mapping of diverse sex work settings. We also worked with local sex work advocacy and support organizations to distribute posters.[45] Women were eligible to participate if they were 19 years of age or older and had engaged in sexual service provision for money or other resources in the previous 6 months. The University of British Columbia's Research Ethics Board provided ethics approval for the project and consent was obtained verbally. Data were transcribed verbatim and checked for accuracy, and identifying information such as names, places, and agencies was removed before entering the data into NVivo™ 10.0 software package for qualitative data management to facilitate analysis.

Initial coding by the authors identified general thematic codes noting the types of health concerns women described and their experiences of, and perspectives about, healthcare encounters. As coding progressed, we refined the codes to reflect a more theoretical approach to examine how women's shared and differing experiences in health and healthcare were situated within relations of power that perpetuated stigma and oppression and contributed to significant ethical issues in access to and receipt of healthcare. To aid in coding women's experiences within the realm of healthcare ethics and relations of power, we drew from the critical perspectives of Collins[46] and Crenshaw,[47] who argued that relations of power are significant factors of all social organizations that regularly operate across various social locations (e.g., age, class, race, gender, occupation) to justify and sustain inequities within society. We specifically employed a framework known as the matrix of domination that encompasses both macro and micro social relations that are historically and socially specific. The hegemonic domain incorporates dominant ideologies (bodies of ideas, assumptions, and beliefs) that represent the interests of a particular social group. The structural domain refers to the organization of social institutions such as healthcare. The disciplinary domain represents the policies and practices of social institutions, and the interpersonal domain comprises people's social interactions and personal relationships.[46] By examining the interrelationships between stigma and women's experiences of access to and receipt of healthcare within a framework of power, we found that stigmatizing ideologies of deviance contributed to significant oversight in ethical healthcare encounters and health service programming. To help illustrate the complex interplay between healthcare ethics and female sex workers' access to and receipt of healthcare, we organized the findings into two overarching analytic categories: (1) stigma, disrespect, and healthcare and (2) inadequate resources. To situate these findings, we first we present an overview of women's general health.

Results

The participants experienced a range of acute and chronic health concerns throughout their lives, although the frequency and severity were not experienced equally. Depression, anxiety, and posttraumatic stress disorder were the most common health concerns, with fewer women identifying problematic substance use, degenerative bone disease, and diabetes as significant issues. Many women were taking prescribed antidepressant and antianxiety medications. All participants were proactive in promoting their health, and many spoke eloquently of the interrelationship between stigma, mental health, and their overall well-being. Sexual health was identified as a key priority in their health promotion, and the prevention of STIs was an active part of their everyday work activities. Most participants reported never having had an STI and engaged in STI testing between two and six times per year. As one participant noted, "I've never had any STDs [sexually transmitted diseases], but I do get tested often to be sure. So I wouldn't say that STDs are the biggest health concerns for us."

Stigma, Disrespect, and Healthcare

Women accessed healthcare for a variety of reasons, some that had very little to do with sex work and some that they considered an essential aspect of promoting and protecting their health in the context of their work. Regardless of the reason, ensuring that they were not "outed"—having their sex work involvement made known to others—was paramount to receiving timely and effective care. Once outed, the impacts of stigma and discrimination were devastating. In some instances, women's capacities and rights as active agents in decision making about their healthcare were completely negated, illustrating substantial ethical practice concerns. Ideologies of deviance that infantilize women engaged in sex work as irresponsible and incapable of taking care of themselves were apparent within these descriptions. Women told numerous stories of being excluded from discussions by care providers despite being present when the providers were talking. They were often completely ignored when someone such as a husband or boyfriend was present, as one woman noted: "Oh, like, doctors and nurses, it's crazy. Especially if you are single and don't have a husband or something like that. They would rather speak to someone in authority—well, someone who has authority over you, not just you."

For women engaged in sex work who were experiencing significant mental health and addiction issues, the ethical issues of disrespect and inappropriate treatment were severe. Women talked openly about having their "basic humanity" ignored and talked about emergency departments as places "to be avoided at all costs." In the following excerpt, a 60-year-old woman discussed her treatment in an emergency department following an assault that occurred while she was working. Stigma and discrimination negatively affected her care and the entire encounter was re-traumatizing. The healthcare providers' actions limited opportunities for the collection of evidence necessary for successful prosecution of her assailant and instead negated that an actual assault had occurred. She was made to feel that she deserved what happened as a consequence of her actions (i.e., sex work). Ultimately, this woman, like many of our participants, chose to avoid the healthcare system, thereby denying women's equal opportunity for care afforded to most Canadians.

> That hospital—so I don't go back. They are very judgmental to women. Once they found out my age group and that I was a working girl—whoa! did they treat me like shit! They didn't even do a rape kit, and that is why I went there. The ambulance people were nice, though. And when they brought me in, she [the emergency medical technician] said, "You take good care of this lady. She is a nice lady." But when she left, boy, things just changed. They thought, "She's just another street person." And then I was told I need to leave and I said, "Do you think maybe you can get a wheelchair for me, 'cause I can barely walk?" And the nurse said, "What, do you want me to walk all the way down there and a bring a wheelchair back for you? Why don't you just walk yourself?" It's all stigma, you know—my age group, a working girl, being raped by a date, and that I use drugs.

Ideologies of risk associated with disease transmission also contributed to significant ethical challenges during clinical encounters. Women repeated numerous stories of having their health concerns denied by a care provider once they were outed, either through communications noted in their medical records or if they chose to tell their care provider. Once outed, most care providers appeared to focus solely on STI testing, reinforcing the group stigma experienced by the participants and the paternalism inherent in their care. Consequently, women's reasons for attending to care were discounted, leaving them with unmet healthcare needs. Women spoke with feeling about the myths and stereotypes about sex work and described healthcare providers as "incredibly ignorant" about sex work. As one woman noted:

> And all this stuff about STIs, that's another thing that pisses me off. There is all this talk [in healthcare] about sex workers being STI-ridden, but sex workers are more safety-conscious that anyone else. Like, how many civilians use condoms for blow jobs? They [non–sex workers] are way less careful. When I am working I get tested every 2 months and I never had an infection.

Accordingly, most participants identified an urgent need for healthcare providers to learn about sex work, with specific recommendations that they work with local sex work advocacy organizations to learn about the diversity of the industry. They explicitly recommended that care providers become knowledgeable about the range of health issues that women can experience and the complexity of circumstances associated with women's health. They argued that healthcare providers must understand that many of the health issues women face are usually not limited to sex work but can be influenced by inequities associated with racism, poverty, ageism, education level, immigration status, and the amount of control they have over their work activities. Ultimately, they noted that being respectful and nonjudgmental was critical. As one woman said, "Don't judge. It could be your daughter one day needing services."

Although the actual incidence of STIs among the participants was low, testing was among the most frequent reasons for engaging in healthcare. Women discussed many positive clinical encounters in attending for sexual healthcare. These positive encounters, however, were something that developed over time as women sought out nonjudgmental places to access these services. It often took women years of experiencing derogatory interactions with clinicians to find a safe place to attend for regular testing. Two sexual health clinics within the city were considered particularly good. Words such as "ethical," "nonjudgmental," "warm," and "respectful" were used to describe the care providers in these settings. The sense of safety supported women to share that they were engaged in sex work, and they found that the physicians and nurses working in these sites were an important resource for referral to seek care for other health concerns, including, for instance, mental health.

Stigma, mental health, and their interrelationships were also evident in all of the women's discussions. As noted earlier, the interactional experience of stigma frequently has significant and negative effects for people's mental health. Sallman posits that stigma normalizes violence against sex workers at a structural level so much so that it becomes embedded in systems and practices, including the larger healthcare system.[48] These concerns were evident in the experiences of the participants. The fear of being outed and the unethical treatment they received by healthcare providers, including the relentless discrediting of their knowledge and expertise about their health and wellness, were incredibly stressful. Women identified mental health problems as the primary health concern facing sex workers and spoke to the complexity of the array of factors that contributed to stress, anxiety, and depression. Isolation due to fear of being outed was significant, and this isolation left people without important social supports. Hiding their identities from friends, family, and care providers exacerbated feelings of loneliness as they felt an inability to be authentic about what was happening in their lives.

As with other health concerns, women expressed that the "shaming and blaming" they experienced when seeking care for their mental health just exacerbated the problem. It seemed that being engaged in sex work became the identifying factor in their care, leaving women with few opportunities to engage in a more holistic approach to addressing their mental health concerns: "If you are feeling stressed out or anxious or depressed and you go to a counselor and then you say, 'I'm a sex worker,' they're probably going to think it's because you are a sex worker that you have all of these issues, when actually it's not that simple."

Women discussed at length the insufficient availability of publicly funded mental health services, noting that these issues were exacerbated by their inability to pay for private services. Moreover, the workers identified their underlying assumptions that the negation of sex workers' humanity at structural levels of healthcare also contributed to this gap:

> You know, government healthcare providers ... they figure if someone chooses to go into the [sex] industry, well, then they are no longer human beings and they shouldn't then be treated as such because they chose to do this ... and if you reveal that piece of information about yourself—people don't realize how traumatic that is for the person revealing, because a lot of time it is flipped against you. And you just know you're going to be judged ... and when you don't have a network of support or counseling that makes you feel legitimate, you feel like, "What's the point [of accessing services]?" And then the people who could probably help, well, they charge me money and I can't afford to pay. But, hey, put your face on national TV and be humiliated, *that*

will pay. But the health system, they don't want to really help, and it's the stigma attached to sex work.

Some women did have what they described as "ethical" encounters with mental health services—a term used to describe respectful and effective receipt of services. Unfortunately, addressing the impact of the previous and ongoing derogatory interactions with other care providers was part of the therapy they received to promote their mental health: "I've suffered depression all my life, and when I go to my doctor's office, the nurse there just made me feel really ashamed. But it took some really good people, some counselors, to show me that I wasn't a bad person or I wasn't doing something totally wrong."

Resource Access and Allocation

Although women did benefit from some excellent resources, there were many barriers to resource access and allocation that illustrated inequitable distribution of services and resources necessary to meet women's health needs. Unfortunately, the primary care clinics that many women used to access STI testing services were not accessible to all women. Women who were relatively new to Canada, who did not speak English fluently, and who worked in the city's massage parlor industry were often at a loss for where to attend for care.

Recent health service cuts included the discontinuation of a nurse outreach program. As part of this program, nurses visited women in their work settings to offer basic primary care services, including STI testing, vaccination, health education, and referrals for other health services, and the loss of these nurses exacerbated many health concerns.[2,10] The nurses were replaced by an online testing system that was completely inaccessible to women as it was described as not addressing the unique needs of sex workers, nor did women feel safe sharing personal information online. The loss of these healthcare services was a further issue for women new to the industry, many of whom begin working in a managed setting such as a massage parlor, as outreach nurses were described as helping women learn about sexual health and condom negotiation with their clients, along with a myriad of other health-promoting practices. Recent estimates indicate that there are over 60 sex work agencies operating in the city of Vancouver similar to those the participants described.[45] The number of women per agency ranges from 4 to 10; thus, the loss of outreach nurses to these settings has been significant.

Sex work advocacy organizations have noted the impact of the loss of these services and in recent forums discussed that although the nurses provided excellent care, the healthcare system has failed to take the health of sex workers seriously, as evidenced by their removal as an outreach service.[2] They noted that the low STI rates were seen as a reason to discontinue this service; thus, they described health services as not meeting women's needs but rather providing services they perceived as protecting the public from sex workers.[2] Women reinforced this argument by stating explicitly that the stigma and resulting devaluing of sex workers worthy of healthcare was the main reason for losing this program. They went further to argue that there are no services that specifically speak to the myriad of issues women face or that are specific to mental health. They discussed the need for greater services, as evidenced in the following quotation:

> There needs to be a resource network. If someone is not ready to exit the industry and they are trying to figure out how to conduct their business safely, there should be a hotline. There should be some resource that we can reach out to where we can ask questions . . . that is what would help our mental health.

Women also spoke to stereotypic assumptions within health service programming that all sex work occurred in a street-based marketplace, despite estimates that over 80% of the North American industry operates indoors.[31,49] Women recognized that services for women working at street level were necessary, particularly given their complex needs and the multiple intersecting factors such as poverty, violence, and unstable housing that were affecting their health. These services did not necessarily fit the unique needs of women in indoor settings, however:

> A lot of the services are for survival sex workers on the streets, and even though I was given the contact information of the [not-for-profit sex workers' organization], I didn't feel like I would be understood. I kind of felt like, you know, they would say, "What the fuck are you complaining about?" I didn't feel like the services were there for someone like me and I didn't feel I deserved them. There are no services for anybody working from home, and services are really necessary for us because the isolation can get so bad. When you are working from home in such an emotionally exhausting setting and such a stigmatized job—it's just hard.

Ultimately, the participants highlighted that the current publicly available services to promote and protect the health of sex workers are significantly under-resourced. What does exist continues to have limited focus in terms of the groups of sex workers served and the scope of services available.

Discussion

The stigma and discrimination experienced by women engaged in sex work raise important ethical concerns for the organization and delivery of health services, including women's experiences in healthcare encounters. Most of what is known about female sex workers' experiences of healthcare in Canada has been limited to access to sexual health services, including testing and treatment for STIs and HIV. Minimal attention has been paid to the ethical context of women's experiences of healthcare or the relations of power in which these encounters are situated. Consequently, there are significant gaps in our understandings of how best to address stigma and its devastating effects for women's health, including their access to and receipt of ethical and effective care. Investigation into the interrelationships between sex work, stigma, discrimination, and healthcare ethics is a critical first step to address this knowledge gap and to identify essential strategies to improve the organization and delivery of health services.

In this chapter we explored a group of Canadian sex workers' experiences of engaging with the healthcare system to identify how stigma and discrimination operated within macro and micro social relations to influence ethical healthcare within both the organization and receipt of health services. Ideologies of sex workers as "disease vectors" for STIs and HIV intersected with care provider practices that infantilized women. Subsequently, women were regularly denied the opportunity to be active agents in their healthcare, a situation that increased the likelihood of unmet healthcare needs, produced significant humiliation and degradation, and reflected a health system that is largely unresponsive to the actual needs of many women working in the Canadian sex industry.

Our findings also reinforce other research that group- and disease-associated stigma intersect to contribute to significant ethical issues in healthcare for women engaged in sex work.[3,32,34,37] An ethical issue of particular concern was unmet mental health needs. As noted in our results and those of other scholars concerned with addressing the negative effects of stigma for sex workers, mental health issues exacerbated by interrelationships between isolation, stigma, discrimination, and women's previous life experiences are a major concern for sex workers in Canada and many other industrialized nations.[32–44] However, all of the participants in this study noted a dearth of accessible and affordable mental health care. The issue of affordable mental health care is indeed an ethical one. In Canada, it is estimated that 20% of the population will experience a mental health issue at some time their life, yet the lack of public funding for mental health remains a barrier to care.[50] Additionally, women continue to be overrepresented among the economically disadvantaged, a situation shared among many female sex workers that renders them less likely to afford private mental health services.[51] When sex workers do access care, it appears that the stigma and related misconceptions position sex work as a woman's identity versus a source of income. The complexity of women's mental health and the stress experienced among a myriad of life experiences are overlooked, and factors that contribute to poor mental health, such as limited social support, social withdrawal, and the stress associated with being stigmatized, remain.[9,28,40,41] These oversights perpetuate power dynamics and oppression of women, which renders both the organization and delivery of services unethical and limits the opportunities for optimal mental wellness.[52]

Disease- and illness-associated stigma further played out in the context of how sex workers were positioned in healthcare more generally. As noted in the introduction, there has been an overemphasis on STI and HIV prevention among female sex workers in Canada, contributing to a perception of these women as vectors of disease.[6,10,31] Our findings illustrated the impact of a limited focus within the health system on sexual health for both services and women's healthcare encounters. Loss of services that considered the range of the social determinants of health (e.g., access to primary services) and health issues (e.g., pregnancy, violence) were reported in settings with low STI rates among workers, the consequences of which could have significant impacts for violence prevention and access to care for young and immigrant sex workers in our locale.

Recommendations to Enhance Ethical Care

This study's findings suggest the need for a series of highly actionable recommendations to reduce stigma and discrimination and promote ethical healthcare:

1. The proper conceptualization of sex work is necessary so that it is understood as a viable economic activity versus a purely sexual activity.[1,53,54]

Positioning sex work as work among adults who engage in the consensual exchange of an array of sexual services for money can support effective occupational health and safety programming.[1] Consequently, the range of health issues and contributing factors that sex workers may experience can become part of publicly funded health services.

2. Healthcare providers and decision makers involved in health service programming must heed the global call by sex work advocacy and support organizations that the health system move beyond "thinking that STI treatment is the primary goal of health care for sex workers."[53(p1)] However, shifting the ideological underpinnings of sex work as deviant is critical to fully develop an ethical healthcare system and providers' practices when providing care to sex workers.[10,57] Education to care providers to address misconceptions is essential and, as has been shown elsewhere, can serve as an effective means of enhancing ethical care encounters, particularly when led by sex worker organizations and their healthcare partners.[10,56,57] Moreover, health policy and programming development are also more effective when informed by the actual knowledge and expertise of the diversity of sex workers whom these policies and programs are intended to serve.[10,32,53,56]

3. The blatant paternalism in health policy and provider practices must change to a more critical healthcare ethic that seeks to limit gender-based power dynamics, oppression, and diminished opportunities for sex workers to be active agents in both program design and their actual healthcare.

Conclusion

This study, to our knowledge, is one of the few that explores the intersections between healthcare, ethics, stigma, and discrimination among female sex workers in a Canadian context. However, there are limitations to the study. The sample is not representative of the population of sex workers in our locale and may have been biased through nonparticipation of those who did not wish to participate. Nevertheless, this chapter does contribute to increasing knowledge about how sex workers experience healthcare and the range of devastating effects that paternalism, oppression, and misconceptions can have for women's health. This information can inform future health programming and provide important insights to healthcare providers who aim to achieve a more ethical health care encounter with the women to whom they provide care.

References

1. Manning E, Bungay V. "Business before pleasure": the golden rule of sex work, payment schedules and gendered experiences of violence. *Cult Health Sex*. 2017;19:338–351. doi:10.1080/13691058.2016.1219767.
2. SPACES Team. Recommendations from the off-street sex industry in Vancouver. https://open.library.ubc.ca/cIRcle/collections/facultyresearchandpublications/52383/items/1.0340040. Published 2016. Accessed March 24, 2018.
3. Jackson L, Bennett C, Sowinski B. Stress in the sex trade and beyond: women working in the sex trade talk about the emotional stressors in their working and home lives. *Crit Public Health*. 2007;17:257–271.
4. Kelly P. *Lydia's Open Door: Inside Mexico's Most Modern Brothel*. Berkeley, CA: University of California Press; 2008.
5. Sanders T, Campbell R. Designing out vulnerability, building in respect: violence, safety and sex work policy. *Br J Sociol*. 2007;58:1–19.
6. Shaver F. Sex work research: methodological and ethical challenges. *J Interpers Viol*. 2005;20:296–319.
7. Bungay V. Health care among street-involved women: the perpetuation of health inequity. *Qual Health Res*. 2013;23:1016–1026.
8. Armstrong P. Health, social policy, social economics and the voluntary sector. In: Raphael D, ed. *Social Determinants of Health: Canadian Perspectives*. 1st ed. Toronto: Canadian Scholars' Press; 2004:331–344.
9. Benoit C, Shumka L. *Gendering the Health Determinants Framework: Why Girls' and Women's Health Matters*. Vancouver: Women's Health Research Network. http://www.cwhn.ca/en/node/43355 Published 2009. Accessed March 24, 2018.
10. Bungay V, Kolar K, Thindal S, Remple V, Johnston C, Ogilvie G. Community-based HIV and STI prevention with women working in indoor sex markets. *Health Promot Pract*. 2013;14:247–255. doi: 10.1177/1524839912447189
11. Ngugi E, Benoit C, Hallgrimsdottir H, Jansson M, Roth EA. Partners and clients of female sex workers in an informal urban settlement in Nairobi, Kenya. *Cult Health Sex*. 2012;14:17–30.
12. Basu A. HIV/AIDS and subaltern autonomous rationality: a call to recenter health communication in marginalized sex worker spaces. *Commun Monogr*. 2011;78:391–408.
13. Spittal P, Bruneau J, Craib K, et al. Surviving the sex trade: a comparison of HIV risk behaviours among street-involved women in two Canadian cities who inject drugs. *AIDS Care*. 2003;15:187–195.
14. Strathdee SA, Crago AL, Butler J, Bekker LG, Beyrer C. Dispelling myths about sex workers and HIV. *Lancet*. 2015;385:4–7.
15. Pruiss-Ustun A, Wolf J, Driscoll T, et al. HIV due to female sex work: regional and global estimates. *PLoS One*. 2013;8(5): e63476. https://doi.org/10.1371/journal.pone.0063476. Published May 23, 2013. Accessed March 24, 2018.

16. Bungay V, Halpin P, Halpin M, Johnston C, Patrick D. Violence in the massage parlour industry: experiences of Canadian-born and immigrant women. *Health Care Women Int*. 2012;33:262–284. doi:10.1080/07399332.2011.
17. Shannon K, Csete P. Violence, condom negotiation, and HIV/STI risk among sex workers. *JAMA*. 2010;304:573–574.
18. Shannon K, Bright V, Duddy J, Tyndall M. Access and utilization of HIV treatment and services among women sex workers in Vancouver's downtown eastside. *J Urban Health*. 2005;82:488–497.
19. Farley M. "Bad for the body, bad for the heart": prostitution harms women even if legalized or decriminalized. *Violence Against Women*. 2004;10(10):1087–1125.
20. Inciardi J, Lockwood D, Pottinger A. *Women and Crack Cocaine*. New York, NY: Macmillan; 1993.
21. Lowman J. Street prostitutes in Canada: an evaluation of the Brannigan-Fleischman opportunity model. *Can J Law Soc*. 1991;6:137–164.
22. Benoit CM. *Team Grant on Contexts of Vulnerabilities, Resiliencies and Care Among People in the Sex Industry*. Ottawa: Canadian Institutes of Health Research; 2012.
23. Kurtz S, Surrat H, Inciardi J, et al. Sex work and "date" violence. *Violence Against Women*. 2004;10:357–385.
24. Raphael J, Shapiro D. Violence in indoor and outdoor prostitution venues. *Violence Against Women*. 2004;10:126–139.
25. Rekart M. Sex-work harm reduction. *Lancet*. 2005;366: 2123–2134.
26. Lewis J, Maticka-Tyndale E, Shaver F, Schreamm H. Managing risk and safety on the job. *J Psychol Human Sex*. 2005;17:146–167.
27. Bungay V, Guta A. Strategies and challenges in preventing violence against Canadian indoor sex workers. *Am J Public Health*. 2018;108:393–398. doi:10.2105/AJPH.2017.304241.
28. Wong W, Holroyd E, Bingham A. Stigma and sex work from the perspective of female sex workers in Hong Kong. *Sociol Health Illn*. 2011;33:50–65.
29. Shaver F, Lewis J, Maticka-Tyndale E. Rising to the challenge: addressing the concerns of people working in the sex industry. *Can Rev Sociol*. 2011;48(1):47–66.
30. Bungay V, Halpin P, Halpin M, Johnston C, Patrick D. Violence in the massage parlour industry: experiences of Canadian-born and immigrant women. *Health Care Women Int*. 2012;33:262–284. doi:10.1080/07399332.2011.
31. Weitzer R. *Legalizing Prostitution: From Illicit Vice to Lawful Business*. New York, NY: NYU Press; 2012.
32. Bowen R, Bungay V. Taint: an examination of the lived experiences of stigma and its lingering effects for eight sex industry experts. *Cult Health Sex*. 2016;18:184–197. doi:10.1080/13691058.2015.1072875.
33. Phillips R, Benoit C. Social determinants of health care access among sex industry workers in Canada. *Res Sociol Health Care*. 2005;23:79–104.
34. Benoit C, Shumka L, Vallance K. *Research Brief 1: Violence as a Determinant of Girls' and Women's Health*. Vancouver: Women's Health Research Network; 2010.

35. Coburn D. Beyond the income inequality hypothesis: class, neo-liberalism, and health inequalities. *Soc Sci Med.* 2004;58:41–56.
36. Camp DL, Finlay WML, Lyons E. Is low self-esteem an inevitable consequence of stigma? An example from women with chronic mental health problems. *Soc Sci Med.* 2002;55:823–834.
37. Link B, Phelan J. Stigma and its public health implications. *Lancet.* 2006;367:528–529.
38. Schulze B, Angermeyer M. Subjective experiences of stigma: a focus group study of schizophrenic patients, their relatives and mental health professionals. *Soc Sci Med.* 2003;56:299–312.
39. Miller C, Kaiser C. A theoretical perspective on coping with stigma. *J Soc Issues.* 2001;57:73–92.
40. Stuber J, Meyer I, Link B. Stigma, prejudice, discrimination and health. *Soc Sci Med.* 2008;67:351–357.
41. Carlarne J. Multi-context engaged learning and ethnographic fieldwork: some notes from the middle of the edge. *Int J Social Res Methodol.* 2011;14(2):135–152.
42. Gibson E, Exner H, Stone R, Lindquis J, Cowen L, Roth EA. A mixed methods approach to delineating and understanding injection practices among clientele of a Victoria, British Columbia, needle exchange program. *Drug Alcohol Rev.* 2011;30:360–365.
43. Frost DM. Social stigma and its consequences for the socially stigmatized. *Social Personal Psychol Compass.* 2011;5:824–839.
44. Lynch J. Income inequality and mortality: importance to health of individual income, psychosocial environment, or material conditions. *BMJ.* 2000;320(7243):1200–1204.
45. Bungay V, Oliffe J, Atchison C. Addressing underrepresentation in sex work research: reflections on designing a purposeful sampling strategy. *Qual Health Res.* 2016;26(7):966–978. doi:10.1177/1049732315613042.
46. Collins PH. *Black Feminist Thought: Knowledge, Consciousness, and the Politics of Empowerment.* New York, NY: Routledge; 2000.
47. Crenshaw K. Mapping the margins: intersectionality, identity politics, and violence against women of color. *Stanford Law Rev.* 1991;43:1241–1299.
48. Sallman J. Living with stigma: women's experiences of prostitution and substance use. *Affilia.* 2010;25:146–159.
49. Hanger MP, Maloney J. *The Challenge of Change: A Study of Canada's Criminal Prostitution.* Report of the Standing Committee on Justice and Human Rights. http://www.ourcommons.ca/DocumentViewer/en/39-1/JUST/report-6. Published 2006. Accessed March 24, 2018.
50. CMHA fact sheet: access to services. https://cmha.ca/documents/access-to-services-2. Accessed March 24, 2018.
51. CMHA fact sheet: women and work. https://cmha.ca/documents/women-and-work. Accessed March 24, 2018.

52. Rogers WA. Feminism and public health ethics. *J Med Ethics*. 2006;32:351–354. doi:10.1136/jme2005.013466.
53. Wolffers I. Sex workers' health, HIV/AIDS, ethical issues in care and research. *Res Sex Work*. 2004;7:1–2.
54. Benoit C, Ouellet N, Jansson M, Magnus S, Smith M. Would you think about doing sex for money? Structure and agency in deciding to sell sex in Canada. *Work Employ Soc*. 2017:1–17. doi:10.1177/0950017016679331.
55. Koken J. Independent female escorts' strategies for coping with sex work–related stigma. *Sex Cult*. 2012;16(3):209–229.
56. World Health Organization, United Nations Population Fund, Joint United Nations Programme on HIV/AIDS, Global Network of Sex Work Projects, The World Bank. Addressing violence against sex workers. In: *Implementing Comprehensive HIV/STI Programmes with Sex Workers: Practical Approaches from Collaborative Interventions*. Geneva: World Health Organization; 2013:19–38.
57. Amnesty International. Amnesty International policy on state obligations to respect, protect and fulfil the human rights of sex workers. https://www.amnesty.org/en/documents/pol30/4062/2016/en/. Published May 26, 2016. Accessed March 24, 2018.

9 PRIMARY HEALTHCARE FOR QUEER WOMEN AND TRANS PEOPLE

CONFRONTING HETERONORMATIVITY AND CISNORMATIVITY

Erin Fredericks and Kelly Baker

Healthcare provision for queer women and trans people must be approached with an understanding of the systematic and historical oppression of these patients in the healthcare system. While it is valuable to consider the unique healthcare needs of queer and trans patients because of their differing health behaviors and risks, most healthcare sought by queer women and trans people is for the same reasons heterosexual and cisgender patients seek healthcare. It is important that we attend to the care provision differences that remain for members of this community, even when seeking care for the same health concerns in a publicly funded system. In this chapter, we conceptualize primary healthcare for queer women and trans people as nonspecialized care that requires structural changes to clinic spaces and procedures, updated clinical language to disentangle gender identity from bodies, and critical reflection on the role of provider biases and assumptions in healthcare provision.

The word *normativity* simply refers to the ways in which particular ways of thinking and acting are assumed and maintained in any given situation. *Heteronormativity*, then, refers to ways that heterosexuality is maintained as standard and "normal," with non-heterosexual sexualities deemed "abnormal" and "deviant." *Cisnormativity*, similarly, is the assumption that all bodies are cisgender—that one's gender identity corresponds with one's sex assigned at birth. If healthcare providers are to provide good-quality care to queer women and trans people, they must dismantle the heteronormativity and cisnormativity that shapes all parts of their practice. We draw on social science research to examine the ways in which these institutionalized forms of oppression shape the patient–provider relationship, the clinic space and practices, clinical language, and provider assumptions, and provide guidance about how best to dismantle them through structural and individual change. We anticipate that what we see and conclude through our social science lens aligns with ethical principles and responsibilities of health professionals and service providers. The purpose of this chapter is to support healthcare providers in understanding and challenging heteronormativity and cisnormativity in their practice. To this end, we provide examples of changes healthcare providers can make to improve the inclusiveness of their services. Throughout this chapter we use the fictional story of Heather and her family to encourage deeper understanding of best practice with queer women and trans patients.

Speaking About the Queer and Trans Community

> Heather is a trans woman in a same-gender relationship with her cisgender partner, Jennifer. They have a two-year-old child named Max. Heather came out as trans 6 years ago, but her family still struggles to accept her. Jennifer came out as a lesbian when she was a teenager and has family support. Heather and Jennifer have discussed moving to an urban center to access healthcare at a clinic that specializes in queer and trans healthcare, but Jennifer's family and their friends live in the rural area where they grew up. They'd like to raise their child with their support network. They are preparing to meet a new primary care provider they hope will be able to provide good care to all members of their family, but they're concerned that this healthcare provider won't be knowledgeable about or know how to respectfully speak about queer and trans health concerns.

The word *queer* was formerly a derogatory term that has been reclaimed by the 2SLGBTQIA+[1] community as an umbrella term for those who are not heterosexual. When we use the phrase *queer women*, we refer to women-identifying or feminine non-binary people who identify as queer, pansexual, polysexual, bisexual, lesbian, or another non-heterosexual sexual orientation. These women are not necessarily in a same-gender relationship, and they may or may not engage in same-gender sexual behaviors. While their sexual and romantic behaviors are diverse, queer women are positioned similarly in a healthcare system that presumes heterosexuality.

It is difficult to estimate the percentage of Canadians who identify as queer women. Statistics Canada cites the Canadian Community Health Survey to state that 1.7% of the population aged 18 to 59 identify as gay or lesbian, and 1.3% identify as bisexual, for a total of 3%.[1] In contrast, a well-publicized research study in the United Kingdom suggested that more than half of youth aged 13 to 20 identify as not entirely heterosexual.[2] Measuring the number of queer people is difficult because survey questions often exclude many queer identities; Statistics Canada uses the words *lesbian* and *bisexual* but no other non-heterosexual sexual orientation, and some queer people may be hesitant to identify themselves in surveys.

Transgender ("trans") people are those whose gender identity does not correlate with the sex assigned to them at birth. Past narratives of transgender people suggested that their brain gender did not match their physical bodies. More recent understandings of trans identities call into question the process of assigning sex at birth. These understandings of trans identities suggest that sex assignment before we know a child's felt gender is the source of this perceived mismatch between gender identity and assigned sex. *Cisgender* people are those whose gender identity does correlate with their sex assigned at birth. Trans people may claim a variety of gender identities, including but not limited to agender (without gender), gender non-binary (an umbrella term for gender identities outside the typical binary of woman and man), woman, or man. Trans people may also identify with a gender expression, including but not limited to transfeminine or transmasculine. We have chosen not to limit our discussion to the healthcare needs of trans women or transfeminine people, because all trans people experience gender-based oppression and marginalization. The experiences of trans people are diverse, but they face many similar challenges in a healthcare system in which they are medicalized, marginalized by cisnormativity, denied care, and exoticized. Best estimates suggest that approximately 0.5% of the population, or 1 in 200 people, are transgender.[3]

Queer women and trans people live in all areas of Canada and other countries. Metronormative narratives dominate our understandings of queer and trans people's lives, leading us to believe that most queer and trans people migrate to urban centers after coming out.[4] The marginalization of rural queer and trans stories and the low population in rural areas often leads to the invisibility of rural queer and trans people,[5,6] which may lead rural healthcare providers to assume they do not need to understand how to provide good-quality care to queer and trans patients. As all healthcare providers will treat queer women and trans patients, we argue that all providers must learn how to provide good-quality care to this population.

For the purposes of this chapter, we will be speaking broadly about queer women and trans people. It is also important to note that these identities are not mutually exclusive—a queer woman may also be trans, for example—and that queer and trans experiences vary significantly for those who also experience racism, ableism, classism, and other forms of oppression. Although the healthcare needs of queer women and trans people vary significantly, both of these communities are marginalized in the healthcare system by institutionalized heteronormativity and cisnormativity that shapes all of their interactions with healthcare providers.

Unique Healthcare Needs of Queer Women and Trans Patients

> Heather came out as trans 6 years ago, before she met Jennifer. After coming out, Heather quickly socially transitioned by dressing in feminine clothing and asking friends and family to call her Heather. Her family refused and she was no longer welcome at family events. Soon after socially transitioning she sought access to hormones to medically transition. When Heather asked her physician for help accessing gender-affirming healthcare, he refused to provide a referral and told her she should just accept her sex assigned at birth. At the same time, Heather was fired from her retail position for wearing feminine clothing. Heather found some queer and trans friends at a bar in a nearby town but soon found she was drinking excessively to cope. When a trans friend offered Heather access to her hormones Heather considered taking them, but she was worried about the effects.

Some studies have shown that queer women and trans people face higher risks of suicide, mental illness, and stress-related illness and are less likely to engage in health-promoting behaviors and preventive care.[7-9] Transgender people specifically experience higher rates of drug and alcohol use, infection with human immunodeficiency virus (HIV), and mental illness.[10] It is important to see these healthcare needs and risks as a result of experiences of marginalization, not a result of differing biology. Increased drug use among trans people, for example, has been correlated with social stigma and exclusion.[11]

When working with queer women and trans people, healthcare providers should shift from seeing these patients as high risk-individuals and instead view risk as the result of long-lasting experiences of oppression that have physiologic effects, as well as shaping coping behavior. Although we will not list all of the unique healthcare needs of queer women and trans people, we would like to highlight the importance of a few of them.

Trans people may socially transition through dress, speech, and behavior and medically transition through the use of hormones and surgery. Although our story of Heather describes a linear transition from sex assigned at birth to "opposite" gender identity, not all trans people's transition stories are this straightforward. Transition is different for all trans people and may not follow a linear move from assigned sex at birth to an "opposite" gender identity.[12] Gender identity and expression can change over time for all people, including trans people. It is important that healthcare providers not expect trans people to act or dress in a particular way to "pass" as their gender identity. Trans women, for example, are women because they identify as women, not because they look or act a particular way.

Although not all will undergo medical transition,[12] access to hormonal and surgical gender-affirming care may be life-saving for those trans people who desire it. For trans people who desire medical transition, access to the hormones and/or surgeries they need decreases suicide attempts.[13,14] When prescribed hormonal treatments are not available to trans people, they may turn to non-medical sources to access these treatments.[15] In the TransPulse survey in Ontario, 43% of respondents were using hormones, and of those 25% had obtained hormones from friends or relatives, on the street, from strangers, or from websites.[15] Nonprescribed hormone use is associated with increased use of shared needles and potential side effects. Lack of support from healthcare providers, negative healthcare experiences, and lack of funding are also associated with increased rates of self-performed surgeries by trans people.[15] Supporting access to gender-affirming care for trans patients who desire medical transition is key to increasing safety for this community.

Many discussions of the healthcare needs of queer women and trans patients focus on sexual health. While this is important, providers must be careful not to reduce all queer and trans healthcare needs to sexual healthcare. However, it is worth stating that the sexual health needs of queer women and trans patients should be based on their actual sexual practices, not their sexual orientations or gender identities. To encourage preventive healthcare practices, providers should also make patients aware that all people with cervixes should have access to Pap tests, and all people with prostates, prostate exams.

Although it is very important for healthcare providers to understand the unique healthcare needs of queer women and trans patients, we argue that it is equally important to view the majority of care provided to queer and trans patients as nonspecialized care. That is, most healthcare visits queer women and trans people make will be for the same healthcare concerns for which their heterosexual and cisgender peers seek care. The differences in care provision and needs for queer women and trans people are most often the result of institutionalized heteronormativity and cisnormativity.

Queer and Trans Marginalization: Introducing Heteronormativity and Cisnormativity

> Days before their healthcare appointment with their new primary care provider, Heather and Jennifer start getting nervous. They meet with queer and trans friends and share stories of awkward healthcare appointments. Heather recounts the time a provider said that trans women were just men trying to access women's spaces. Jennifer describes her experience trying to explain to a provider that her partner is a woman with a penis. Their friends share their own stories of feeling out of place in a healthcare system that assumes all patients are heterosexual and cisgender.

Queer women and trans people are marginalized in the healthcare system due to institutionalized heteronormativity and cisnormativity. These forms of oppression are complex and manifest in individual assumptions, interpersonal interactions, policies and practices, and clinic spaces. Heteronormativity, cisnormativity, and cissexism function in connection with gender normativity to make queer women and trans people invisible in the healthcare system.[9,16–24] And when queer women and trans people do become visible in a heteronormative and cisnormative healthcare system, their presence is often experienced as disruptive of regular practices or interactions.[18,19]

We want to be clear that heteronormative and cisnormative assumptions are *learned* as we are socialized into a heteronormative and cisnormative culture. While individuals cannot be blamed for being socialized in a way that leads to acceptance of these widespread beliefs, it is the responsibility of individuals with privilege, including healthcare providers, to acknowledge, critically reflect on, and challenge these assumptions within themselves. To support healthcare providers in understanding and challenging heteronormativity and cisnormativity in their practice, in this section we explore the ways that heteronormativity and cisnormativity can be embedded within various elements of the healthcare setting and offer ways for healthcare providers to challenge this in their practice.

Although most people have heard the word *homophobia*, meaning fear or hatred of queer people, fewer are aware of the importance of acknowledging the ways in which less hateful but more common beliefs about heterosexuality shape the lives of queer people. Queer women's healthcare experiences are shaped by providers' heteronormative assumptions. Heteronormativity manifests as a set of assumptions that heterosexuality is the norm and that individuals are heterosexual until proven otherwise.[25] In heteronormative settings, queer women must "come out" because they are presumed heterosexual. Some healthcare providers recognize that they presume patients' heterosexuality,[26] while others are unaware of the influence of their heteronormative assumptions.[27–30] Institutionalized heteronormativity creates a context in which "heterosexuality is descriptively normative (statistically 'normal') as well as prescriptively normative."[25(p48)] Due to these pervasive assumptions, queer women's presence as patients in the healthcare system is often experienced as disruptive of regular practices or interactions.[18,19]

Transphobia describes fear or hatred of trans people. Unlike homophobia, which is widely viewed as unacceptable in Canadian society, transphobia remains widespread and accepted in our culture and negatively shapes the lives of trans people, who are more likely than cisgender people to experience violence, suicide, and abuse.[13,31,32] It is clear that healthcare providers must not be transphobic, as this would make it impossible to provide good care to their trans patients. In addition to challenging transphobia, providers must also question whether taken-for-granted cisnormative, cissexist, and transmisogynist beliefs shape their practice.

Cisnormativity describes the expectation that people's assigned sex at birth should align with their gender identities. For example, from a cisnormative perspective we would assume that people assigned "female" at birth will identify as women.[17] This assumption is so pervasive that it is taken for granted for most people, including healthcare providers. Cisnormativity disallows the possibility of trans existence or trans visibility. As such, the existence of an actual trans person within systems such as healthcare is too often unanticipated and produces a social emergency of sorts because both staff and systems are unprepared for this reality.[17] Thus, trans patients are invisible to healthcare providers until they make themselves visible. This visibility disrupts normal practices and is often experienced as a burden by healthcare providers, who then need to adapt cisnormative practices to make space for trans patients.

Cisnormativity functions in tandem with *cissexism*, which further marginalizes trans people. Serano, a trans activist and biologist, coined the word *cissexism* to describe "the set of beliefs and resulting actions that privilege, validate, and essentialize cis identities to the exclusion of trans identities; cissexism formulates trans identities and trans bodies as less real, valid, and desirable than cis identities or bodies."[17(p356)] These experiences may be even more pronounced for trans women who experience transmisogyny, which manifests as hatred, suspicion, or negative attitudes about transfeminine people.[33] Trans patients report experiences of their identities being questioned, criticized, or undermined by healthcare providers who view trans identities and bodies as less valid or real.

Contextualizing the Patient–Provider Relationship

> Later in their conversation with their friends, Heather and Jennifer have finished sharing personal stories and start talking about stories they've heard from other members of the community. Jennifer speaks about an older lesbian in the community who was sent to a conversion camp. Heather shares a story of a trans woman who thought she was going to a psychologist for gender-affirming care but was instead told that being trans was a disorder that could be "fixed" with therapy. Heather and Jennifer know these things happened recently and are still happening. Although it was nice to express their fears openly, their discussion with friends has not decreased their fear of their upcoming appointment. Until they had a child, Heather and Jennifer just avoided building relationships with primary care providers by accessing healthcare at walk-in clinics, but now they need the continuity of care provided by a primary care provider. Their friends suggest they go see a physician in the next town who is a gay man, but they've been trying to get into his clinic for years and they know he's not taking any more patients.

In 1968, the *Diagnostic and Statistical Manual of Mental Disorders (DSM) II* classified homosexuality as a mental disorder.[34] In 1973, homosexuality was removed from the *DSM* and replaced by the diagnosis *sexual orientation disturbance*, which pathologized individuals who were "in conflict" with their sexual orientation, essentially medicalizing the effects of homophobia and justifying the use of conversion therapy.[34] Sexual orientation disturbance was later replaced with *ego-dystonic homosexuality*, which wasn't removed until 1987.[34] Some healthcare providers, even in Canada, continue to practice "conversion therapy" (sometimes referred to as "reparative therapy"), which has the goal of converting queer people into heterosexual people. This homophobic practice has been shown to be both extremely damaging and ineffective, but it has not been banned in Canada or the United States.[35] Queerness is yet to be fully recognized by medicine as a form of human diversity worth protecting.

Trans people continue to be pathologized. Until 2013, the *DSM* listed *gender identity disorder*—disparity between sex assigned at birth and gender identity—as a mental disorder, essentially defining being transgender as a disorder. In 2010, the Canadian Professional Association for Transgender Health issued a statement regarding the *DSM* that gender variance and gender non-conforming behavior does not "constitute a psychological disorder."[36] In 2013, *gender identity disorder* was replaced with *gender dysphoria*, defined as discomfort with one's assigned sex that results in distress. While the definition of gender dysphoria is an improvement because it views being transgender as an expression of human diversity,[37] the focus on the distress experienced by some transgender people may pathologize the effects of transphobia. Transgender people often require a medical diagnosis to access necessary gender-affirming medical care. Despite progress, more changes to the medical system are required to understand trans existence as a manifestation of human diversity.

Healthcare providers must understand the context in which they are providing care to queer women and trans patients. An understanding of how queer women and trans patients have historically been and continue to be marginalized will shape a more ethical engagement in the clinic. These historical and recent experiences of being medicalized as "deviant" shape all queer women and trans people's engagement with the healthcare system. Overcoming these histories and changing future practice requires understanding the barriers queer and trans patients face in accessing healthcare.

Barriers to quality care are popularly defined in financial terms. Within public healthcare contexts such as Canada, the complex non-monetary barriers to good healthcare for queer women and trans people may be overlooked. Due to institutionalized heteronormativity and cisnormativity, and complex histories and presents of medicalization and pathologization, queer women and trans people often express fear about seeking healthcare or disclosing their identities to healthcare providers. It is important to recognize that all queer women and trans people are affected by the ways their identities have been and continue to be understood by medicine, even if they have never experienced homophobia or transphobia in the healthcare system. We also know that many queer and trans patients have negative healthcare experiences because of their identities. Bauer and colleagues,[38,39] for example, found that 38% of transfeminine and 37% of transmasculine people had at least one trans-related negative healthcare experience, and 52% of trans people report negative experiences accessing emergency care.

Due to fear of identity-based negative care reactions, some queer women and trans patients are uncomfortable discussing health issues with their providers or avoid accessing healthcare. Care avoidance negatively affects queer women and trans people's health.[17,19] Some queer and trans people avoid healthcare or access healthcare through walk-in clinics to avoid the fear of building healthcare relationships with a provider or "pass" so they do not have to disclose their gender identity or sexual orientation.[17,19] Yet, continuity of care requires an ongoing and open healthcare relationship. Those who avoid care or seek care from many different providers or emergency departments may be less likely to engage in preventive healthcare.

Queer women and trans people often negotiate around these barriers by seeking health advice from other members of the community. Anecdotally, social media groups feature frequent posts from community members requesting recommendations for safe healthcare providers and how to access gender-affirming or other treatments. While this informal navigation of the system is helpful in that it may provide access to safe providers, many negative stories about healthcare experiences are also shared through community networks, and queer- or trans-safe healthcare providers may become overburdened by the number of patients seeking care. Some healthcare jurisdictions have formalized this community referral process by hiring a patient navigator for LGBTQ+ patients. prideHealth in Halifax, Nova Scotia, for example, answers patient questions, provides referrals, and provides education for healthcare providers.[40] These formalized networks help to alleviate the stress queer and trans patients face in navigating healthcare access. Individual healthcare providers can also help alleviate the fear that is a barrier for healthcare access for queer and trans patients by making structural changes to clinic spaces and procedures, updating clinical language, and reflecting on the role of their own biases and assumptions in healthcare provision.

Structural Changes to Clinic Spaces and Procedures

> Heather, Jennifer, and Max arrive for their first appointment with their new primary care provider. The receptionist seems confused that they're Max's parents and has to scratch out "Father" on the form to write "Mother 2." Max gets bored during the long time at the reception desk and starts noisily trying to get out of Jennifer's arms. Heather and Jennifer feel like everyone in the waiting room is looking at them. When they finally take a seat, Heather jokingly passes Jennifer a *Women's Health* magazine, pointing to the article titled "10 ways to please your man." The receptionist calls "Jennifer and Robert" into the waiting room. Heather wishes she could disappear as she gets up and everyone in the waiting room watches them walk with Max into the provider's office. Sitting and waiting in the office, both Heather and Jennifer look for signs that this provider will be safe.

When queer and trans patients enter a clinic space, they are hypervigilant as they look for signs that their provider will be open and accepting.[19] Heteronormativity and cisnormativity are institutionalized in clinic spaces and procedures, including forms, washrooms, brochures, and interactions with healthcare providers and administrative staff.[41,42] As a consequence, queer and trans patients entering heteronormative and cisnormative clinics disrupt usual practices. In response, clinic staff and healthcare providers must often make one-time changes to regular practices to quickly accommodate visible queer and trans patients. These one-time changes may include hand-editing forms, changing language after being corrected, or reluctantly allowing access to gendered spaces after confusion about where someone is allowed. This process of adapting heteronormative and cisnormative practices only after queer and trans patients enter the clinic is exclusionary as it suggests queer women and trans patients should not be treated as all other patients. In addition, this ignores the needs of queer and trans patients who are not visible because they have not disclosed their sexual orientation or gender identity to their providers. In contrast, preemptive changes to clinical spaces and procedures support the development of trusting patient–provider relationships, which may decrease care avoidance and increase open communication.[42]

Healthcare providers are often unaware of the attention queer and trans patients pay to the physical space of the clinic in making a determination about safety. Many queer and trans patients enter clinic spaces looking for signs that this will be a safe space to receive care. If care providers know they are providing good-quality care for queer and trans patients, pride (rainbow) and trans (pink, white, and blue) flag stickers may be used to convey a sense of safety and inclusion to patients.

Healthcare providers are less aware of the taken-for-granted elements of their clinic space that may be seen as heteronormative and cisnormative by patients.[19] Family photos, for example, are intended by healthcare providers to humanize the provider and make the space less clinical, but when featuring families that all look the same, photos may convey an unintended normative judgment about what a family should look like.[19] Magazines and brochures also convey inclusion or exclusion to those in the waiting room. Healthcare providers can convey safety by including magazines and brochures that feature queer and trans content.

Changes to forms completed before appointments can also signal inclusion to queer and trans patients. Asking all patients to indicate if they are transgender or cisgender, sex assigned at birth, gender identity, sexual orientation, pronoun, legal name, name, and partner's name (if applicable) may seem insignificant to other patients, but these questions signify inclusion to queer and trans patients who are looking for signs of inclusion. We acknowledge that there is debate about whether or not healthcare providers should ask all patients their sexual orientation[43] and gender identity. It is important to note that deciding how and when to disclose is stressful for queer and trans patients. Queer women and trans patients feel a sense of responsibility to disclose their identities in a way that does not upset providers.[19] At the same time, remaining invisible or "passing" is also a lot of work because it requires altering one's stories, dress, and body language.[19] Explicitly asking all patients if they identify as transgender or queer is required to provide inclusion for all patients.[19]

Given that sexual orientation and gender identity influence healthcare experiences and that disclosing or not disclosing is a burden for queer women and trans patients, we believe healthcare providers should ask this question. Bauer and colleagues[17] similarly argue that all patients should be prompted to indicate if they are transgender or cisgender. Some providers express concern that asking everyone their sexual orientation is potentially "weird."[43] We agree with Ma[43] that many people do not see their sexual orientation as more private than other topics discussed with healthcare providers, and that the benefits outweigh the risks. Asking for sexual orientation and gender identity on forms or during a standard list of oral questions makes this process more straightforward. Electronic health records will facilitate this process by making this information available to all providers treating a patient.[38]

That said, during appointments, providers should not request more information about gender identity and sexual orientation than is required. Trans people, for example, have reported being asked personal questions about their intentions for transition during unrelated appointments. *Exoticization* is the practice of viewing someone different from oneself as exotic. In healthcare practice with trans patients, healthcare providers may be fascinated by trans patients and inquire about transition or trans identities in a way that is objectifying. Although less common, healthcare providers may also exoticize queer women patients when asking about their gender expression, relationships, or sexual practices. Healthcare providers should be careful to ask questions that are relevant to the care being provided in a professional manner.

In another article, with Harbin,[19] we argued that providers' efforts to build rapport with patients through humor, display of personal photos, and telling personal stories sometimes resulted in patients assessing spaces of providers as heteronormative and actually increasing fear. For example, a physician who joked with a woman patient about being in relationships with men was clearly trying to bond with the patient, but the patient expressed fear about coming out as bisexual because the provider assumed she was heterosexual.[19] In building rapport with patients, healthcare providers should avoid drawing on heteronormative and cisnormative humor and make visible their openness to queer and trans patients.

Trans people express fear about being outed by medical receptionists who call their "dead name" (name assigned at birth) instead of their name into the waiting room, or who express confusion when they call a "male" name or pronoun, for example, and a feminine person stands up. "Dead naming" trans people in a healthcare space makes them feel unwelcome and invisible. In addition, trans people are at high risk of violence, and outing them to a crowded room may result in violence or fear of violence from those who overhear the exchange. Trans people may have a name that is different from their legal name on health cards, as changing documents is expensive and complex. Calling patients by last names or asking patients to indicate when their names differ from their documents creates a more inclusive space.

Gendered spaces are also exclusionary for trans patients. Trans patients report being placed in sex-segregated wards that are not appropriate for their gender identity.[17] Trans patients should be placed in the ward that is most comfortable for them. All gender washrooms should be available for all patients.

Lastly, healthcare providers should be mindful of the fear queer women and trans people often have in meeting new healthcare providers. Referrals should be made to providers who can provide good-quality care to these patients. Assuring patients who appear fearful that this is being considered in referral practices may alleviate these concerns. Communicating the gender identity and sexual orientation of patients to new providers will also support good-quality care.

The needs of queer and trans patients should be considered in the design of these spaces and practices. Overcoming heteronormativity and cisnormativity requires dismantling the ways queer and trans patients are excluded from or deemed exceptional in healthcare systems. Queer and trans patients are often anxious entering new clinics; visible symbols of inclusion should be used to quickly communicate safety for this community.

Updating Clinical Language and Knowledge

As with clinic spaces and procedures, heteronormativity and cisnormativity are institutionalized in clinical language and knowledge, leading to the exclusion of queer and trans patients. We outline the importance of differentiating specialized from general care and removing gendered assumptions from clinical language. It is also important to consider all of the discussions conducted with patients to ensure that casual conversations are also not heteronormative or cisnormative.

From a cisnormative and cissexist perspective, knowing someone's gender identity tells us about their body. We assume, for example, that all men have penises. However, we know that this is not true: gender identity is distinct from sex assigned at birth and from bodies. Cisnormative assumptions infuse clinical language, and healthcare providers must work to disentangle language about bodies from language about gender. Heteronormative assumptions also manifest in questions about the bodies of sexual partners.

Phrasing their questions in an inclusive manner is one way that healthcare providers can improve their practice. To do so, healthcare providers will want to reflect on why the question is being asked, and then phrase their questions using body-focused language. In a sexual health screening, for example, a healthcare provider may ask the body-focused question "In the last year have you had sex with anyone with semen?" rather than the gender-focused question "In the last year have you had sex with men?" Similarly, body-focused language like "people who can become pregnant" replaces gender-focused language about women. While gendered language is often used as a shortcut, specific words that focus on the body are more accurate, less cisnormative or heteronormative, and therefore preferred.

Bauer and colleagues[17,38] report that trans patients often encounter physicians who state they do not know about trans people and trans healthcare. This occurs when healthcare providers do not know how to support gender-affirming care access, and when healthcare providers mistakenly assume that knowledge of trans-specific care is necessary to provide primary healthcare. Regarding gender-affirming care provision, many guidelines exist to support healthcare providers in providing gender-affirming care or referrals. The World Professional Association for Transgender Health, for example, offer Standards of Care on its website. Familiarity with these standards will support healthcare providers in making referrals and better understanding how to support patients through medical transition. That said, most of the care provided to trans patients will be primary healthcare, so healthcare providers should not overstate the complexity of providing healthcare to trans patients.

Critical Reflection on the Role of Provider Biases and Assumptions in Healthcare Provision

Cultural humility describes "a lifelong process of self-examination and critique of the biases and assumptions that may perpetuate health disparities."[44(n.p.)] Scholars studying healthcare provision for queer women and trans patients recommend this model.[38,41] This model is preferred to cultural competence models of care that emphasize memorization of information about a culture and can perpetuate stereotypes.[28] In contrast, cultural humility requires healthcare providers to continually recognize and examine their own assumptions, understand the effects of power relations, and examine the role of medicine and healthcare providers in perpetuating inequality.[41]

Engaging in the practice of cultural humility while providing care for queer and trans patients requires dismantling institutionalized heteronormativity and cisnormativity to make space for these patients, not memorizing facts about the community.[41] When confronted with the realities of the institutionalization of cisnormativity and heteronormativity in their practice, healthcare providers often retreat to a place of neutrality and comfort. However, research on care provision for queer and trans patients suggests that professional neutrality[41] and seeking comfortable interactions[18] often reproduces these and other forms of normativity and hinders critical reflexivity.

Baker and Beagan argue that "there is no magical state of neutrality, no view from nowhere."[41(p16)] As heteronormativity and cisnormativity are taken-for-granted perspectives, this "neutral" perspective often reproduces the assumptions that all people are heterosexual and cisgender, and further entrenches attitudes and practices that normalize these ways of being. Instead of seeking to remain neutral or treat everyone the same, healthcare providers should be aware of power relations in the clinic and use informed generalizations about queer women and trans people to guide their discussions.[45] Unlike stereotypes, generalizations provide a starting point for clinical discussions:

> Generalisations allow physicians to take into account the possible effects of shared experiences that arise from marginalisation and discrimination. They bring together group-specific observations and experiences. They suggest difference, not deficit. Stereotypes are an end point for understanding a person, limiting rather than broadening understanding, and applying group tendencies inflexibly to all members of the group. Generalisations are a starting point for understanding an individual, sensitising physicians to possible patterns, and potentially valuable questions.[45(p. e20)]

For example, a family physician working with a pregnant queer woman and her woman partner may anticipate that these patients may have concerns about the maternity ward being a queer-friendly space. The physician may inquire to see if this is a concern and what they could do to create a sense of safety for the patient and her partner.

For health professionals, comfort, like neutrality, is often seen as a sign that a clinical interaction is going well. However, health professionals' comfort in the context of institutionalized heteronormativity and cisnormativity may be a sign that the dominant ways of thinking and organizing are not being challenged to make space for queer women and trans patients.[18] When queer women and trans patients enter the clinic and disrupt taken-for-granted practices, they create an opportunity to critically reflect on institutionalized forms of oppression. Avoiding discomfort undermines the potential of these moments for creating safer spaces and practices for queer women and trans patients.[18] Healthcare providers may view moments of discomfort or disorientation as opportunities for learning and change.

Conclusions

Queer women's and trans people's experiences as patients in the healthcare system are negatively shaped by histories and presents of pathologization, and subtle assertions of cisnormativity and heteronormativity. While queer women and trans patients will not always visit the clinic with concerns related to their gender identities or sexual orientations, their identities as queer and trans people will shape all of their healthcare experiences in a system that is disrupted by their presence. In a healthcare system that has pathologized, and continues to pathologize, queer women and especially trans people, supporting the health and well-being of these patients requires healthcare providers to work to dismantle the heteronormativity and cisnormativity that further entrenches the oppression of members of this community. Making structural changes to clinic forms, procedures, spaces, language, and knowledge can begin to dismantle institutionalized heteronormativity and cisnormativity. Changes within the healthcare interaction that focus less on maintaining healthcare providers' neutrality and comfort, or, alternatively, on the exoticized aspects of queer and trans identities, will further disrupt cisnormativity and heteronormativity within the patient–provider interaction, build trusting provider–patient relationships, and increase access to quality healthcare for this community.

Note

1. 2S stands for Two-spirit, an identity claimed by many Indigenous LGBTQ+ people. LGB stands for lesbian, gay, and bisexual. T represents the transgender community. Q is for queer, an umbrella term for people who are non-heterosexual or gender nonconforming. I is for intersex people. A represents those who identify as asexual. This diverse community is united by their experiences of marginalization on the basis of gender and/or sexual orientation.

References

1. Statistics Canada. Same-sex couples and sexual orientation . . . by the numbers. 2015. https://www.statcan.gc.ca/eng/dai/smr08/2015/smr08_203_2015.
2. YouGov. 1 in 2 young people say they're not 100% heterosexual. 2015. https://yougov.co.uk/news/2015/08/16/half-young-not-heterosexual/.
3. Conron KJ, Scott G, Stowell GS, Landers SJ. Transgender health in Massachusetts: results from a household probability sample of adults. *Am J Public Health*. 2012;102(1):118–122.
4. Halberstam J. *In a Queer Time and Place: Transgender Bodies, Subcultural Lives.* New York, NY: New York University Press; 2005.

5. Gray ML. *Out in the Country: Youth, Media, and Queer Visibility in Rural America.* New York, NY: New York University Press; 2009.
6. Gray ML, Gilley BJ, Johnson, CR, eds. *Queering the Countryside: New Frontiers in Rural Queer Studies.* New York, NY: NYU Press; 2017.
7. Fredriksen-Goldsen KI, Kim H-J, Barkan SE, Muraco A, Hoy-Ellis CP. Health disparities among lesbian, gay, and bisexual older adults: results from a population-based study. *Am J Public Health.* 2013;103(10):1802–1809.
8. Polonijo AN, Hollister BA. Normalcy, boundaries, and heterosexism: an exploration of online lesbian health queries. *J Gay Lesbian Soc Serv.* 2011;23(2):165–187.
9. Steele LS, Tinmouth JM, Lu A. Regular health care use by lesbians: a path analysis of predictive factors. *Fam Pract.* 2006;23(6):631–636.
10. Clements-Nolle K, Marx R, Guzman R, Katz, M. HIV prevalence, risk behaviors, health care use, and mental health status of transgender persons: implications for public health intervention. *Am J Public Health.* 2001;91(6):915–921.
11. Scheim AI, Bauer GR, Shokoohi M. Drug use among transgender people in Ontario, Canada: disparities and associations with social exclusion. *Addict Behav.* 2017;72:151–158.
12. Scheim AI, Bauer G. Sex and gender diversity among transgender persons in Ontario, Canada: results from a respondent-driven sample. *J Sex Res.* 2015;52(1):1–14.
13. Bauer GR, Pyne J, Caron Francino M, Hammond R. Suicidality among trans people in Ontario: implications for social work and social justice. *Serv Soc.* 2013;59(1):35–62.
14. Bauer GR, Scheim AI, Pyne J, Travers R, Hammond R. Intervenable factors associated with suicide risk in transgender persons: a respondent driven sampling study in Ontario, Canada. *BMC Public Health.* 2015;15(1):525–540.
15. Rotondi NK, Bauer GR, Scanlon K, Kaay M, Travers R, Travers A. Nonprescribed hormone use and self-performed surgeries: "do-it-yourself" transitions in transgender communities in Ontario, Canada. *Am J Public Health.* 2013;103(10):1830–1836.
16. Barbara AM, Quandt SA, Anderson RT. Experiences of lesbians in the health care environment. *Women Health.* 2001;34(1):45–62.
17. Bauer GR, Hammond R, Travers R, Kaay M, Hohenadel KM, Boyce M. "I don't think this is theoretical; this is our lives": how erasure impacts health care for transgender people. *J Assoc Nurses AIDS Care.* 2009;20(5):348–361.
18. Harbin A, Beagan B, Goldberg L. Discomfort, judgment and health care for queers. *J Bioethic Inq.* 2012;9(2):149–160.
19. Fredericks E, Harbin A, Baker K. Being (in)visible in the clinic: a qualitative study of queer, lesbian, and bisexual women's health care experiences in Eastern Canada. *Health Care Women Int.* 2017;38(4):394–408.
20. Goldberg L, Ryan A, Sawchyn J. Feminist and queer phenomenology: a framework for perinatal nursing practice, research, and education for advancing lesbian health. *Health Care Women Int.* 2009;30(6):536–549.

21. Goldberg L, Harbin A, Campbell S. Queering the birthing space: phenomenological interpretations of the relationships between lesbian couples and perinatal nurses in the context of birthing care. *Sexualities*. 2011;14(2):173–192.
22. Ryan-Flood R. *Lesbian Motherhood: Gender, Families and Sexual Citizenship*. New York, NY: Palgrave Macmillan; 2009.
23. Salamon G. The sexual schema: transposition and transgender. In: Shrage LJ, ed. *You've Changed: Sex Reassignment and Personal Identity*. Oxford, UK: Oxford University Press; 2009:81–97.
24. Valanis BG, Bowen DJ, Bassford T, Whitlock E, Charney P, Carter RA. Sexual orientation and health: comparisons in the Women's Health Initiative sample. *Arch Fam Med*. 2000;9(9):843–853.
25. Beagan BL, Fredericks E, Goldberg L. Nurses' work with LGBTQ patients: "they're just like everybody else, so what's the difference?" *Can J Nurs Res*. 2012;44(3):44–63.
26. Westerstahl A, Bjorkelund C. Challenging heteronormativity in the consultation: a focus group study among general practitioners. *Scand J Prim Health Care*. 2003;21(4):205–208.
27. Beagan BL. Teaching social and cultural awareness to medical students: "it's all very nice to talk about it in theory, but ultimately it makes no difference." *Acad Med*. 2003;78(6):605–614.
28. Beagan BL, Kumas-Tan Z. Approaches to diversity in family medicine: "I have always tried to be colour blind." *Can Fam Physician*. 2009;55(8):e21–e28.
29. Berger JT. The influence of physicians' demographic characteristics and their patients' demographic characteristics on physician practice: implications for education and research. *Acad Med*. 2008;83(1):100–105.
30. Hinchliff S, Gott M, Galena E. "I daresay I might find it embarrassing": general practitioners' perspectives on discussing sexual health issues with lesbian and gay patients. *Health Soc Care Community*. 2005;13(4):345–353.
31. Kenagy GP. Transgender health: findings from two needs assessment studies in Philadelphia. *Health Soc Work*. 2005;30(1):19–26.
32. Melendez RM, Pinto R. "It's really a hard life": love, gender and HIV risk among male-to-female transgender persons. *Cult Health Sex*. 2007;9(3):233–245.
33. Serano J. *Whipping Girl: A Transsexual Woman on Sexism and the Scapegoating of Femininity*. Emeryville, CA: Seal Press; 2007.
34. Drescher J. Queer diagnoses revisited: the past and future of homosexuality and gender diagnoses in DSM and ICD. *Int Rev Psychiatry*. 2015;27(5):386–395.
35. Drescher J, Scwartz A, Casoy F, et al. The growing regulation of conversion therapy. *J Med Regul*. 2016;102(2):7–12.
36. Canadian Professional Association for Transgender Health. CPATH Position Statement DSM and ICD, March 2010. http://www.cpath.ca/wpcontent/uploads/2010/05/CPATH_PS_Dx_0310-1.pdf.

37. Bockting WO. Transforming the paradigm of transgender health: a field in transition. *Sex Relation Ther*. 2009;24(2):103–107.
38. Bauer G, Zong X, Scheim AI, Hammond R, Thind A. Factors impacting transgender patients' discomfort with their family physicians: a respondent-driven sampling survey. *PLoS ONE*. 2015;10(12):e0145046.
39. Bauer G, Scheim AI, Deutsch MB, Massarella C. Reported emergency department avoidance, use, and experiences of transgender people in Ontario, Canada: results from a respondent-driven sampling survey. *Ann Emerg Med*. 2014;63(6):713–720.
40. Nova Scotia Health Authority. prideHealth. 2017. http://www.nshealth.ca/content/pridehealth.
41. Baker K, Beagan B. Making assumptions, making space: an anthropological critique of cultural competency and its relevance to queer patients. *Med Anthropol Q*. 2014;28(4):578–598.
42. Wilkerson JM, Rybicki S, Barber CA, Smolenski DJ. Creating a culturally competent clinical environment for LGBT patients. *J Gay Lesbian Soc Serv*. 2011;23(3):376–394.
43. Ma R, Dixon M. Should all patients be asked about their sexual orientation? *Br Med J*. 2018:360:k52. http://www.bmj.com/content/360/bmj.k52.
44. Grubb H, Hutcherson H, Amiel J, Bogart J, Laird J. Cultural humility with lesbian, gay, bisexual, and transgender populations: a novel curriculum in LGBT health for clinical medical students. *MedEdPortal*. 2013;9:9542.
45. Beagan B, Fredericks E, Bryson M. Family physician perceptions of working with LGBTQ patients: physician training needs. *Can Med Educ J*. 2015;6(1): e14–e22.

III REPRODUCTIVE HEALTHCARE

REPRODUCTIVE BEHAVIOUR

10 THE MORAL AGENCY OF ABORTION PROVIDERS

CONSCIENTIOUS PROVISION, DANGERTALK, AND THE LIVED EXPERIENCE OF DOING STIGMATIZED WORK

Lisa Harris

Introduction

In medical school, I still got excited when mail arrived—it wasn't yet mostly bills or loan repayment notices. Perhaps the anticipation of something lovely in the thick white envelope in my mailbox one Friday morning made it all the more startling when I found the *Bottom Feeders* pamphlet inside. I began flipping through it:

What has an IQ of 7?
Eight Abortionists.
How do you tell if an abortionist is lying?
His mouth is moving.
What would you do if you found yourself in a room with Hitler, Mussolini and an abortionist, and you had a gun with only two bullets?
Shoot the abortionist twice.
Did you hear about the abortionist who refused to listen to his conscience?
He didn't want to take advice from a stranger.[1(p1–16)]

This pamphlet was my first exposure to the efforts of antiabortion activists to deploy stigma to deter future doctors from including abortion care in their practice. In my case, the effort surely backfired, as abortion became an important part of the full spectrum of reproductive health care I provide, and that I teach young doctors to provide. Indeed, others were similarly affected by receiving *Bottom Feeders*, and Medical Students for Choice was launched by Jody Steinauer in 1993 in part as a response to it.[2] While the pamphlet may have paradoxically contributed to my commitment to provide abortion care, I nevertheless understood from the very earliest part of my medical career that performing abortions would "mark" me in a range of ways the pamphlet described: as dishonest, stupid, evil, and—my focus here—lacking conscience.

In this chapter I tell several stories of abortion provision and conscience. First is the conventional narrative of their relationship—in which abortion provision is immoral and unconscionable, and in which abortion providers do their work because they lack conscience, moral agency, and moral standing. This is the narrative deployed by antiabortion advocates to stigmatize abortion providers, to justify violence against them, to generate restrictive abortion legislation, and to provoke fear and uncertainty among women considering abortion. However, antiabortion advocates are not alone in their promotion of this idea of the incompatibility of conscience and abortion provision. I will briefly review scholarly work in bioethics, which has a similar focus; that is, bioethics scholarship consistently depicts conscience as something that leads to objection to, and therefore non-provision of, certain kinds of medical care, especially abortion. There is a regrettable dearth of literature on the idea that conscience may *compel* provision of that very same care. I will review what we know about conscience as a motivator for abortion provision, which comes largely from the sociologic work of Carole Joffe and from a burgeoning newer scholarly and advocacy literature on the idea of "conscientious provision." Indeed, a handful of abortion providers are now speaking and writing about the moral and religious basis for abortion provision. I will consider reasons for this historical neglect of conscientious provision as both a concept and a lived experience, suggesting that it has largely to do with the historical silence of abortion providers about their work, due to fear of stigma, harassment, and violence.

I will end by recouping a point that has gotten a bit lost in the deployment of conscience arguments in the US abortion wars: that my own articulation of a conscientious provision argument in 2012[3] was not at its heart a pro-choice political argument, though it was partly that, and is certainly deployed by pro-choice advocates as that. My articulation of conscience as a motivator for abortion care was a story of my *lived experience*: my lived experience of being a doctor, my lived experience of my commitment to accompany women through all (not selective) moments in their reproductive lives, and my lived experience of knowing the compassion, kindness, and *goodness* of my abortion provider colleagues around the country and around the world. When I honor my lived experience of conscientious provision, and understand its contributions to the ethics of abortion, I must also honor that my lived experience of abortion work also includes experiencing it as violent, as something that really does "stop a beating heart," as something morally complicated, and which for me raises real questions about human life, and what it means to be a person. This part of my lived experience is usually felt to be threatening to pro-choice advocacy and messaging, and in fact is usually coopted by *antiabortion* activists to advance their case for legal restriction of abortion, or even elimination of abortion from the US healthcare landscape. To put it another way, advocates on both sides of the abortion issue generally are willing to recognize only selected parts of my experience, in order to make the case that abortion is either right or wrong, a fundamental right or an affront to humanity, and they neglect the parts of my experience that do not fit neatly with their side of this polarized contemporary US abortion debate. However, I do not experience abortion as straightforward, or as simply "good" or "bad." I experience it as both vitally important and morally fraught. I hold both ideas of, and feelings about, abortion at the same time, and I do not feel the need—in fact cannot—make it simply one or the other. And it turns out that, based upon a decade of focus group work with over a thousand abortion providers on four continents, many abortion providers are experts not only in the technical skills required to provide safe abortion but in holding this tension—this tension of opposites, if you will.[4,5] So I will end by considering the significance of honoring lived experience, and the significance of holding the "tension of opposites" for the moral life of an individual and for communities, at a time when it appears that social polarization is deepening and poisoning many arenas of social life.

Conventional Narratives: Abortion Work and Conscience as Incompatible

As the *Bottom Feeders* pamphlet illustrated, anti-choice stories about morality and abortion typically focus on abortion providers as being devoid of conscience. In some versions of this narrative, abortion providers do not understand what they do, morally speaking, when they perform an abortion, because they are lacking any moral foundations, any ability to discern right from wrong. Alternatively, if the narrative is that they in fact know what they are doing, then they are monsters. In either case, some kind of moral deficiency or failure leads to abortion provision. Indeed, I have been described as (accused of?) having a "malleable conscience" at best and being like Nazi doctor Josef Mengele at worst.[6]

These negative stereotypes are powerful and may be shared by patients seeking abortion care and internalized by providers themselves. As summarized by one caregiver in a focus group workshop, "I feel very judged. . . . Patients think *we're* bad people even though we're doing what they want us to do." Another caregiver wondered, "Do other people drive home crying, upset that you had this negativity . . . and stereotypes pushed at you [by clients]?"[7(p1066)]

Stereotypes of abortion providers as morally deficient have origins in historical discourse and persist in the rhetoric of contemporary public life as well. Both pro-life *and* pro-choice forces for two centuries have deployed the image of the stereotypical abortion "butcher" to advance their political agendas. The butcher is of course the immoral, dirty, inadequately skilled provider who provides unsafe abortions and gets rich doing so. Antiabortion forces used this image in the 1800s in their (successful) quest to make abortion illegal.[8] Pro-choice forces recycled it in the 1970s to make the case for the legalization of safe abortion.[9,10] In contemporary times, antiabortion advocates continue to invoke these images to justify restrictive state-level abortion laws. For example, Texas's House Bill 15,[11] which mandates pre-procedure ultrasound viewing by patients, relied on depictions of abortion providers as predatory and untrustworthy. Supporters of the bill argued that it was necessary to "protect the integrity and ethical standards of the medical profession."[12(p16)] Legislation in other states, such as Michigan's House Bill 5711[13] and Virginia's Senate Bill 924[14], which essentially require abortion clinics to be regulated as hospitals, rely on depictions of abortion providers as more dangerous and requiring more state oversight than other doctors, to prevent harm to patients.[15] In the rare cases in which an abortion provider (most famously, Kermit Gosnell) does engage in practices that are clearly unconscionable, not to mention illegal, his transgressions are depicted by abortion foes as routine, as typical of the "abortion industry."[16] Pro-choice forces have reinvested in this stereotype as well, relying on it to make the case for not going back to the "bad old days" of illegal and unsafe abortion. For example, prominent advocacy organizations such as Planned Parenthood Action Fund and Center for Reproductive Rights commonly cite death and complication rates from illegal abortion as a warning against what may happen should *Roe v. Wade* be overturned.[17,18] So, the unsafe, ill-motivated, and immoral provider is very much alive in the public imagination and has been for many decades.

Scholarly Narratives of Conscientious Objection, Not Provision

Scholars in philosophy and bioethics, without explicitly calling abortion providers immoral as antiabortion advocates do, nevertheless implicitly reinforce the idea that high moral ground is occupied only by those healthcare providers who refuse to provide abortion or other contested care. Specifically, there is quite a sea of literature on conscientious objection to care provision. Conscientious objection describes situations in which conscience—generally based in religious beliefs or moral values—tells someone *not* to do something. Philosophers and bioethicists call this a negative claim of conscience; that is, the conscience says, "don't." There is an enormous scholarly literature on conscientious objection and negative claims of conscience, much of that centered on abortion, as well as more recently on medical aid in dying, care of sexual minority and transgender patients, and care in a range of other contested arenas.[19-25] Within this literature there is a great deal of disagreement on whether conscientious objections are ever ethically permissible, and if they are, their limits, including whether providers who exercise a conscience claim must nevertheless refer for the care they will not provide, how direct the care provision must be in order to make a legitimate claim of conscience, and whether referral or participation in care even very indirectly brings moral complicity. Despite debate and disagreement on particular dimensions of refusal, the overall body of conscientious refusal literature relies on the idea that the central problem of "conscience" in healthcare, and especially in abortion care, is that provision of care—and perhaps even any association with that care—is antithetical to conscientious action, creating and reinforcing a dichotomy between conscience-based care and abortion provision.

In contrast, there is quite a dearth of literature on conscientious *provision* of abortion care, and indeed in the entire arena of positive claims of conscience. A positive claim of conscience in medicine is one in which conscience compels, or requires, that a healthcare provider offer care. In other words, one's conscience says, "do." In an article in 2012, I called for recognition of conscience in *provision* of contested care, and especially in abortion provision. I argued that abortion care can come from a deep moral concern for women's well-being. I used the voices of abortion providers solicited and documented by Joffe, as well as several contemporary voices, to make my case. In Joffe's 1996 book *Doctors of Conscience*,[10] she describes doctors' motivations for abortion provision both before and after the US Supreme Court's decision in *Roe v. Wade* in 1973, which invalidated state bans on abortion. Joffe found that before *Roe*, when abortion was illegal in the US, abortion providers were motivated by a commitment to ensuring that safe services were available, so that women could be treated without risk to their lives or future fertility. While legal threats to doctors were removed after *Roe*, doctors faced harassment and threats to their life from antiabortion extremists. Indeed, in the 40 years since *Roe*, 11 physicians and clinic workers have been killed, and there have been 26 attempted murders.[26] Most recently in 2016 in Colorado, three people were killed in a clinic shooting. In addition, doctors across the country continue to describe the heavy burden of stigma—feeling the need to keep their work in abortion a secret and recognizing the impact of secrecy on their relationships with family, friends, acquaintances, and strangers. Joffe described that doctors in both eras—before and after *Roe*—did their work in different kinds of adverse conditions but shared a common motivation: compassion for women, and a deep desire to help when most others turned their backs.[10] Doctors in her study provided abortion care out of their firmly held belief that it was the right—morally right—thing to do. Joffe understood this motivation to be conscience, hence the title of her book.

Other memoirs of abortion providers over the past decade echo Joffe's findings. Suzanne Poppema, in her 1996 memoir *Why I Am an Abortion Doctor*, described that she included abortion in her practice because it felt "right and good and important."[27(p11)] More recently, Dr. Willie Parker wrote eloquently about abortion work as a moral calling in his memoir *Life's Work*.[28] He describes that his religious upbringing led him for most of his career in obstetrics and gynecology to refuse to provide abortion care. After two decades as a physician it was religious teachings in compassion, nonjudgment, and the importance of being a Good Samaritan in the lives of women that led him to seek out training in abortion care, and to devote the latter half of his career to abortion provision in the US South.[28]

The bottom line, as I concluded in 2012, is that there is a case to be made for positive claims of conscience around abortion—for conscientious provision. To focus on conscience only insofar as it leads to objection to care provision is what I called "moral hemi-neglect"; that is, it neglects half of the way conscience might work in healthcare provision. And indeed, in the past several years, other authors—writing from clinical, legal, public health, and philosophical perspectives, have endorsed the idea that conscience indeed motivates provision of contested care.[29-31]

Conscientious Objection/Provision in Law and Policy

Though we appear to be witnessing the beginning of a shift in our understanding of conscience and healthcare provision, law and policy remain imbalanced, focusing on protecting conscientious objections (refusals) to provide care. Since the 1973 Church Amendment (named for the legislator who proposed it, Frank Church, not the religious institution), federal law has protected healthcare workers from being required to participate in, or from being discriminated against if they decline to, "any sterilization procedure or abortion if his [sic] performance or assistance in the performance of such procedure or abortion would be contrary to his [sic] religious beliefs or moral convictions."[32] Since then, 24 other federal statutes have further articulated conscientious objection protections, including the Coats-Snowe and Weldon Amendments, and Section 1553 of the Affordable Care Act, which protected objections to participation in aid in dying.[33] While the Church Amendment also forbids discrimination against healthcare providers who *do* provide sterilization or abortion care, this part of the amendment is typically neglected in public discourse, and there has yet to be a clear legal strategy built around positive claims of conscience, though there have been calls for one. A recent *New York Times* op-ed piece called for more balanced protection of conscience claims, protecting those whose conscience compels them to provide care, not just compels them not to.[34]

As a case in point, in January 2018, the US Department of Health and Human Services (HHS) announced the creation of a new body to protect religious freedom and conscientious objection. This new Conscience and Religious Freedom Division within its Office of Civil Rights (OCR) was established to "restore federal enforcement of our nation's laws that protect the fundamental and unalienable rights of conscience and religious freedom."[35] According to HHS, "The creation of the new division will provide HHS with the focus it needs to more vigorously and effectively enforce existing laws protecting the rights of conscience and religious freedom, the first freedom protected in the Bill of Rights." As the OCR director described, "The new division will help guarantee that victims of unlawful discrimination find justice. For too long, governments big and small have treated conscience claims with hostility instead of protection, but change is coming and it begins here and now." The acting HHS secretary added, "President Trump promised the American people that his administration would vigorously uphold the rights of conscience and religious freedom. That promise is being kept today." The focus of the new office is to ensure that "no one is compelled to participate in procedures such as abortion, sterilization and assisted suicide when it would violate their religious beliefs or moral convictions."[35] In other words, the new administration appears to be interested only in protecting conscientious objection, not conscientious provision, despite the fact that those who do provide care are routinely discriminated against when they are denied hospital admitting privileges, targeted for restrictive legislation, and denied training and care opportunities, for example.[34] The division also appears to have little interest in collecting reports of harm to patients caused by care refusals.

Why Has It Been So Hard to Recognize (and Protect) Conscientious Provision of Abortion Care?

In the face of stereotypes of abortion providers as immoral, greedy, and dangerous, it may feel jarring or counterintuitive to advance an argument about the abortion provider as a moral agent, a conscientious actor. This idea does not fit decades (even centuries) of negative stereotypes. There are reasons for this lopsided understanding of conscientious action, coming largely from the intense stigmatization of abortion. Stigma and conscience, as I will show, intersect in ways that undermine full understanding of what it means to act with conscience in healthcare settings.

By "stigma" I mean what the sociologist Erving Goffman first described in 1963 as the way in which people become "marked" or devalued as the result of an attribute they have—or, rather, as a result of the meanings that other people assign to that attribute; stigma is always an interpersonal process.[36,37] Sometimes that stigmatized attribute is one's work, as in the case of abortion provision. Sociologist C. Everett Hughes called stigmatized work "dirty work" and the people who do it "dirty workers." Classic examples are garbage collectors and gravediggers.[38] Abortion workers are also "dirty workers" who do work that is looked down upon and that carries physical, social, and moral taint.

The relative stability of negative stereotypes of abortion providers comes in part from of a phenomenon that I have come to call a "legitimacy paradox" for abortion providers, in which stigma and silence work together in a vicious cycle.[39] The paradox is that abortion providers are skilled, "real" physicians, but they are often portrayed as unskilled, illegitimate healthcare providers. The gap between perception and reality comes in large part from the reluctance of abortion providers to speak openly about their work. In focus group research with abortion providers around the world, I have heard over and over that, while abortion providers do their work for reasons of moral or ethical commitment, they often do not speak about it, or their motivations for doing it, with others—even their own family members. They remain silent for a range of reasons: the topic of abortion is a "conversation stopper," meaning that people do not know how to respond to a disclosure of abortion work at, say, a cocktail party or Thanksgiving dinner; disclosures of abortion work can be disruptive to family and friend relationships; and speaking openly about abortion can lead to harassment and violence. The result is a vicious cycle of stigma and silence: abortion providers do not disclose their abortion work in everyday conversations and do not share their reasons for doing it, including their reasons of conscience and ethical commitment. Absent providers speaking for themselves about their motivations, antiabortion activists fill in the blanks, and abortion work is depicted as a product of *deficiencies* in conscience. This further stigmatizes abortion provision, and that stigma in turn leads to more silence on the part of providers. That abortion providers do their work because of a moral calling remains hidden.

So, stigma interferes with recognizing conscientious *provision* of abortion care. It is worth also pointing out that stigma may interfere with robust understanding of conscientious *objection*, insofar as refusals to provide care are not assessed for their origins in conscience versus stigma. That is to say, there are many reasons besides conscience that healthcare providers might object to participating in abortion care (or any contested service). For example, they may not want to be "marked" as an abortion provider, associated with negative stigmatizing stereotypes. Other reasons for declining to participate in abortion care might include not wanting to be bothered or harassed by protesters, family objection, potential discord in their practice or among their office staff, habit, erroneous understanding of medical evidence for the safety of abortion care, insufficient training, and so forth. We do not have a good way to sort out the origins of objection, and there are no tools available to help distinguish claims of conscience from the other reasons healthcare providers might not want to do something, especially something as stigmatized as abortion. Even among obstetrician-gynecologists who train in abortion care as residents, and are committed to supporting abortion access for women, half ultimately do not provide it. They have no conscience-based objection but decline to provide abortion care largely due to stigma and institutional logistical barriers. Lori Freedman has called these doctors "willing but unable."[40] In other words, non-provision of abortion cannot be automatically equated with conscientious objection to abortion provision, though in current practice, and perhaps increasingly likely under new HHS protections, it may be treated as such.

My Journey to Recognition of Conscientious Provision

When I first articulated the idea and necessity of recognizing conscience in abortion provision, I did so in an academic journal, and by framing my argument for a scholarly audience it was necessarily a theoretical argument, grounded in literature in philosophy, bioethics, and sociology. But in actuality, it was not literature that brought me to the idea of conscientious provision. Instead, it was my lived experience of being a doctor, and of being part of a national and international community of doctors and advanced practice clinicians who provided abortion care around the world.

In my practice, I delivered babies, provided general gynecologic care, ran a miscarriage clinic, and continued to include abortion in the spectrum of clinical care I offered. To have excluded abortion care from my practice would have needed to be a deliberate decision, since I had been well trained in residency, and since I—like 97% of all US obstetricians-gynecologists—saw women seeking abortion in the course of everyday practice.[41]

It was my feeling that it would be wrong—morally wrong—for me to selectively pick and choose which moments in a woman's reproductive life I wanted to participate in. It felt morally wrong for me to abandon a woman at moment of crisis, which abortion is for some women. It felt morally wrong to put a barrier to care in her way. And in particular it felt very wrong to substitute my judgment of what was best for a woman facing undesired pregnancy in place of her own. I had the training and skills to provide abortion care, and my crisis of conscience would have come from denying that care to a woman who requested it. I felt called—morally called—to the work. And given harassment, threats, stigmatization, and marginalization within medicine that I and many others have faced, I was not sure why I or anyone *would* provide that care, if not called to it.

And when I looked around me at my colleagues also providing abortion care in the US and Canada, and in Africa and Latin America—regions of the world where my research had taken me—I saw a similar phenomenon. Caregivers are *called to* this work, often in adverse conditions, where providing abortion care brings intense stigmatization, threat of legal prosecution, the wrath and admonition of religious leaders, and ostracism from families and communities. In my lived experience, the people who did this work did not fit the negative, unidimensional stereotypes promulgated by antiabortion activists. It was on the whole a group that I found to be devoted to their patients, to compassionate care, to public health, to practicing evidence-based medicine, to generating the research base for evidence-based practice, and to women's civil and human rights. And the abortion providers I knew had a kind of expertise not just in the technical aspects of abortion but in structural competency.[42] That is, abortion providers knew how to get patients the care they needed even when there were enormous local structural constraints. Here I am thinking of the many instances in which, for example, abortion providers are able to arrange care even when patients have no transportation, no health insurance or means of paying, when there are no sympathetic subspecialist colleagues with whom to consult in medically complicated patients, when there are barriers to in-hospital care if needed, and when it is difficult to transport a patient to a hospital in rare cases of emergency. Around the globe I have seen how abortion providers figure out how to get people cared for against the most difficult odds.

I have observed abortion providers to be, as a group, people called to this work from their deepest core ethical beliefs, who feel a duty to take on care that most others—even other staunchly pro-choice colleagues—will not. And that is how my conscience argument arose. I felt and saw and heard conscience—moral and ethical calling and duty—in my own work and that of my colleagues. It was my lived experience. Pro-choice advocates embraced the argument because it aligned squarely with the needs of their movement to defend and advance abortion rights. But it is important to understand that it was not an argument that came from politics or advocacy or a desire to fulfill pro-choice movement needs. It came from simply paying attention to my experience, and that of the people around me.

Dangertalk and an Ethics of Lived Experience

However, my lived experience of abortion is not simple, and I observe this to be true for many of my colleagues as well. When I, at a woman's request, end a pregnancy, I often wonder who that unborn human would have turned out to be, had they been born. When I examine fetal tissue after a procedure, as I must do to confirm complete removal of the pregnancy, I marvel at the intricacies of human anatomy. I am sad that in different circumstances, many women would continue their pregnancy, in particular if poverty and economic strain were not issues. I do know that abortion "stops a beating heart" because I see it happen on ultrasound during a procedure. When I am with my friends and family members who are adopted, I am grateful that the women who gave birth to them chose to continue their pregnancies. These feelings coexist with my conviction that I must make myself available to provide abortion care for women.

When pressed, there is usually a point at which I, and many of my most ardently pro-choice colleagues, become uncomfortable with abortion provision—not simply because of technical or training issues, but because it "feels wrong" to do an abortion in the circumstances. For some, it is a matter of gestational age, meaning that after some point in pregnancy abortion begins to feel too violent or gruesome. Sometimes discomfort comes when a very minor fetal anomaly leads a woman or couple to end a pregnancy. Some providers, indeed most, according to the best evidence are uncomfortable with abortion for sex selection. Indeed, in a survey of obstetrician-gynecologists, 65% of those who provided abortion services had a moral objection to abortion for reasons of sex selection, in contrast to their feelings about abortion in other circumstances, such as failed contraception, or in the setting of breast cancer, diabetes, or rape, where fewer than 10% object.[43]

I am, in fact, sympathetic to many of the moral arguments against abortion. I do see fetuses as human organisms. I understand them to be entities with moral significance. And I am sympathetic to those whose hearts break when they think of all of the people who will not be born, and whose unbornness leaves all kinds of questions: Who would they have become? How would our world be different if they had been born? Isn't there something sacred in that potential human-ness? I wonder all of these things too.

I have come to call these kinds of experiences, when expressed, "dangertalk."[5] By dangertalk I mean acknowledging and giving voice to things that are fully true to one's lived experience, but at the same time potentially dangerous to a movement that one is part of and supports, even loves. These experiences are dangerous because extreme social and political polarization around abortion demands unambiguous support for, or objection to, abortion rights and access. Because policy and law are the potential outcome of public opinion on abortion, unwavering commitment or opposition to abortion rights feels urgent. As a result, abortion providers are well aware of the potential danger of speaking about their full experiences of their work. In focus groups around the world they share that they feel that their speaking is policed by pro-choice advocates, and that experiences that are "off message" vis-à-vis conventional pro-choice messaging are unwelcome. In other words, the silence in which abortion providers routinely engage is not only rooted in their fear of stigmatization, harassment, and violence; it is also in part self-imposed silence, self-censorship, that comes from the fear that giving voice to their full experiences—including moral conflict, judgmental feelings about patients, feelings that abortion is violent, among others—would be harmful to pro-choice causes.

Lived experience is complicated and does not always fit movement scripts. My own lived experience of abortion work fits some pro-choice movement needs, but not others. My experience of conscientious provision clearly supports a pro-choice political position. However, my experience of dangertalk may be threatening to it. I want to be very clear, though: I could not have articulated "conscientious provision" without also articulating "dangertalk." Both came from reflections and engagement with my lived experience of abortion work, and both are true. Abortion provision comes from a moral place in me, and simultaneously, I understand abortion as morally fraught. Pro-choice advocates might prefer conscientious provision without dangertalk. Anti-abortion advocates might like dangertalk without conscientious provision. However, they are both true to my lived experience and are, in fact, inseparable.

Holding the Tension of Opposites

So how can it be true that I experience abortion provision simultaneously as a moral calling, a duty, and as morally fraught and complex at times? The answer is actually quite simple: It is both. And I have no will, or ability, to make it be simply one or the other. Scholar and activist Jeannie Ludlow described this in a beautiful essay, borrowing from anti-abortion rhetoric to say about women's abortion experiences that "Sometimes it is a child and a choice."[44]

The abortion clinic is full of ambiguities, complexity, tensions of seemingly opposite things. They are tensions for me, my colleagues, and my patients. Some patients ask for copies of ultrasound pictures as keepsakes or ask to see the baby (often their word) after their procedure is over. It means something to some, even as they abort it. Some patients might share that their abortion was sad and difficult, and that they were so glad they could have one. During their procedure, many patients talk lovingly about the children they already have; patients and caregivers often exchange stories about their children even as the abortion procedure is under way. Often the biggest stress of the day for patients (as well as caregivers) is getting out in time to pick up kids after school or childcare. Abortion and parenthood go hand in hand; loving children and preventing them from being born are fully compatible in lived experience, though perhaps not in rhetoric. So is loving abortion work and feeling disturbed by it: abortion clinic workers might tell you that they have an enormous sense of purpose and fulfillment from their work, and that they became weak-kneed the first time they viewed fetal parts in a second-trimester abortion. In the abortion clinic space, patients and caregivers hold all kinds of tensions, sometimes of seemingly opposite things. In lived experience, there are nuances and complexities in abortion that do not find a comfortable home in the pro-choice movement's (or the pro-life movement's) rhetoric.

The idea that one might not need to choose between seemingly opposite ideas is not a common one in contemporary polarized social life, but it is well described in psychology, especially in the work of Jungian psychoanalyst Marian Woodman. She calls this holding of seemingly opposite ideas holding a "tension of opposites."[45] Holding the tension of opposites is the capacity to hold and engage with seemingly opposite, incompatible things, and that wholeness as a human comes only when we can accept, hold, engage with, and befriend the very opposing things we hold within ourselves. In Jungian theory that might be the spiritual and material parts of ourselves, or our "dark" and "light" sides—we are always both. Jung and his followers describe that there is a new kind of consciousness that arises when we engage both faces of dualistic thinking and embrace and integrate seemingly opposing things. In abortion those "opposites" might be that abortion "stops a beating heart" and "is vital for women's agency." Holding the tension of opposites here would mean that rather than feel the need to make it one or the other, we could recognize *and accept* that it is both. For many, maybe even most, people, it is difficult to hold seemingly incompatible ideas like these together. We like things to be clear-cut, unambiguous, when choices feel incompatible. Therefore, we habitually privilege one set of beliefs or feelings over the other to avoid inner turmoil, or we live conflicted lives.

It turns out that holding this tension of opposites appears to be an important capacity of abortion providers generally. In focus group work they describe this phenomenon as a central part of their experience. For example, some providers acknowledge there is uncertainty in their work. Said one, "I still to this day say to myself, 'I hope I'm doing the right thing.' That never goes away. I embrace [this uncertainty] because . . . it lets me know that certainty about being right is not necessary to move forward." Another shared, "Abortion is life and death, and I think for me it's about providers being able to say 'yes, we end lives here,' and being okay with that." Many providers have a capacity to tolerate nuance and ambiguity, to see abortion as an important service they provide, and to see it as ending a potential human life. They are willing to reflect on complex issues and resist the pro-life/pro-choice divides that dominate public discourse. In other words, they appear to be able to do the work of "holding the tension of opposites." There is no way to know which came first—do people with this capacity get drawn to abortion work because they are intrigued by its complexities, or is it a capacity that develops in the course of involvement with abortion work? It may be both.

What I long for is a space and place in public discourse and life for a robust, whole honoring of lived experience, in all of its complexity. It may not fit squarely with either pro-choice or antiabortion rhetoric. That—as I see it—is where real moral engagement happens. Reflexive "pro-choice" or "pro-life" positions do not actually require moral engagement, since we know the answer before we start. I see engagement—real engagement—as seeing multiple faces, honoring inconsistencies, expressing doubt, having empathy for those who believe differently. That is where moral work is happening.

The Moral Necessity of Holding the Tension of Opposites in a World of Extreme Social Polarization

The capacity to truly engage with lived experience requires the capacity to hold the tension of opposites—because lived experience is messy. It does not always match politicized messaging. We are living in an ugly, polarized time for abortion, and a wide range of other issues. When issues are polarized, it feels urgent that all experiences to which we give voice are filtered through movement lenses. Extreme social polarization asks us—perhaps coerces us—to squeeze our lived experiences into political boxes that may or may not be a good fit. There is a horrible, tragic loss there—the loss of expression of, and perhaps even awareness of, one's full lived experience. The extreme social polarization in which we find ourselves means that we are, in some respects, in a struggle for reality. And no one should have to fight to acknowledge their own lived experience.

The ability to hold the tension of opposites feels like a *moral* issue to me, because it is hard moral work to wrestle, consider, look from all sides, widen our gaze, consider not only the strengths but the limitations of our beliefs. Holding the tension of opposites requires a full, 360-degree view of an issue. It does not allow for selective picking of different aspects of an issue in order to fit a predetermined view. Engaging with complexity can be uncomfortable. It may be difficult to reckon with the fact that there may be only bumpy, uneven moral ground, not clear high and low ground. Engaging with complexity is a needed moral skill.

The ability to hold the tension of opposites also feels like a moral issue because there is a certain dehumanization of others that comes with our current state of social and political polarization. We think we "know" people when we learn who they voted for in the 2016 US election, or when we learn their view on abortion or other contested issues. If we are unwilling to engage in the tension of opposites, we are likely unable to see people who believe differently from us as full, complex humans. I do not see another way out of our current extreme social polarization, and the dehumanization that comes with it, besides embracing, tolerating, and engaging with moral complexities.

As Columbia University psychologist and researcher Peter Coleman has found, in a world of oversimplification, it takes moral courage to see things in a complex way.[46] In his work he has shown that complexity is an antidote to conflict. Oversimplification of issues leads to vilification of people who we understand to be on the other side of an issue. In Coleman's words, "nuanced understanding of the issues can lead to better solutions, stronger relationships, and a more unified society."[46(para.3)] It turns out that when we hold, tolerate, and engage with contradictions within ourselves, we are more tolerant and open to other people. In other words, the ability to hold the tension of opposites within ourselves would appear to be required for a humane, peaceful society and, by extension, democracy.

Conclusion

Polarization may be good for some purposes—it no doubt "mobilizes the base" on both the political right and left, and perhaps can be strategically deployed for fundraising for issue-oriented advocacy groups. But social polarization may not be good for the soul, to the extent that it disconnects us from others—even our own family members—and circumscribes the limits of what we are able to authentically claim as our true lived experience. So, I would like to consider the possibilities that open up when we, collectively, are able to hold the tension of opposites.

When it comes to the issue of abortion, it is at least worth exploring if people with opposing views on abortion might otherwise share views on a range of other issues on the reproductive life spectrum. For example, perhaps they envision a world without sexual coercion, harassment, or violence. Alternatively, some might wish to work for support and skill-building for parents. Some may feel that wide access to a contraception is vital. Others might want to work toward humane, patient-centered birthing options. Yet others might want to focus on helping young people learn how to have fulfilling relationships. Indeed, the reproductive justice movement was birthed by women of color advocates in the 1990s, out of recognition that a focus on abortion alone was much too narrow a way of understanding what it meant to have reproductive rights.[47] Some groups, like SisterSong,[46] work towards a shared vision of reproductive justice, even as its members do not all explicitly endorse pro-choice views. However, there are limited avenues for people who disagree about abortion yet agree on other dimensions of reproductive rights and justice to collaborate toward a shared vision. If people on both sides of the abortion issue approached each other while engaging with the tension of opposites—meaning with access to and acceptance of the limitations and ambiguities in their own beliefs and experiences—there might be more opportunities for collaboration across what currently appear to be insurmountable ideological divides.

In my own scholarly life, some of my most important collaborations have been with people with whom I disagree on a wide range of issues, including the acceptability of abortion, contraception, in vitro fertilization, sex outside of marriage, among other issues. However, these collaborations—full of intellectual honesty and bravery—have helped me to clarify my own thinking. Most relevant to my comments here, I would not have been able to articulate a vision of "conscientious provision" if it were not for the central importance of conscience to one of these particular colleagues. In fact, polarization around conscience protections is so deep that many abortion rights supporters were hesitant to elevate and validate conscience protections as an important concept, or to make a moral claim for abortion provision; "morality" and "conscience" had for so long been enemies of abortion rights. Ironically, I needed the support and intellectual contributions of people who value conscience deeply—who believe in its importance as a "witness" to life. Those colleagues turned out to be deeply religious and opposed to abortion. But their strong commitments to the exercise of conscience in healthcare helped me see my own expression of it, and eventually to articulate my argument for recognizing positive claims of conscience with respect to abortion. My experience is one piece of evidence supporting the need for collaboration across ideological divides. What the "tension of opposites" means for law and policy is unclear, given that the law is adversarial in its design, and that our nation is governed through a two-party system that seems particularly vulnerable to dualistic, polarized approaches. I can optimistically (some might say naively) hope that with more nuance and complexity, bipartisanship might be a more realistic goal.

I am making an argument for engaging with the tension of opposites and, even further, am arguing for the social and moral necessity of doing so. And I am making a fairly bold suggestion that abortion providers, rather than embodying a stereotype of moral vacancy, may actually offer moral guidance in a time when, in US contexts, there appears to be a growing tendency to see the world in only black-and-white, polarized, toxic, terms. Real life unfolds in many in nuanced shades of gray, and it turns out that *is* the world of abortion provision. I am arguing for understanding the moral agency of abortion providers in a new way—in a way that resists the dualistic, polarized nature of contemporary abortion discourse and rhetoric, and that might honor the full range of their lived experiences. On a personal note, I am tired of my experiences being selectively curated for political ends. And on a political note, I do not see another way to preserve a robust democracy.

References

1. *Bottom Feeders: The Abortionists' Jokebook*. Denton, TX: Life Dynamics, Inc.; 1992.
2. Platt L. Making choice real. *American Prospect*. December 19, 2001. http://prospect.org/article/making-choice-real. Accessed February 24, 2018.
3. Harris L. Recognizing conscience in abortion provision. *N Engl J Med*. 2012;367:981–983.
4. Debbink M, Hassinger J, Martin LA, Maniere E, Youatt E, Harris LH. Experiences with the Providers Share Workshop method: abortion worker support and research in tandem. *Qual Health Res*. 2016;26(13):1823–1827.
5. Martin LA, Hassinger J, Debbink M, Harris LH. Dangertalk: voices of abortion providers. *Soc Sci Med*. 2017;184:75–83.
6. Hall AK. Abortion and the malleable conscience. *Stand to Reason*. October 20, 2009. https://www.str.org/blog/abortion-and-the-malleable-conscience#.WpIXBLQ-e-s.
7. Harris LH, Debbink M, Martin L, Hassinger J. Dynamics of stigma in abortion work: a pilot study of the Providers Share Workshop. *Soc Sci Med*. 2011;73(7):1062–1070.
8. Smith-Rosenberg C. The abortion movement and the AMA. In: *Disorderly Conduct: Visions of Gender in Victorian America*. New York, NY: Oxford University Press; 1985.
9. Joffe C. Abortion and medicine: a sociopolitical history. In: *Management of Unintended and Abnormal Pregnancy: Comprehensive Abortion Care*. Blackwell Publishing, Ltd.; 2009.
10. Joffe C. *Doctors of Conscience: The Struggle to Provide Abortion Before and After Roe v. Wade*. New York, NY: Beacon Press; 1996.
11. Texas Legislative Session 85R. House Bill 15 (2017). http://www.legis.state.tx.us/BillLookup/History.aspx?LegSess=85R&Bill=HB15.
12. Weitz T, Kimport K. The discursive production of abortion stigma in the Texas ultrasound viewing law. *Berkeley J Gender Law Justice*. 2015;30(1):6–21.
13. Michigan Legislature House Bill 5711. http://legislature.mi.gov/doc.aspx?2016-HB-5711.

14. Senate Bill No. 924. 2011, p. 1–3. https://lis.virginia.gov/cgi-bin/legp604.exe?111+ful+SB924+pdf.
15. Harris LH, Martin LA, Youatt E, et al. Michigan's HB5711: a case study of the role of abortion provider stigma in anti-abortion legislation. *Contraception*. 2013;88(3):443.
16. PAFamily.org. After Gosnell: What the Abortion Industry unashamedly fought (and thankfully failed) to stop. https://pafamily.org/2018/10/aftergosnellstory/
17. *Roe v. Wade*. Planned Parenthood Action Fund. https://www.plannedparenthoodaction.org/issues/abortion/roe-v-wade.
18. What If *Roe* Fell? Center for Reproductive Rights. https://www.reproductiverights.org/what-if-roe-fell.
19. Chavkin W, Leitman L, Polin K. Conscientious objection and refusal to provide reproductive healthcare: a white paper examining prevalence, health consequences, and policy responses. *Int J Gynecol Obstet*. 2013;123:S41–56.
20. Dickens B, Cook R. The scope and limits of conscientious objection. *Int J Gynecol Obstet*. 2000;71(1):71–77.
21. Cook R, Olaya M, Dickens B. Healthcare responsibilities and conscientious objection. *Int J Gynecol Obstet*. 2009;104(3):249–252.
22. Gerrard J. Is it ethical for a general practitioner to claim a conscientious objection when asked to refer for abortion? *J Med Ethics*. 2009;35(10):599–602.
23. ACOG Committee on Ethics. The limits of conscientious refusal in reproductive medicine. ACOG Committee Opinion #385, November 2007. https://www.acog.org/Clinical-Guidance-and-Publications/Committee-Opinions/Committee-on-Ethics/The-Limits-of-Conscientious-Refusal-in-Reproductive-Medicine.
24. Holm S. The debate about physician assistance in dying: 40 years of unrivalled progress in medical ethics? *J Med Ethics*. 2015;41:40–43.
25. Green E. When doctors refuse to treat LGBT patients. *The Atlantic*. April 19, 2016. https://www.theatlantic.com/health/archive/2016/04/medical-religious-exemptions-doctors-therapists-mississippi-tennessee/478797/.
26. Violence Statistics and History. National Abortion Federation. https://prochoice.org/education-and-advocacy/violence/violence-statistics-and-history/.
27. Poppema S. *Why I Am an Abortion Doctor*. Amherst, NY: Prometheus Books; 1996.
28. Parker W. *Life's Work: A Moral Argument for Choice*. New York, NY: Atria; 2017.
29. Dickens B, Cook R. Conscientious commitment to women's health. *Int J Gynecol Obstet*. 2011;113(2):163–166.
30. Harris LH, Shaffer E. Capsules from the Medical Care Section of APHA: Call to the public health clinical community to practice conscientious provision of abortion care. *Med Care*. 2016;54(12):1033–1034.
31. Buchbinder M, Lassiter D, Mercier R, Bryant A, Drapkin Lyerly A. Reframing conscientious care: providing abortion care when law and conscience collide. *Hastings Center Rep*. 2016;46:22–30.

32. 42 U.S.C. 300a-7(b)(1)(2015). http://uscode.house.gov/view.xhtml?req=(title: 42%20section:300a-7%20edition:prelim).
33. Conscience Protections for Health Care Providers. US Department of Health and Human Services. 2017. https://www.hhs.gov/conscience/conscience-protections/index.html.
34. Fernandez Lynch H, Stahl RY. Protecting conscientious providers of healthcare. *New York Times*. January 26, 2018. https://www.nytimes.com/2018/01/26/opinion/protecting-conscientious-providers-of-health-care.html.
35. HHS Announces New Conscience and Religious Freedom Division. US Department of Health and Human Services. January 18, 2018. https://www.hhs.gov/about/news/2018/01/18/hhs-ocr-announces-new-conscience-and-religious-freedom-division.html.
36. Goffman E. *Stigma: Notes on the Management of Spoiled Identity*. New York, NY: Simon & Schuster, Inc.; 1963.
37. Link BG, Phelan JC. Conceptualizing stigma. *Ann Rev Sociol*. 2001;27:363–385.
38. Hughes EC. Work and self. In: *The Sociological Eye: Selected Papers*. Piscataway, NJ: Transaction Publishers; 1971.
39. Harris LH, Martin L, Debbink MP, Hassinger J. Physicians, abortion provision and the legitimacy paradox. *Contraception*. 2013;87(1):11–16.
40. Freedman LR. *Willing and Unable: Doctors' Constraints in Abortion Care*. Nashville, TN: Vanderbilt University Press; 2010.
41. Stulberg D, Dude A, Dahlquist I, Curlin F. Abortion provision among practicing obstetrician–gynecologists. *Obstet Gynecol*. 2011;118(3):609–614.
42. Metzl JM, Hansen H. Structural competency: theorizing a new medical engagement with stigma and inequality. *Soc Sci Med*. 2014;103:126–133.
43. Harris LH, Cooper A, Rasinski K, Curlin FA, Drapkin Lyerly A. Obstetrician-gynecologists' objections to and willingness to help patients obtain an abortion. *Obstet Gynecol*. 2011;118(4):905–912.
44. Ludlow J. Sometimes it's a child and a choice: toward an embodied abortion praxis. *NWSA J*. 2008;20(1):26–50.
45. Woodman M. *Holding the Tension of the Opposites*. Louisville, CO: Sounds True, Inc; 1994.
46. Coleman P. The power of moral complexity. *Psychology Today*. 2014. https://www.psychologytoday.com/blog/the-five-percent/201409/the-power-moral-complexity.
47. Ross, Loretta. Keynote address at the Reproductive Justice—A3 in A2 Conference, Ann Arbor, Michigan, May 29th, 2013.

11

PERINATAL MENTAL HEALTH

THE LENS OF RELATIONAL ETHICS

Lori d'Agincourt-Canning and Deirdre Ryan

Introduction

Family planning and reproductive decision making are important issues for women with mental illness, just as they are for any woman. However, when considering a family, managing a pregnancy, or caring for a newborn, women with chronic depression, anxiety, or psychotic illness constitute a particularly vulnerable group. Ethical challenges may include uncertain or impaired decision-making capacity, being controlled or exploited by others, unrecognized medical problems, and fragile social circumstances. Historically, pregnancy has been associated with women's supposed mental instability. While feminist bioethics and women's health have argued against the pathologizing of women during pregnancy, there has been inadequate attention paid to the intersection of mental health concerns and perinatal care in the women's health and feminist bioethics literature.

Perinatal mental health spans the period from pregnancy to the postpartum period. Treatment is complex; both the needs of the woman and her fetus, and later the mother and newborn, should be considered carefully. Unfortunately, ethical precedents and legal judgments have tended to view mother and fetus as adversaries. Society's protectiveness toward the fetus results frequently in management decisions that elevate concerns for the fetus or the future child over maternal preferences and well-being. Too often "maternal–fetal conflict" is the model through which reproductive decisions about women with mental illness are framed. Yet, the most important factor for a child's well-being is the mother's mental health. Ensuring the mother's optimal health lays the foundation for the child's optimal development.

This chapter reviews ethical issues pertaining to the care of perinatal women with mental illness. Like Miller,[1] we take the position that the relationship between a mother and fetus/child is not an adversarial one: rather, the interests and well-being of both are intimately intertwined. Miller cites relational ethics as an important concept in guiding reproductive management of women with mental illness. We build on this work and argue that the ethical basis of mental health practice can be strengthened further by incorporating a feminist view of relational autonomy into decision making with patients.

In the sections that follow, we will (1) describe the incidence of mental illness during the perinatal period and respective treatments; (2) introduce and propose relational autonomy as a key principle in guiding treatment decisions for perinatal women experiencing mental illness; and (3) illustrate the value of relational autonomy in addressing ethical challenges related to three cases in reproductive mental health: psychotropic medication decisions during pregnancy; enforced treatment; and disclosure of medication use to fathers. For the fourth case, we broaden the discussion to address social justice considerations regarding mother–baby units for women experiencing a perinatal mental health crisis.

Perinatal Mental Health: How Many Are Affected?

As many scholars have noted, pregnancy is a time when women experience profound psychological changes.[2,3] The emotional "tasks" of pregnancy include accepting the pregnant state, constructing a sense of self as a mother, and beginning a relationship with the unborn child.[2] Some cultures, recognizing the importance of pregnancy and the postpartum period, have implemented rituals to support and educate women through this transition.[4]

Depression and Anxiety

Depression and anxiety are the most common mental health problems during pregnancy, with 10% to 15% of women experiencing major depression and 13% anxiety.[5] Depression and anxiety also affect 15% to 20% of women in the first year after childbirth. Other mental health disorders that can occur on their own or coexist with depression during the perinatal period include obsessive-compulsive disorder, posttraumatic stress disorder, adjustment disorders, and eating disorders.[5-7] Bipolar disorder is characterized by depressive and manic episodes and occurs at a rate of 0.5% to 1.5% in the general population. The typical age at onset is late adolescence or early adulthood, putting women at risk for illness throughout their reproductive years.[5,8]

The first year after delivery is a vulnerable time for the development of a psychiatric illness, but social disadvantage increases the risk of perinatal mental illness or can exacerbate its effects. For instance, the risk of depression is higher for teenage mothers and for women living in poverty, poor housing, or homelessness.[9] Migration, extreme stress, exposure to violence, emergency and conflict situations, natural disasters, and low social support also increase risks for specific disorders.[10]

Psychotic Disorders

Psychotic symptoms can occur in a number of different psychiatric conditions, including schizophrenia, bipolar disorders, and severe major depressive disorders. Women who are experiencing psychotic symptoms have lost touch with reality. They may be delusional and believe that other people are trying to harm them. They may hallucinate, hear voices, and/or behave in a very disorganized way.

Risk factors associated with schizophrenia make pregnancy particularly challenging for this group. Psychosis during pregnancy can lead to denial of pregnancy, failure to access prenatal care, and failure to recognize the signs of labor.[11] Compared to "healthy" women of the same socioeconomic status, pregnant women with schizophrenia have more unplanned pregnancies and experience a higher incidence of stillbirth and neonatal death.[12] Social risks include poverty, lack of partner support, substance misuse, vulnerability to violence, and poor nutrition.[4,13,14] The rate of child apprehension is also disproportionately high for this group. That said, approximately 50% all women with a diagnosis of schizophrenia are mothers.[6] "Most women with schizophrenia value their roles as mothers, and their adult children remain attached to them."[15(p51)]

Some women with bipolar disorder experience mental illness for the first time following childbirth; other women with preexisting bipolar disorder experience a recurrence or exacerbation at this time. The risk of developing a psychiatric illness is greater for all women during the early postpartum period than at any other in their lives because of hormonal changes, sleep deprivation, and the psychological and emotional stress of infant care.

Postpartum psychosis, although rare, is the most serious postpartum psychiatric illness. It affects around 2 in 1,000 new mothers, and onset is rapid, most often occurring 72 hours to 4 weeks after delivery.[6] It causes confusion, severe mood disturbance, paranoia, and erratic or disorganized behavior.[9] Delusional thinking is common and often involves the infant. Auditory or visual hallucinations may compel the mother to harm herself or her infant. Risk for suicide, as well as infanticide, is a critical concern. Women with a personal or family history of postpartum psychosis, bipolar disorder, and schizophrenia are at particular risk for developing psychosis. The majority of women who experience their first psychotic episode after delivery will go on to be diagnosed with a bipolar disorder.[6]

Treatment

Depression and Anxiety

Depending on the severity of the mental health issue, there are a range of options for treating perinatal mental illness. Many women have mild cases of depression and anxiety, for which cognitive-behavior therapy (CBT), mindfulness training, or interpersonal therapy can be quite effective. Education also plays a large role in helping women to manage their symptoms. However, a significant number of pregnant women and new mothers suffer from more severe illness that calls for referral to specialist services and possibly medication.

"Perinatal mental health disorders are unique in the sense that they affect a group of people who are already connected to the health service at the time they develop symptoms."[9(p5)] Despite this, detection and treatment rates remain low. Research shows that women with perinatal depression face a range of barriers in accessing care that meets their needs.[16] In a study conducted at the University of Michigan,[17] 1,837 pregnant women from several hospital-based obstetrics clinics were screened using a standardized questionnaire for depression. Among the women found to be at high risk for depression, only 20% received some type of depression treatment. Further, among women meeting criteria for major depression at the time of the study, only 11% received adequate treatment with an antidepressant. Having a current episode of depression did not alter these findings.

These results indicate that while depression is relatively common during pregnancy, most women do not receive any type of treatment. Of significant concern is the finding that even when depression *is* known, most women do not receive adequate treatment. Given the uncertain and often contradictory information about the safety of antidepressants on fetal development, physicians frequently recommend against medication use and women elect to discontinue medications during pregnancy.[16]

Yet, untreated depression may actually be riskier for women during pregnancy than at other times in their life.[18] Studies[19] show that women with unipolar depression who discontinue their medication have significantly higher rates of relapse compared to those who continue their medication. Likewise, in study of women with bipolar disorder, Viguera and colleagues[20] found that women who discontinued mood stabilizers spent over 40% of their pregnancy in an illness episode, versus only 8.8% among subjects who maintained treatment. This is concerning as suicide is a leading cause of death for women in the first year after birth. Women who commit suicide after the delivery often do so in a violent way.

Psychotic Disorders

Women with schizophrenia need considerable support during the perinatal period. Those treating women with schizophrenia who are pregnant, or wish to conceive, emphasize the importance of "wraparound care," which involves close collaboration between obstetric, psychiatric, public health, and case management services.[14,15]

The risks and impacts of bipolar disorder can also be successfully managed through preconception counseling and perinatal planning that takes into consideration the severity of the woman's illness, previous response to medication, and available supports.[6] While postpartum psychosis is rare, those who have experienced psychosis have a greater than 50% risk of developing another postpartum psychotic episode after subsequent deliveries. Any woman who experiences an episode of postpartum psychosis needs to be educated about her risk and plan for early postpartum psychiatric management.[6]

As with depressive conditions, pharmacologic intervention is a major facet of treatment for schizophrenia and other psychotic disorders. There is again a lack of data about the reproductive safety of these medications. As a result, women with psychotic illness may choose to discontinue their medications when trying to conceive or upon learning they are pregnant, rendering them highly vulnerable to their illness.[11]

Ethics Guiding Reproductive Care

In an opinion paper, the American College of Obstetrics and Gynecology Ethics Committee[21] recommends that its practitioners adopt a "toolbox" approach to ethical decision making. It stresses that clinical problems are too complex to be using simple rules or applying principles in rigid ways. The different frameworks the committee recommends in guiding ethical decision making are principle-based ethics, virtue ethics, care-based ethics, and feminist ethics, among others.

Harris[22] and Miller[1] draw on relational perspectives in considering, respectively, issues in perinatal ethics and reproductive care of women with mental illness. Previously, McCullough and Chervenak[23] established a framework of obstetrical decision making using principle-based obligations. They argued that clinicians have both autonomy- and beneficence-based obligations to the pregnant woman and beneficence-based obligations to the fetus once it reaches viability (approximately 24 weeks gestation). If an ethical dilemma arises, they advised that practitioners determine the relative weights of the component obligations to the pregnant woman and fetus separately and make a decision based on the weightiest obligation. Here, mother and fetus are treated as two distinct and unconnected beings whose interests can be weighed and judged on opposite ends of a scale.

Harris[22] identifies three important limitations to principle-based ethics based on feminist scholarship. The first limitation claims that principles are too abstract and too removed from the everyday realities in which moral choices are made. Rather than viewing ethics as the rational deliberation of universal rules, she calls for a relational conception of moral life that recognizes the interdependency of human relations, and the responsibilities that ensue from these. The second limitation speaks to the notion that people approach ethical dilemmas from their own standpoint and that certain standpoints (e.g., a clinician's standpoint) are more privileged than others.

A third limitation is that a principle-based approach typically ignores the broader social and structural context in which clinical care occurs and decisions are made. Yet, inherent to the broader context are unjust social practices and power relations that result in certain groups being disadvantaged over others. As an example, Harris cites a study examining drug and alcohol use during pregnancy in Florida.[24] It showed that despite the rates of drug use being equally prevalent among Caucasian and minority women, African-American women were 10 times more likely to be reported to authorities. This example makes explicit how clinicians' actions may serve to entrench or extend existing social biases and structural inequalities.[25]

In appealing to a relational view of ethics, Harris[22] calls for a broader gaze in assessing situations where maternal and fetal interests appear to conflict. She considers the case study of a woman who is in preterm labor but ignores medical recommendations for bed rest. Harris calls attention to context and how social and family relationships might shape the pregnant woman's response to medical concerns about preterm labor. For example, she posits the woman may need to care for other children at home or have other responsibilities that take priority over her clinician's recommendations for bed rest. Simply "blaming" the woman and viewing her response as evidence of maternal–fetal conflict is unlikely to help clinicians or the woman identify choices that align with her needs.

Harris also asks clinicians to reflect on their own life circumstance and how this might influence their perceptions of ethical dilemmas. For example, she noted it might be difficult for physicians or other clinicians with material resources to imagine a situation where they could not afford childcare, yet financial factors translate into access barriers for many people. Lastly, Harris asks clinicians to consider whether the woman's prior interactions with healthcare providers, such as discrimination, would cause her to mistrust the recommendations made to her.

Relational ethics, together with the four principles, figure prominently in Miller's[1] discussion of ethical issues concerning prenatal and postpartum care of women with mental illness. Rather than considering the moral weight of obligations owed to the pregnant woman and fetus separately, Miller views their interests as intricately linked. She presents a case involving a pregnant woman with bipolar disorder who, in a psychotic manic phase, has the delusional belief that her fetus is an evil spirit that must be removed. The woman is brought to hospital after attempting unsuccessfully to puncture her abdomen with a knitting needle and now refuses treatment. Miller observes that women who harm their babies because of delusions suffer profoundly later when they come to realize what they have done. From this vantage point, treating the woman for her own well-being is as important as treating her for fetal well-being. At the same time, Miller recognizes that informed consent necessitates a surrogate decision maker, preferably someone who understands the patient's values.

Relational Autonomy

The principle of respect for autonomy dominates many areas of bioethics. The core concept sustaining the principle is "the simple but compelling idea that as moral agents we have the right to make important decisions about our lives and to determine what happens in and to our bodies."[26(p71)]

Closely linked to respect for autonomy is capacity, the ability of patients to make their own treatment decisions. This ability is viewed largely as a cognitive skill, based on elements of understanding (nature of health problem, treatment and non-treatment options), reasoning (weighing the pros and cons of each option), appreciation (considering the consequences of each option), and expressing choice.[27] The emphasis placed on capacity and, in turn, the liberty to make decisions is exercised through informed consent. Informed refusal mandates the same elements and capacity as informed consent.

Traditional accounts of respect for autonomy in healthcare have emphasized an ideology of individualism and independent choice.[28,29] Feminist theorists have long held this view to be inadequate and sought to reconceptualize the concept of autonomy in ways that reflect the social dimensions of agency and selfhood. Relational autonomy is an umbrella term, referring to a range of related perspectives that share the conviction that persons are socially embedded and that their identities are formed through relationships of interdependence. Relational autonomy also brings into account how intersecting social factors (e.g., race, class, gender, ethnicity) are integral to one's sense of identity.[28(p4)] Like other feminist scholars, Jennifer Nedelsky rejects the notion that relationships deter autonomy, arguing instead that autonomy emerges within and because of relationships:

> I see autonomy as the core of a capacity to engage in the ongoing, interactive creation of our selves—our relational selves, our selves that are constituted, yet not determined, by the web of nested relations within which we live. . . . As we act (usually partially) autonomously, we are always in interaction with the relationships (intimate and social-structural) that enable our autonomy. Relations are then constitutive of autonomy rather than conditions for it.[29(p45–46)]

A key feature of feminist and relational theories is that a woman does not exist in isolation but is defined through her social roles, relationships, and history.[30,31] Another hallmark is its focus on power relations and the effect these impart on individuals' choices, opportunities, and capacities. Social relationships can enhance autonomy, fostering its development if enacted within the context of respectful and reciprocal relationships.[26] However, social and familial relationships can also be coercive, manipulative, and abusive, resulting in harmful treatment that impairs an individual's ability for autonomous action.

In a similar vein, relational autonomy draws attention to structural issues that shape and restrict individuals' choices and opportunities for choice.

Numerous examples exist where economic or social constraints prevent individuals from having access to care based on race, ethnicity, class, sex or sexual preference, and religion. By attending to material, economic, and occupational circumstances, educational and social resources, social institutions, and cultural norms, relational theory examines the true availability of options that permit self-determining choices.[32] A commitment to relational autonomy also goes beyond offering a critical perspective to developing strategies that could potentially reverse these constraints.

A relational approach to autonomy has ethical significance for marginalized persons, such as those with severe mental illness, whose capacity for self-determination may be limited not only by their condition but by their social circumstances. It would begin with careful consideration of the relational dimensions of the patient's life (social and structural) that may be addressed or acted upon to support the patient's autonomy and well-being. However, features of mental illness may limit what autonomy alone can achieve. By definition, mental health disorders are characterized by their impact on a person's emotional state, cognition, and subsequent behavior. For example, delusions and hallucinations are symptoms of schizophrenia, affecting how a person thinks, feels, and behaves.[6] Those with bipolar illness may also experience delusions during the manic phase. At times, severe depression, anxiety, or compulsive disorders may distort a woman's perception of her own goods, harms, interests, values, and goals.

While decision-making capacity is impaired only in the most severe cases of mental illness, attention to relational autonomy may help practitioners better address the vulnerabilities their patients face. It can be drawn upon to guide a commitment to supportive relationships, fostering a collaborative approach between the woman and significant others as well as the woman and her health professionals. Further, it recognizes the importance of contextual and social factors for mediating autonomous action. Lastly, a relational conception of autonomy considers an individual's relationship to prevailing social norms, beliefs, and practices and their effect on self-identity. The way a pregnant women or new mother experiences mental illness is influenced by the way others see and understand her. Stigmatization and discriminatory attitudes (e.g., rejection, humiliation) toward those with mental illness can affect the woman's self-worth as a person, new mother, and partner.

In the next section, in four different situations, we apply the concept of relational autonomy to consider the needs and clinical decision making of women who have perinatal mental illness.

Relational Autonomy in Practice
Medication Use

Maria had a history of recurrent depressive episodes dating back to her early 20s. She experienced some improvement with CBT but achieved a complete remission of her symptoms only after being prescribed a selective serotonin reuptake inhibitor (SSRI) for her depression. Maria remained on the antidepressant for a number of years. Every time she stopped the antidepressant, she experienced a relapse. She was taking the antidepressant when she became pregnant. Maria immediately stopped her medication because she had read on the internet that her baby might develop a heart defect if exposed to this antidepressant during pregnancy. In spite of starting a course of CBT, by 16 weeks gestation, her mood had deteriorated. She was crying every day, isolating in bed, and became convinced that she would be an awful mother. She even briefly contemplated terminating the pregnancy. She had no interest in eating and lost a significant amount of weight. Her obstetrician became concerned about the baby's growth. She was referred to a reproductive psychiatrist for assessment.

The decision on whether to stop or continue antidepressant treatment in pregnancy, or later when breastfeeding, remains a dilemma for many women. Treatment is "complicated by the fact that few studies have been conducted to determine which medications are efficacious, how changes in body weight and metabolism may affect dosing, and what alternatives to medications are available that successfully treat psychiatric illness during pregnancy."[33(p218)] Thus, decisions must be made with limited quality evidence (see Chapter 14 for further exploration of this issue).

Unfortunately, medication use during pregnancy is often framed in terms of weighing maternal interests versus fetal interests. It is not uncommon for medical professionals to advise women about the risks of antidepressants to the fetus without providing comparative information about the risk of untreated depression to the mother, fetus, and later newborn.[1] Studies show that physicians worry more about risks of commission (actively doing something, such as performing a procedure or prescribing medication) than of omission (not doing something).[34] The main reason for this seems to be that physicians view themselves as more responsible for causing harm if the harm results from something they do or recommend, in contrast to something they do not do.[35] Yet, untreated depression also adversely affects fetal health. Evidence shows depressive symptoms in pregnancy are associated with poor nutrition, smoking, poor prenatal care, increased risk of substance use, low-birthweight infants, impaired mother–infant bonding, and suicidality.[6,36]

Respect for relational autonomy goes beyond recognizing the interrelated interests of mother and fetus to broadening the scope of what autonomy requires. Providers can draw on the principle of relational autonomy to justify exploring a patient's beliefs about medication use during pregnancy, and to create the groundwork for a careful discussion of the pros and cons of antidepressants within the particular context of that woman's life and illness. Addressing misperceptions about the risk of antidepressants is consistent with the promotion of autonomy. Rather than automatically agreeing to any choice a competent patient makes, relational autonomy asks providers to consider the particular contextual features that shape and constrain options for the woman. This may include addressing how social expectations about pregnancy and being a "good mother," coupled with stigma toward mental illness, may make it difficult for the patient to accept treatment. Indeed, depression is still seen by many as a character flaw rather than a serious medical illness with a potentially fatal outcome.

Respect for relational autonomy is consistent with a shared responsibility between the healthcare provider and patient for shaping and promoting the autonomy of the patient.[37] In this case, it is particularly important that the provider probes with Maria the meaning and perceived consequences of various options and how these shape her understanding of fetal risk. It is also important that Maria understands the rates of relapse and consequences of depression on her pregnancy and fetal development. At the same time, relational autonomy reminds us that attention to power differentials is essential when exploring a patient's values. This attention can guide providers to consider how the assumptions and values they hold about pregnancy, medication risk, and mental health influence the ways in which they advise the patient.

By attending to the particularity of the woman's life, the provider can engage in a process with the patient in which they consider available effective treatment, the comparative benefits and risks of each, and then work together to develop a plan of what works best for the patient.[38] If, after thoughtful discussion, Maria remains strongly against taking medication during pregnancy, her clinician should pursue a course of close follow-up and offer nonpharmacological treatment, like CBT, during and after the pregnancy. A partnership based on good communication is important to maintain so if the patient experiences a relapse of her condition, she will be engaged in care and hopefully more likely to seek treatment.

Enforced Treatment and Hospitalization

> Ann was diagnosed with schizophrenia when she was 25. She attended a mental health clinic and was prescribed an antipsychotic medication. She did well but did not like the weight that she gained as a side effect of her medication. Her boyfriend was also critical of her weight gain. Subsequently, Ann decided to stop taking her medication. Three months later, Ann returned to the clinic in a state of severe agitation. She told her worker that she was unable to sleep and was not eating. She reported that she was hearing male voices telling her not to go home. She was convinced that someone was "bugging" her rented room and trying to harm her. She had begun to sleep on the street. Her psychiatrist was concerned that she could be pregnant because her abdomen was clearly distended. Ann did not know if she was pregnant. She was very frightened and refused to consider returning to her rented room. She refused to restart her medication because she did not believe that she needed it. Her psychiatrist committed her involuntarily to psychiatric treatment because it was clear that she was at risk of harming herself.

Relational autonomy, like other bioethical theories, recognizes that not everyone has an equal opportunity or capacity for autonomous decision making. This patient exhibits vulnerabilities that cut across several dimensions. First, Ann is vulnerable because her psychosis distorts her view of reality, judgment, and, accordingly, capacity for voluntary choice. The nature of this illness is such that she does not recognize her illness and medical help is shunned. Second, Ann is vulnerable because of her possible pregnancy; until now, she has not received any prenatal care. Third, living on the streets leaves her susceptible to violence, exploitation, and abuse.

Because of her schizophrenia, Ann's capacity to make decisions and her ability to protect both herself and her fetus are severely compromised. A vulnerable person's diminished autonomy requires a delicate balance between empowering the person to make decisions of which she is capable and protecting her (and, in the case of pregnancy, the developing fetus) from excessive harm.[39] For vulnerable patients with severe mental illness, empowerment may be achieved "through social support, collaboration, education, and by encouraging relationships that help patients manage discrete aspects of their lives."[39(p.W2)] This includes collaborative relationships with healthcare providers and hospitalization as a safeguard when the individual is at risk of considerable harm. Vulnerable patients need advocacy, and Ann is no exception in this regard.

The same standards for inpatient psychiatric admission and use of emergency involuntary medication apply to pregnant women with psychotic disorders as for those who are not pregnant.[40] Specific pregnancy-related indications include a psychotic woman who does not recognize she is pregnant or in labor, refuses treatment, and therefore is at risk for unassisted delivery. In this case, Ann's paranoia and agitation pose a risk for continued inability to manage the multiple stresses of her pregnancy. Her clinician is faced with the need to balance the patient's interests (de-escalating acute psychotic symptoms with medications) with potential harm toward the patient (enforcing treatment against her will) and fetus (fetal exposure to medications with unknown risks). Relational ethics underscores the complexity of the situation because harm to the fetus (based on the mother's current behavior or psychiatric medication exposure) might prove ultimately harmful to the mother's mental health if she regrets the actions taken once her mental health improves.

In keeping with Dudzinski[39] and concepts of relational autonomy, we argue for an approach that supports the patient in her vulnerability through interdependence with others. This begins with her healthcare team. Healthcare providers can show respect for a person's impaired autonomy by restoring decisional capacity through treatment, by engaging the patient to voice preferences and participate in decision making, and by involving a surrogate. There is no harm-free intervention, but as Dudzinski and Sullivan observe: "In this way, we minimize some harm, accept that the patient may still suffer, and assuage that suffering through an ongoing therapeutic relationship."[41(p480)]

After the patient has regained capacity, she can participate more meaningfully in decisions regarding which antipsychotic medication to use. Eliciting a life narrative, which includes the women's identity, her relational style and coping mechanisms, and a reproductive history, can be therapeutic.[40] Through a collaborative process, the patient's values, strengths, and areas in which she needs support, as well as barriers and facilitators to her well-being, can be identified. Based on these features, a tailored relational approach can be developed to facilitate conditions that allow greater recognition and uptake of the patient's contributions in collaborative decisions regarding her pregnancy and upcoming birth.[42]

While this kind of approach may be similar to assisted decision making,[13,23] a relational perspective contributes to the understanding that interdependency is not autonomy-depriving but rather a form of empowerment for vulnerable persons whose judgment may be impaired due to mental illness. Further, it promotes the view that capacity is not only a cognitive skill alone but includes the ability to form and depend on important relationships. In other words, relational capacity is a skill that can be developed. It starts with an awareness of one's own limitations, and includes the ability to seek, find, and accept help in the context of positive and caring relationships. At the same time, a relational approach reminds us that not all relationships are positive, and some may disempower or harm vulnerable patients.

Disclosure to Fathers

> Betty was referred to a reproductive psychiatrist when she was 4 months pregnant to discuss her diagnosis and treatment plan. She was told that her partner was welcome to join the discussion, but Betty declined this offer. Betty had a long history of major depression and had responded well to her antidepressant medication. She did not want to make any changes to her medication because she was afraid that her mood would deteriorate. She was informed that she was at risk of experiencing a deterioration in her mood postpartum and that her medication dose might need to be increased after the delivery. It was recommended that her partner could provide her with both practical and emotional support after the delivery and monitor her mood for signs of a relapse. Betty was opposed to involving her partner, as she had not told him about her diagnosis. She was ashamed of her psychiatric history and was afraid that he would reject her because of it.

The decision on whether to share information about medication use with fathers (against the mother's wishes) is a common ethical issue arising in reproductive psychiatry. Disclosure reveals sensitive information about the mother and possibly about other family members. Clinicians may face the dilemma of who the information belongs to, especially if there is a possibility that the newborn may experience withdrawal symptoms from the medications taken during pregnancy.

Some clinicians would take the position that informing the partner about Betty's medical history and medication use would constitute a violation of trust and breach of confidentiality. Another possible harmful consequence of disclosure is that her partner may pressure Betty to stop taking medications during her pregnancy out of concern for the unborn child. A third possible harmful consequence may be the undermining of the family itself. The revelation that Betty has a mental illness may put pressure on the relationship and cause the couple to split up.

Considering the other side, the central arguments that would favor disclosure are (1) the father has a right to know, (2) physicians have a duty to truthful disclosure, and (3) disclosure may benefit the child. For example, studies indicate that exposure to SSRIs late in pregnancy may cause mild neonatal withdrawal symptoms (tremor, restlessness and increased crying, increased muscle tone). Knowledge that their baby's irritability is a transient symptom may ease the father's potential concerns and help him to care for the baby through this period.

Rather than a benefit–risk analysis, respect for relational autonomy turns our attention to Betty's relational and social context. Doing so reinforces the active role of the patient and the collaborative partnership between Betty and her clinician.

In this case, communication with Betty should include exploration of the rationale for her wishes and the nature of her concerns. Asking "why" is critical to understanding and assessing the situation, as well as building trust in the therapeutic relationship. Shared deliberation may include a deeper discussion of the impact that mental illness has had on Betty's relationships, friendships, and extended family. It may help reveal other aspects of home life that raise concern and, in turn, lead to a better understanding of the meaning and context shaping Betty's choice.

This collaborative approach also creates the opportunity for the psychiatrist to provide education and support to help Betty gain a better understanding of her own mental health. This may include a discussion of how stigma can become internalized, causing people to blame themselves for their condition and lead to self-imposed harms. By acknowledging the ways Betty and her partner are interdependent for support and emotional well-being, the psychiatrist can attend to the relational dimensions of Betty's life. This attention may guide the psychiatrist to raising the possibility of including the partner in future appointments so together they could discuss Betty's strengths and areas where she might need support. Likewise, clinicians committed to relational autonomy will be prepared to help address circumstances that hinder the patient's autonomy. Ultimately, however, if Betty refuses to share personal medical information with her partner, then her wishes should be respected.

Mother–Baby Units

> Patricia was delighted when her first son, Luke, was born after a protracted labor. However, she did not sleep for 3 days and was exhausted. That night, she lay awake, unable to sleep, thinking that the birth of her son was "a miracle." He was "a perfect baby, very special and destined for greatness." Because she couldn't sleep, she decided to clean the house and cook some meals to put in the freezer. Her husband became concerned that she was running around and talking nonstop. She shouted at him when he suggested that she return to bed. He was alarmed, as he had never seen Patricia act like this before. He called his mother, who suggested that he call 911. Patricia was taken to the emergency department and diagnosed with an acute manic episode, peripartum onset. She was hospitalized for psychiatric treatment under mental health legislation. She remained on a general psychiatric ward for 2 weeks and started on treatment. Her husband visited every day and brought Luke to visit for short periods of time. Her milk supply dried up in the hospital, and Patricia felt very guilty about not being able to breastfeed and being separated from Luke. She felt that she had "let my son down." When she was discharged from the hospital, she continued to bottle-feed Luke. She worried that he was not attached to her and appeared to prefer other family members. She was devastated if she could not console him.

Clinical strategizing, coupled with a model of preventive ethics, includes anticipating that some women with severe mental illness will need to be hospitalized. Women experiencing a mental health crisis are considered to be those who pose a severe threat to themselves, to others, or to their own or another's child. Indeed, all women are at risk for psychotic illness during the postpartum period, and those with bipolar illness are particularly vulnerable.[43] "The effect of these illnesses can be devastating if they are not recognized and treated promptly."[44(p10)]

Until fairly recently, mothers with postpartum mental illness were separated from their newborns out of concern for the baby's safety. The practice of separating mothers and babies began to shift, however, when research showed what many women knew intuitively: keeping mothers and babies together was best for forming a secure mother–child relationship. This led to the creation of mother–baby units (MBUs) where mother and baby are admitted jointly on the same ward.[45] The aim of joint admission and mother–baby treatment is not only to treat the mother's mental health disorder but to facilitate mother–infant interaction, foster a secure attachment between baby and mother, support parenting, and promote child development.[46,47] Without appropriate support, problems in the mother–baby relationship in the first year after childbirth are associated with increased maternal mental health problems and a range of problems for the baby, including delayed cognitive and emotional development.[5]

MBUs have been recommended in clinical guidelines internationally. In setting out practice standards for perinatal mental health, the National Institute for Health and Care Excellence (NICE) advises that women who need inpatient care should be admitted to a specialist MBU "unless there are specific reasons for not doing" (NICE Guideline. Antenatal and Postnatal Mental Health (2014). p. 79. https://www.nice.org.uk/guidance/cg192). Similarly, the Scottish Intercollegiate Guidelines Network recommends mothers have the option of joint MBU admission.[48] As early as 1992, the Royal College of Psychiatrists (UK) recommended MBUs as best practice for women with severe perinatal mental illness.[47]

Yet, as Brockington and colleagues point out, "no nation has come near to meeting the needs of mothers and their infants,"[49(p114)] and this is particularly true with respect to mothers with perinatal mental illness. MBU provision varies internationally. The countries that have most actively promoted specialized inpatient MBUs include the UK, Australia, France, and Belgium, which is reflected by the higher number of MBUs in those countries. The US has one and Canada none (to the best of our knowledge). While England leads the way—approximately 18 MBUs in total—delivery remains patchy and inconsistent and is some way from meeting the standards identified through NICE and the Royal Colleges.[16] A quality review of perinatal mental health services in England found that lack of support for perinatal mental health MBUs is "more often due to lack of funding and resources rather than lack of recognition of its importance."[16(p7)]

Feminist relational theory brings attention to how broader social, cultural, and historical contexts are ethically significant and thus subject to moral examination. This includes reflecting on entrenched cultural and political patterns that restrict options for socially disadvantaged groups. In relation to MBU funding, a critical theme that deserves attention is stigma, discrimination, and the devaluing of those with mental illness.

As Hinshaw[50] observed in 2007, stigma against people with mental disorders is universal. Despite the increasing recognition of the prevalence of mental illness, stigma and discriminatory attitudes prevail worldwide. Stigma occurs when elements of labeling, stereotyping, separation, status loss, and discrimination coexist within power relations that are unequal.[51] Indeed, persons with mental health disorders are commonly perceived as unpredictable, unfixable, and dangerous.[52] They are frequently blamed for their illness as being brought on by themselves.

Stigma and the ensuing discrimination create inequities at multiple levels. In comparison with physical diseases, mental illness predicts low levels of employment and independent housing and poor access to healthcare. Research funding regarding the causes and treatments for mental disorders lags far behind resources for physical illnesses, and the disparity in insurance coverage for mental disorders compared to coverage for other conditions is stark.[53] Those who divulge mental illness histories may face restrictions on the right to vote or the ability to obtain a driver's license or to maintain child custody.[50] Further, the media's association of mental illness with violence is pervasive and widely accepted. Yet research shows the contrary—that is, persons with mental illness are far more likely to be victims of violence than offenders.[54]

Governments have historically failed to respond appropriately to diseases that primarily afflict socially undesirable groups. On a systemic level, this is clearly seen through governments' unwillingness to invest in mental health services, fueling the myth that mental illness is untreatable and hopeless.[50] Notably, research shows that both patients and providers see a lack of resources for mental health as contributing to stigma.[52] This finding appears to be particularly apt with respect to the funding of MBUs. Not only do pregnant women or new mothers face discriminatory attitudes because of their mental disorder, but they may be further judged as being mentally, and thus also morally, unfit to care for their child. Indeed, many women are deterred from seeking help because of stigma or fear of losing their child, putting their and potentially their child's health at further risk.[16,44]

Promoting the mental health of pregnant women and new mothers should be a public health priority given the risks to both mothers and infants when mental illness is not treated.[49] Recognition of the unique harm inflicted on the mother–infant relationship by separation is essential for justice. Mother–infant separation threatens to diminish or destroy a woman's capacity to participate in activities that define what it means to be a mother, endangering her self-identity, notions of personhood, and ability to bond with her child. Further, poor mother–baby attachment has profoundly negative effects on the emotional and physical well-being of the child.[5]

A key strength of MBUs is that they allow mothers and infants to stay together. Different levels of supervision and support may be offered, depending on individual circumstances and risk. Patricia's story illustrates the psychological and emotional harms that can occur when mothers are separated from their babies. Further, these harms often persist, affecting the future relationship between mother and child and influencing other pregnancies she may have as well.

Conclusion

Feminist relational theory provides a powerful way of understanding the multiple challenges faced by women with perinatal mental illness and their providers. Women with perinatal mental health problems experience intense feelings of guilt and failure, stigma, and worries about being perceived unfit to care for their child. Rather than treating mother and infant as distinct and separate entities, relational theory highlights their mutual interdependency. A feminist concept of relational autonomy does not deny individuality or the importance of individual choice, but rather redirects our attention to context and relationships as necessary for human flourishing. It also brings attention to how ethical issues and illness processes are linked to the broader social and structural contexts of women, their clinicians, and their communities.

Indeed, any approach to improving care for women with perinatal mental illness must be multifaceted and multilevel. Sustainable solutions to maternal mental health require a mix of system-based strategies, changes to organizational and mental health practices, consistent guidelines for practitioners, as well as improving access to evidence-based treatments for women and their families. It is important to engage all stakeholders—professionals and the public alike—in creating awareness about perinatal mental health and in making a concerted effort to challenge the stereotypes that the media impose on persons with mental illness. As others have highlighted, stigma is a form of social injustice.[50] It not only thwarts recovery but affects personal agency. Further, recognizing the profound harm that separation inflicts on the mother–infant relationship is a necessary first step in developing adequate crisis support for women.

References

1. Miller L. Ethical issues in perinatal mental health. *Psychiatr Clin North Am.* 2009;32:259–270.

2. Antonucci T, Mikus K. The power of parenthood: personality and attitudinal changes during the transition to parenthood. In: Michaels G, Goldberg W, eds. *The Transition to Parenthood*. Cambridge, UK: Cambridge University Press; 1988:62–84.
3. Côté-Arsenault D, Denney-Koelsch E. "Have no regrets:" parents' experiences and developmental tasks in pregnancy with a lethal fetal diagnosis. *Soc Sci Med*. 2016;154:100–109. doi:10.1016/j.socscimed.2016.02.033
4. Miller L. Psychotherapy for pregnant women with schizophrenia. *Curr Womens Health Rev*. 2010;6:39–43.
5. National Institute for Health and Care Excellence (NICE). *Antenatal and Postnatal Mental Health*. National Institute for Health and Care Excellence; 2014:923.
6. British Columbia Reproductive Mental Health Program. *Best Practice Guidelines for Mental Health Disorders in the Perinatal Period*. British Columbia: BC Mental Health & Substance Use Services and Perinatal Services BC; 2014:1–118. www.perinatalservicesbc.ca/Documents/Maternal/MentalHealthDisordersGuidelin.
7. Howard LM, Ryan EG, Trevillion K, et al. Accuracy of the Whooley questions and the Edinburgh Postnatal Depression Scale in identifying depression and other mental disorders in early pregnancy. *Br J Psychiatry J Ment Sci*. 2018;212(1):50–56. doi:10.1192/bjp.2017.9
8. ACOG Practice Bulletin No. 92: Use of psychiatric medications during pregnancy and lactation. *Obstet Gynecol*. 2008;111(4):1001–1020. doi:10.1097/AOG.0b013e31816fd910
9. Galloway S, Hogg S. *Getting It Right for Mothers and Babies: Closing the Gaps in Community Perinatal Mental Health Services*. NSPCC Scotland; 2015. www.nspcc.org.uk/globalassets/documents/research-reports/getting-it-right.
10. World Health Organization. *Maternal Mental Health*. 2016. www.who.int/mental_health/maternal-child/maternal_mental_health/.
11. Frieder A. Preconception counseling for women with schizophrenia. *Curr Women's Health Rev*. 2010;6:12–16.
12. King-Hele S, Webb RT, Mortensen PB, Appleby L, Pickles A, Abel KM. Risk of stillbirth and neonatal death linked with maternal mental illness: a national cohort study. *Arch Dis Child Fetal Neonatal Ed*. 2009;94(2):F105–110. doi:10.1136/adc.2007.135459
13. Coverdale J, McCullough L, Chervenak F. Ethical issues in managing the pregnancies of patients with schizophrenia. *Curr Womens Health Rev*. 2010;6:63–67.
14. Shah A, Christophersen R. Prenatal care for women with schizophrenia. *Curr Women's Health Rev*. 2010;6:28–33.
15. Seeman M. Parenting issues in mothers with schizophrenia. *Curr Women's Health Rev*. 2010;6:51–57.

16. NHS Improving Quality. *Improving Access to Perinatal Mental Health Services in England. A Review.* NHS Improving Quality; 2015.
17. Flynn H, Blow F, Marcus S. Rates and predictors of depression treatment among pregnant women in hospital-affiliated obstetrics practices. *Gen Hosp Psychiatry.* 2006;28(4):289–295.
18. Friedman SH, Resnick P. Postpartum depression: an update. *Womens Health.* 2009;5(3):287–295.
19. Cohen LS, Altshuler LL, Harlow BL, et al. Relapse of major depression during pregnancy in women who maintain or discontinue antidepressant treatment. *JAMA.* 2006;295(5):499–507. doi:10.1001/jama.295.5.499
20. Viguera AC, Whitfield T, Baldessarini RJ, et al. Risk of recurrence in women with bipolar disorder during pregnancy: prospective study of mood stabilizer discontinuation. *Am J Psychiatry.* 2007;164(12):1817–1824; quiz 1923. doi:10.1176/appi.ajp.2007.06101639
21. ACOG Committee Opinion No. 390: Ethical decision making in obstetrics and gynecology. *Obstet Gynecol.* 2007;110(6):1479–1487. doi:10.1097/01.AOG.0000291573.09193.36
22. Harris LH. Rethinking maternal-fetal conflict: gender and equality in perinatal ethics. *Obstet Gynecol.* 2000;96(5 Pt 1):786–791.
23. McCullough L, Chervenak F. *Ethics in Obstetrics and Gynecology.* New York, NY: Oxford University Press; 1994.
24. Chasnoff IJ, Landress HJ, Barrett ME. The prevalence of illicit-drug or alcohol use during pregnancy and discrepancies in mandatory reporting in Pinellas County, Florida. *N Engl J Med.* 1990;322(17):1202–1206. doi:10.1056/NEJM199004263221706
25. Metzl J, Roberts D. Structural competency meets structural racism: race, politics, and the structure of medical knowledge. *JAMA J Med Ethics Virtual Mentor.* 2014;16(9):674–690.
26. MacKenzie C. Conceptions of autonomy and conceptions of the body in bioethics. In: Scully J, Baldwin-Ragaven L, Fitzpatrick M, eds. *Feminist Bioethics: At the Center, On the Margins.* Baltimore, MD: Johns Hopkins University Press; 2010:71–90.
27. Grisso T, Appelbaum PS. Appreciating anorexia: decisional capacity and the role of values. *Philos Psychiatry Amp Psychol.* 2007;13(4):293–297. doi:10.1353/ppp.2007.0030
28. MacKenzie C, Stoljar N, eds. *Relational Autonomy: Feminist Perspectives on Autonomy, Agency and the Social Self.* New York, NY: Oxford University Press; 2000.
29. Nedelsky J. *Law's Relations: A Relational Theory of Self, Autonomy and Law.* New York, NY: Oxford University Press; 2011.
30. Sherwin S. *No Longer Patient: Feminist Ethics and Health Care.* Philadelphia, PA: Temple University Press; 1992.

31. Walker MU. *Moral Understandings*. New York, NY: Routledge; 1998.
32. Fitzpatrick P, Scully J. Theory in feminist bioethics. In: Scully J, Baldwin-Ragaven L, Fitzpatrick P, eds. *Feminist Bioethics: At the Center, On the Margins*. Baltimore, MD: Johns Hopkins University Press; 2010:61–70.
33. Payne JL. Psychopharmacology in pregnancy and breastfeeding. *Psychiatr Clin North Am*. 2017;40(2):217–238. doi:10.1016/j.psc.2017.01.001
34. Kordes-de Vaal JH. Intention and the omission bias: omissions perceived as nondecisions. *Acta Psychol (Amst)*. 1996;93(1-3):161–172.
35. Wand APF. Making decisions in the management of perinatal depression and anxiety. *Adv Psychiatr Treat*. 2014;20(03):175–183. doi:10.1192/apt.bp.113.011866
36. Friedman SH. The ethics of treating depression in pregnancy. *J Prim Health Care*. 2015;7(1):81–83.
37. Ells C, Hunt MR, Chambers-Evans J. Relational autonomy as an essential component of patient-centered care. *Int J Fem Approaches Bioeth*. 2011;4(2):79–101.
38. Hunt MR, Ells C. A patient-centered care ethics analysis model for rehabilitation. *Am J Phys Med Rehabil*. 2013;92(9):818–827. doi:10.1097/PHM.0b013e318292309b
39. Dudzinski DM. Compounding vulnerability: pregnancy and schizophrenia. *Am J Bioeth AJOB*. 2006;6(2):W1–14. doi:10.1080/15265160500506191
40. Spielvogel A, Lee E. Indication for psychiatric inpatient hospitalization for pregnant psychotic women. *Curr Womens Health Rev*. 2010;6:44–58.
41. Dudzinski DM, Sullivan M. When agreeing with the patient is not enough: a schizophrenic woman requests pregnancy termination. *Gen Hosp Psychiatry*. 2004;26(6):475–480. doi:10.1016/j.genhosppsych.2004.07.002
42. Durocher E, Kinsella EA, Ells C, Hunt M. Contradictions in client-centred discharge planning: through the lens of relational autonomy. *Scand J Occup Ther*. 2015;22(4):293–301. doi:10.3109/11038128.2015.1017531
43. O'Hara MW, Wisner KL. Perinatal mental illness: definition, description and aetiology. *Best Pract Res Clin Obstet Gynaecol*. 2014;28(1):3–12. doi:10.1016/j.bpobgyn.2013.09.002
44. Mental Welfare Commission of Scotland. *Perinatal Themed Visit Report: Keeping Mothers and Babies in Mind*. 2016:1–77. www.mwcscot.org.uk/media/320718/perinatal_report_final.pdf.
45. Howard LM. The separation of mothers and babies in the treatment of postpartum psychotic disorders in Britain 1900–1960. *Arch Womens Ment Health*. 2000;3(1):1–5. doi:10.1007/PL00010323
46. Connellan K, Bartholomaeus C, Due C, Riggs DW. A systematic review of research on psychiatric mother-baby units. *Arch Womens Ment Health*. 2017;20(3):373–388. doi:10.1007/s00737-017-0718-9
47. Glangeaud-Freudenthal NMC, Howard LM, Sutter-Dallay A-L. Treatment—mother-infant inpatient units. *Best Pract Res Clin Obstet Gynaecol*. 2014;28(1):147–157. doi:10.1016/j.bpobgyn.2013.08.015

48. Scottish Intercollegiate Guidelines Network. *Management of Perinatal Mood Disorders.* https://www.sign.ac.uk/sign-127-management-of-perinatal-mood-disorders.html
49. Brockington I, Butterworth R, Glangeaud-Freudenthal N. An international position paper on mother-infant (perinatal) mental health, with guidelines for clinical practice. *Arch Womens Ment Health.* 2017;20(1):113–120. doi:10.1007/s00737-016-0684-7
50. Hinshaw S. *The Mark of Shame: Stigma of Mental Illness and an Agenda for Change.* New York, NY: Oxford University Press; 2007.
51. Link BG, Phelan JC. Conceptualizing stigma. *Annu Rev Sociol.* 2001;27(1):363–385. doi:10.1146/annurev.soc.27.1.363
52. Sukhera J, Miller K, Milne A, et al. Labelling of mental illness in a paediatric emergency department and its implications for stigma reduction education. *Perspect Med Educ.* 2017;6(3):165–172. doi:10.1007/s40037-017-0333-5
53. Hinshaw S, Stier A. Stigma in relation to mental disorders. *Annu Rev Clin Psychol.* 2008;2008(4):269–293.
54. Teplin LA, McClelland GM, Abram KM, Weiner DA. Crime victimization in adults with severe mental illness: comparison with the National Crime Victimization Survey. *Arch Gen Psychiatry.* 2005;62(8):911–921. doi:10.1001/archpsyc.62.8.911

12 TECHNOLOGY AND THE ETHICAL PRACTICE OF REPRODUCTIVE CARE

A WOMAN-CENTERED LENS

Laura A. Sturgill, Sara G. Shields, and Lucy M. Candib

Introduction

> Despite our best efforts, technology, supposedly the handmaiden to clinical care, has diverted our attention away from the pregnant woman herself, toward representations of the fetus—biochemical, visual, and electrical. . . . Make no mistake: women desperately want and demand these technologies. But the overall impact is to make each pregnancy and birth less woman-centered and more focused on the fetus.[1(p3)]

Reproductive ethics today often concerns itself with various aspects of assisted reproduction: embryo transfer/preservation/reduction, sex selection, reproductive cloning, surrogacy, and a variety of other thorny topics. However, this framework represents only one point of departure on a huge landscape of the world of women and their bodies in the context of technology, the world of "technomaternity."[2] Maternity has become dominated by the technological process that may start or prevent it (fertility treatments, contraception, abortion), the tests that document and evaluate it (blood tests and ultrasounds), and the tests that "invade it" (chorionic villi sampling and amniocentesis). These tests lead to further ultrasounds that increasingly project a larger and more complete image of the fetus, while reducing the actuality of the mother, whose role becomes the house in a play where the lead actor is on the stage in the living room. Finally, the contemporary practice of continuous fetal monitoring during labor makes clear that technological indicators reflect what is important in labor, not the mother's experience.

Turning the mother into the dwelling (or landlady? or vehicle?) of the inhabitant removes her subjectivity; she becomes a transparent object valuable only for bringing the treasured inhabitant into focus both physically and technically,[2] and she is often devalued because her body—the vehicle—may be uncooperative, unwieldy, even risky for the fetus (e.g., Is she obese? Will her body habitus be a problem in labor? Did she drink alcohol or use other substances during the pregnancy?).

Mothers today (and their partners and families) certainly want and even demand elements of technology (e.g., blood tests, ultrasounds, monitoring). Reproductive technology has become the new normal just as motor vehicles became the standard locomotion method in developed nations during the 20th century. But adoption of technology as the standard of measuring and describing pregnancy creates an ethical distortion of how women and their pregnancies are viewed—by clinicians, institutions, the media, and culture itself. In this chapter we examine techno-maternity through the lens of woman-centered care. This model offers us an ethical standpoint from which to view women and their pregnancies.

Beginnings

Pregnancy is a time of profound physical changes that inevitably alter a woman's sense of control over her body. Early symptoms, sometimes occurring before the pregnancy is suspected, may include nausea, vomiting, overwhelming fatigue, breast tenderness, change in body shape, back pain, bloating, and swelling. A woman's increasingly unrecognizable size and shape in later trimesters, together with poor sleep and increasing physical discomfort, make it entirely clear that she has limited control over this process. Meanwhile, techno-maternity tells the woman that her pregnant body (and the way she lives in it) puts the fetus "at risk," justifying a variety of restrictions and imposing Foucauldian surveillance.[2] Increasingly, the medical world and much of society consider a woman's pregnancy through this sense of persistent possibility of risk.

Global Issues

Before addressing how technology dominates maternity care in industrialized settings, we wish to situate the discussion within an international perspective.

Pregnancy is still a highly risky state *globally* for women, especially in resource-poor settings where the most basic technology is lacking. The greatest biomedical threats from pregnancy and childbirth—hemorrhage, infection, unsafe abortion, hypertension and eclampsia, and obstructed labor—can happen to pregnant women in the best of circumstances. However, around the world, pregnant women in low-resource locations face higher risks in pregnancy than women elsewhere *due to lack of access* to basic safe maternity care, including abortion, though the means to address the problems are known and affordable.

Unsafe abortions cause *one of every eight maternal deaths worldwide* each year (about 50,000 deaths), especially in Africa and Latin America.[3,4] The United Nations (UN) defines unsafe abortion as "a procedure for terminating an unintended pregnancy carried out either by persons lacking the necessary skills or in an environment that does not conform to minimal medical standards, or both."[3] The technology for safe medical, suction, and surgical abortion is well known but poorly available in most low- and middle-income countries. As Regan and Glasier point out in a recent editorial in *The Lancet*, "Liberalizing abortion laws saves women's lives."[5(p.1936)] They report that the 1989 loosening of abortion laws in Romania led to a drop in maternal mortality by more than 50% in less than a year. These authors estimate that if countries with restrictive abortion laws had passed legislation fifty years ago, as did the UK, permitting abortion, even with some restrictions (e.g., a woman seeking abortion in the UK must get two physicians to sign off on the procedure), millions of women's lives would have been saved.[5]

The UN Human Rights Council reaffirms women's right to abortion and deems denial of a therapeutic abortion to be a form of torture; in other words,

> a violation of the individual's right to be free from ill-treatment. . . . The Committee against Torture has repeatedly expressed concerns about restrictions on access to abortion and about absolute bans on abortion as violating the prohibition of torture and ill-treatment.[6]

Thus, despite the visibility of conflict about abortion in the US today, the key contemporary problem in reproductive ethics is not about the morality of legal abortion services and the need for such services extending beyond the first trimester of pregnancy. Rather, the entirely immoral reality today is that basic life-saving maternity care technology and personnel already exist to reduce the unacceptable maternal and infant mortality rates, even in low-resource settings. Likewise, safe, simple abortion strategies exist but are unavailable to the hundreds of thousands of women who now must seek dangerous procedures to end a pregnancy, sometimes ending their own lives. Moreover, a variety of existing effective and safe contraceptive methods, if made fully available, could limit the need for women to seek abortions. These are the overarching ethical challenges in reproductive healthcare that we are setting aside now when we speak of the problems introduced by highly technologized care.

A morally responsible, contemporary approach to ethical matters pertaining to women's reproductive lives must also recognize the legacy of shameful abusive practices that characterized historical attempts to manage women's fertility. This history is relevant because the power of medicine, like other forms of power and control, is *always* vulnerable to abuse, and disadvantaged and disenfranchised persons, often women and often people of color, are always the most at risk.

Sterilization abuse of women, primarily minorities, psychiatric patients, disabled persons, prisoners, and persons considered unfit for reproduction (because of their sexual behavior), has a long history in the US, and to a lesser extent in Canada. African Americans, Mexican Americans, and Puerto Ricans were the main racial and ethnic targets of forced sterilization starting in the 1920s. Puerto Rico was a special showcase of sterilization policies, resulting in 34% of Puerto Rican women having been sterilized by 1965.[7] At one point the rate of postpartum sterilization was so high that the Joint Committee for Hospital Accreditation insisted that the hospitals in Puerto Rico limit sterilization to a maximum of 10% of deliveries to stay accredited.[8] Grounded initially in the eugenics movements of the early 20th century, the abusive practices diminished after the exposures of the Nazis' large-scale sterilizations but nevertheless continued even until the 1980s in California, when legal challenges and public exposures finally ended large-scale abuses in the US.[9] In Canada, sterilization abuse was aggressively practiced in Alberta from 1929 until 1971, when the Sterilization Act was overturned. Although initially promoted to prevent pregnancies among mentally disabled people, by the 1940s the law was used to justify sterilization of women based on their moral and personal behaviors ("promiscuity").[10] Of the 2,834 persons sterilized under this law, about 7.5% were First Nations people at a time when they represented only 3.4% of the Alberta's population.[11] Although these events occurred decades ago, the history remains lodged in the collective memory of many communities, leading to cross-generational mistrust of medical systems.

Forced sterilization of women persists in some countries and institutions today: coerced sterilization and abortion persist in China,[12] and coerced sterilization of HIV-positive women continues in Latin America and Africa.[13] The UN Human Rights Council reports:

> Targeting ethnic and racial minorities, women from marginalized communities and women with disabilities for involuntary sterilization because of discriminatory notions that they are "unfit" to bear children is an increasingly global problem. Forced sterilization is an act of violence, a form of social control, and a violation of the right to be free from torture and other cruel, inhuman, or degrading treatment or punishment . . . forced abortions or sterilizations carried out by State officials in accordance with coercive family planning laws or policies may amount to torture.[6]

Even in the US, nearly 150 female California prison inmates were sterilized between 2006 and 2010, many without informed consent. This prompted Governor Jerry Brown to sign a bill in 2014 prohibiting forced sterilizations in prisons.[14] Thus, an ethical approach to women's reproductive lives must begin with an acknowledgment of women's vulnerability to abuse globally from both within and outside the world of healthcare.

Woman-Centered Care

Woman-centered care (WCC) is the ethical strategy to approach a woman considering reproductive options and decisions. This model does the following:[1]

- Identifies a woman's feelings, ideas, and expectations about the situation
- Recognizes and attempts to reduce the often immense power differential between clinician and patient
- Provides intelligible information about options
- Accepts the woman's values even if different from the provider's own
- Admits uncertainty
- Supports the woman within her chosen relationships with supportive others, yet reminds her she is a valuable person who can make independent choices
- Recognizes the frequency, severity, and probability of violence in women's lives and therefore addresses the woman's experience of past and present abuse (physical, sexual, and emotional)

This is time-consuming work and often yields a conflict between ethical care and the economic realities of contemporary medical practice. Going forward, we will address some of the challenges of trying to provide this model of WCC in today's technological world of reproduction. We review ethical issues in reproductive care that routinely emerge during key periods: adolescence (e.g., access to and choice of contraception; access to and decisions about abortion); desired pregnancy (making decisions about genetic screening); labor and delivery (maintaining WCC in a feto-centric environment); and the postpartum period (promoting breastfeeding in the technological world of breast milk substitutes [formula] and breast pumps). This sampling of potential ethical difficulties involving technology in reproductive care is not comprehensive but rather representative of the situations woman-centered clinicians face daily.

Contraception and Adolescence

> Beth is a 16-year-old girl who recently became sexually active. She uses condoms most of the time but worries about pregnancy. She has read about birth control online and talked with friends who use different methods. She decides to visit her family doctor to ask for Depo-Provera™ shots. She does not want her parents to find out that she is sexually active. Her doctor has told her in private that she can have confidential services for birth control if needed. When she calls the office to schedule an appointment, the receptionist questions why she is calling rather than her parent. She explains that it is a confidential visit, but she feels so embarrassed that she almost skips the appointment. At the visit, her doctor supports her decision to prevent pregnancy but strongly encourages her to consider an intrauterine device (IUD) or contraceptive implant. Beth doesn't want a procedure or something that stays in her body, so she persists in asking for "Depo." About a month later, her parents confront her with the summary they received from their insurance company, indicating her visit at their doctor's office and contraceptive treatment.
>
> Six months later, after missing a "Depo" shot a few months earlier, Beth finds out she is pregnant. Devastated, she feels strongly that she is not able to carry a pregnancy or parent a child at this time. She goes to her local Planned Parenthood clinic to find out about terminating the pregnancy and learns that her state requires parental consent for minors to terminate pregnancy. Again she has to have hard conversations with her parents before getting the care she wants.

As family doctors adhering to the ideals of WCC, we like to think the process starts with the woman's expressed intentions to pursue or prevent pregnancy. Beth, the teen who recently became sexually active, understands her potential fertility and clearly does not want to become a mother now. This degree of clarity is not always present at the beginning of the conversation. Some women do not have the health literacy to understand their fertility or the connection between sexual intercourse and pregnancy, and some women feel ambivalent toward a possible pregnancy. Accurate assessment of the woman's starting place is vital to knowing how to frame the conversation.

The US Centers for Disease Control and Prevention (CDC) recommends preconception planning and counseling to improve the health of women and families.[15] Multiple medical groups have endorsed various approaches to reproductive goal setting, including the One Key Question model (pregnancy intention for the coming year) and reproductive life plan model.[16,17] The goal of these approaches is noble: if a woman expresses clear intentions NOT to have a baby, the clinician should work with her to meet her goal of avoiding pregnancy, and vice versa with positive pregnancy intention. However, up to 30% of women are ambivalent about the idea of pregnancy, and that ambivalence may manifest as changeable intentions.[18]

We might more accurately reframe ambivalence as flexibility. Its origins may lie in culture, religion, and difference between personal and partner or family expectations. Some women feel it more acceptable to "accidentally" become pregnant if their life circumstances are not stable enough to admit they would like to have a baby. In the clinician–patient relationship, a woman may withhold this ambivalence, or withhold truth and present ambivalence, in an effort to provide the answer she thinks the clinician wants to hear. In our often well-planned lives, we as clinicians may find it hard to imagine that someone may be undecided about having a baby, even if she cannot express that ambivalence. Unfortunately, these assumptions and judgments can create a "mismatch between a focus on dichotomous intention and a woman's own perspectives regarding future pregnancy," impairing the clinical relationship and the woman's ability to get needed care.[18(p130)] So the questions then become transformed: What really is an unplanned pregnancy? Should we judge it as a negative thing based on data about outcomes, or should we work to improve outcomes based on all of the possibilities? How do we truly elicit women's intentions, even if they are not clear, or when we do not understand the underlying motivations?

Motivational interviewing (MI) provides one possible framework for approaching these complex conversations. Designed to help move patients from ambivalence to clarity, with their permission, MI starts with deep listening to the patient's starting place, followed by reflecting back to the patient her statements in a nonjudgmental, affirming attitude. Carefully crafted questions and reflective statements can define the ambivalence and invite the patient to grapple with it. In this style of contraceptive counseling, we listen carefully to what is most important to the woman and then reflect that back with suggestions meaningful to that particular woman at that particular time.[19] Though we as providers are approaching this with the goal of movement from ambivalence to clarity and toward greater feelings of self-efficacy, this approach requires patience; we should approach it with the expectation that the ambivalence may not be resolved in a single or even several sessions.

One of the largest growth areas in contraception is long-acting reversible contraception (LARC). Feminist proponents of LARC tout it as being liberating, in that it finally removes the stresses of worrying about accidental conception and of remembering responsibly about daily pills, weekly patches, or condoms and so forth. (Condoms are still essential, however, for protection from sexually transmitted infections, an important risk for sexually active teens.) For adolescents, LARC has been promoted as first-line contraception by both the American Academy of Pediatrics and the American College of Obstetrics and Gynecologists.[20,21] However, LARC requires a provider to perform a procedure for both insertion and removal. If we promote LARC and provide easy access to insertion without access to removal that is just as reliable, effortless, rapid, and affordable, LARC runs the risk of becoming one more example of coercive reproductive technology, in the same arena as forced sterilization. This risk is especially worrisome if LARC is being heavily promoted in those same populations who are traditionally disenfranchised or otherwise underserved, as we have discussed. We should pay close attention to attempts to coerce women into using LARC, and we should pay just as much attention to access for removal as access to insertion. When a woman requests LARC removal, we should remember that she has a right to have the device removed from her body, even if she does not have a clear reason, or one that we agree with, or one that she can express.

Adolescents counseled with MI techniques are more likely to choose and appropriately use highly effective birth control, including LARC, and report significantly higher satisfaction with the encounter.[19,22] Contraception choice is not a goal but rather a process, and what is right for a woman at one time may not be right later. Her priorities may change. If a woman states avoiding pregnancy is her highest priority, she may be counseled toward LARC, but the clinician also must elicit how she feels about indwelling devices and about being dependent on a medical provider for discontinuation. While the woman brings her assumptions and experiences to the discussion, providers also bring cultural, moral, logical, and personal experiences to the table but often do not name them for women (or for ourselves, for that matter). Thus, clinicians need to cultivate insight into our own biases and judgments to prevent them from interfering with the patient's process.

Supported decision making is only the first step in the process of ensuring that women get the care they need and deserve. Multiple barriers interfere with enacting reproductive health plans: finances, geography, accessibility and training of providers, system requirements for visits, and availability of medications and contraceptive devices. Some providers require pelvic exams, multiple pregnancy tests, or other non–evidence-based measures prior to providing contraception. In a study of British women who chose telemedicine-provided medical abortions rather than the widely available surgical abortions through the National Health Service, women cited a barrier of too many required visits prior to abortion.[23] Ulipristal is an effective hormonal emergency contraception, but a survey of pharmacies in major cities across the US revealed that fewer than 10% of pharmacies stocked the medication.[24] For a method that requires timely use, such unavailability, when a woman and her clinician decide that this treatment is best for her, is unethical.

So-called conscience-based barriers significantly reduce access to effective contraception and abortion care for women. Individual providers may refuse to counsel, provide, and/or refer for services they find personally objectionable. In the US, providers are legally protected in this refusal (even the refusal to refer) by federal statute.[25] Hospitals and other healthcare systems limit services provided because of institutional or leadership views of morality. Throughout the world, legal barriers to contraception and abortion are grounded in such moralism. The extent of this barrier loosely masks discrimination against women: "By being refused the means of gaining control over their reproductive lives women are deprived of the attendant benefits." Quoting directly from *Roe v. Wade*, Card is referring to the benefit of women's ability "to participate equally in the economic and social life of the Nation."[26(p2)] International ethics guidelines state that individual providers have the right to abstain from practices they find morally objectionable, but they should provide access for the patient to obtain the care by other means. When the patient's health or life is at stake, if there is no one else to provide the care, providers' first responsibility is to the patient. Manipulation of information to guide women toward a choice the provider feels is more morally acceptable is unethical and antithetical to WCC.

Adolescent access to birth control carries specific ethical dilemmas, in particular respect for the principle of autonomy. In the US, in contrast to Canada and Europe, adolescents are not traditionally considered autonomous, meaning that, legally, only their parents can make decisions regarding their medical care. Most states in the US have legal provisions for exceptions to this rule, enabling adolescents to function as autonomous decision makers for certain aspects of their care, usually limited to reproductive health and addiction care. One impetus for this increased legal autonomy is evidence that teens seek care for these concerns more often if guaranteed privacy.[27] Thus, legally, in many locations, adolescents can seek birth control without their parents' knowledge or permission. Despite this legal right, as illustrated in the vignette about Beth, multiple barriers exist. For organizations to maintain confidentiality, all their staff and clinicians must both understand the importance of and prioritize systems to protect adolescents' privacy so they will seek the reproductive healthcare that they have the right (and desire) to receive.[27]

Ethical Considerations of Genetic Screening in Pregnancy

> Pat and Mike had each had negative experiences with doctors during their formative years and shared a persisting distrust of the medical profession. After a distressing miscarriage in their early 30s, they finally became pregnant again when Pat was 35. They wanted to know about genetic testing for chromosome problems but did not want any intervention that could harm the fetus. They were adamant that no matter what might go wrong, they would under no circumstance terminate a pregnancy. When Pat's integrated screening tests at 16 weeks suggested an increased risk of 1 in 50 of a fetus with trisomy 21 (Down syndrome) and her anatomy ultrasound showed a mild abnormality that could be present in a fetus with Down syndrome, her provider advised that amniocentesis was the only sure way to ascertain if the fetus truly was affected. Upset and worried, she and Mike read about the cell-free DNA blood test and requested it instead to see if they could get any clearer answer without the procedure. They were relieved when the cell-free DNA results were normal.

Genetic screening of the fetus during pregnancy is routine in countries with highly developed medical systems. Multiple complex tests are available with varying timing and differing levels of accuracy as the pregnancy progresses. Some testing only requires blood specimens; some link serial blood tests with ultrasound; and some are invasive, can be painful, and pose some direct risk to the fetus (less so to the mother). Explaining prenatal genetic screening well requires understanding of the limitations and risks of each test, time to explain this information to the woman and her partner or support person, and skill in making sure that she or they understand the explanation.

Providers themselves may have their own limitations, such as bias about patients having screening and expectations that patients will conform to "ordinary" standards, without exploring unique factors that might lead to alternative decisions. In addition, interpreting the tests is complex, as they have uncertainty and variation within them. Many obstetrical providers (family physicians, obstetricians, and midwives) have difficulty describing test accuracy and reveal poor understandings of the biostatistical aspects of the tests (e.g., false positive, false negative, positive predictive value).[28,29] And in the medical culture in general, across nations, clinicians tend to overestimate the benefits of treatments, tests, and screening and to underestimate the harms.[30,31]

Specific skills are needed to adequately counsel about testing and to explain the meaning and limitations of test results. The first step involves exploring the woman's values. Then the clinician can explain the procedures involved and ask the woman (and her partner, if present) whether she wants to pursue testing. Further challenges arise if the woman has limited education and literacy (poor understanding may lead to refusing or accepting the test but not understanding what she has agreed to or declined). Already anxious about doing the right thing for her pregnancy, a woman may struggle to understand these complex subjects and may not hear, understand, or retain what a clinician tells her. A huge gap can result between what a woman thinks the test is for and what it really determines. For non–English-speaking patients, interpreter style is also important in whether a woman will accept screening (e.g., an interview in which the interpreter has a "distant" style is less likely to result in a woman accepting amniocentesis compared with the outcome when the interpreter has a more empathic style).[32] Culture also plays a role in how women interpret information. In one studied situation, genetic counselors tried to give Mexican-American women a balanced picture about amniocentesis in the face of an abnormal alpha-fetoprotein test; many women chose not to have the amniocentesis done. Returning to the women later to explore this choice, the investigators learned that the women concluded that if the test was a good thing to do, then the counselor *would have recommended* it; when she did not recommend it, they concluded that it was not necessary or indicated.[33]

Culture and setting also affect decisions about prenatal testing. Time pressures in outpatient office settings often preclude lengthy discussion. Most clinical settings lack dedicated personnel to review the pros and cons of genetic screening with women and couples in educationally and culturally appropriate ways. At the same time, most women are not routinely referred to genetic counseling for the routine testing; indeed, in many regions, genetic counselors are not readily available even for high-risk women. As a result, maternity providers may end up being their patients' principal resource for genetic screening information. Clinicians may also lack education or experience in the social and cultural context of genetic screening for their patients. For instance, women and their partners from communities of color may distrust testing from a fear that recommendations about an abnormal fetus might carry racist bias. Provider ignorance of the history of forced sterilization in US history (see the beginning of this chapter) can exacerbate the misunderstanding.

WCC in Childbirth

Childbirth is one of the most common areas in women's reproductive health where patient values and the culture of medicine intersect and even clash. Labor is often considered the most painful experience of a woman's life. Accordingly, she may not be able to engage in complicated decision making, and the traditional power hierarchy between doctor and patient can become a slippery slope to provider-centered choices rather than truly informed consent.

The "techno-maternity" model of labor practiced in the US, Canada, the UK, and other high-resource countries relies on the technologies and techniques of labor induction, epidural analgesia, continuous electronic fetal monitoring, and cesarean delivery. These interventions are touted as part of a roadmap for improved safety in maternity care, yet this medicalization has made little headway in improving certain perinatal health outcomes and has actually worsened others (e.g., the soaring cesarean rates in low-risk women). Around the world, providers, pregnant women, and their families falsely interpret this evolving technology as better and safer.[1]

Healy describes this contradiction as the "double-edged sword" of the benefit of technology in reducing infant and maternal mortality with the risks of overuse without clinical indication.[34(p368)] Modern obstetrics emphasizes risk rather than health in pregnancy and childbirth, leading to the perception that safe birth requires intense medical surveillance with technology.[34,35] Even midwives, traditionally viewed as the maternity providers with the most emphasis on health and normality, "increasingly view birth as abnormal with normality now defined by the absence of abnormality."[34(p368)] In the last trimester of pregnancy, this mindset of the womb as a dangerous place leads both providers and patients alike to seek reassurance from the technology of repeated ultrasounds and measuring amniotic fluid and fetal breathing, without fully recognizing how such overuse further fosters the "maxi-min" approach of contemporary obstetrics.[36]

Meta-analysis suggests that midwifery models of care may improve outcomes for women and their infants, but in the US not all insurers cover these options, or women may not be able to find these models in their communities.[37] Thus, since the techno-maternity system "overwhelmingly favors medicalized birth," women who seek midwifery care may not have fully autonomous choices or access to truly shared decision making.[38(p2)]

Women with a prior cesarean section may face similar roadblocks to autonomy in their choices for subsequent labor and birthing location or method. Since the American College of Obstetricians and Gynecologists' 1999 recommendations about the safety of vaginal birth after cesarean (VBAC),[39] the number of rural hospitals in the US that offer women the option of a trial of labor after cesarean has plummeted.[40,41] Women in some areas must either undergo repeat cesarean or travel sometimes great distances to have the option for VBAC. Similarly, a woman with a breech presentation at term may not have the option of attempting vaginal breech birth (which is considered a reasonable, evidence-based option)[42] because no provider in her area has the technical skills or knowledge to attend her.[42,43] This lack of available providers is the downstream effect of the increased emphasis on cesarean delivery, which resulted in a generation of obstetrical providers not trained in vaginal breech delivery. Thus, the technological medical model has limited a woman's autonomy and decision making for her childbirth; indeed, the guidelines of national organizations do not include patient preferences for choices about vaginal breech delivery.[44] Furthermore, as some have noted, instead of perseverating about "cesarean upon maternal request,"[45] providers and health systems should focus on being able to provide "vaginal birth upon maternal request" for those women who are now forced to have operative deliveries for breech presentations. Thus, as Healy elaborates,

Despite the high level of policy support for alternative birth settings there continues to be limited opportunity for women to avail of them and this may be a result of contemporary discourse that emphasizes risk, blame and responsibility, ultimately constraining women's decisions and choice.[34(p368)]

Technology in Labor: Induction

To highlight how technology takes over in one common labor scenario, consider the story of Pat, having her first baby:

> At 38 weeks, Pat noticed a gush of fluid from her vagina without any contractions; Pat and Mike headed to the hospital, where the resident on call confirmed that her waters had broken. Pat wanted to talk to her own maternity provider, Dr. G, before starting any induction of labor, but she agreed to start an antibiotic for her group B streptococcus infection. After discussion with Dr. G once he arrived, the couple decided that they wanted whatever would work fastest and most safely for the baby, with as few vaginal exams as possible and attempting to go as long as possible without pain medication. The initial medication helped Pat progress to 4 cm dilated with just one dose, while she chose different positions with a telemetry monitor attached, with her own music, pillow, and nightgown all helping her to cope. When her contractions became less frequent, Dr. G recommended an oxytocin drip; however, even with regular contractions, her cervix still did not progress beyond 6 cm, and the doctor recommended an intrauterine pressure monitor (IUPC). Pat began thinking that everything was going in the wrong direction: induction, IUPC, what next?

The widespread use of labor induction illustrates how the misuse or overuse of technology in maternity settings can lead to potentially unnecessary intervention, especially for low-risk women. In the US in 2015, nearly one-fourth of women giving birth underwent labor induction, and in an earlier study, selecting just for women planning vaginal birth, nearly half of first-time mothers (47%) and 40% of women with prior births experienced induction.[46] Often the decision to recommend labor induction stems from the technological determination of accurate gestational age dating (using routine early trimester ultrasound) or later-term ultrasound measure of fluid or fetal breathing movements to assess fetal health, or particular patterns of electronic fetal monitoring that are known to inaccurately predict fetal intolerance of labor. During an induction or augmentation of labor such as Pat undergoes, the use of medications and interventions labels a woman as being at higher risk, thus further pathologizing the normal process of birth and leading to continuous electronic fetal monitoring and fewer choices for the woman about ambulation in labor or other nonpharmacologic, "natural" methods for coping with labor pain.

Newer national obstetrical guidelines emphasize avoiding "elective" induction, following safety "bundles" during inductions, and recognizing that induced labor takes longer than spontaneous labor. Such bundles can be described as structured sets of evidence-based interventions that improve outcomes when applied systematically. However, in front-line practice, many busy providers and hospitals are less patient with slowly progressing labor than the guidelines recommend, leading to more cesarean sections for "failed" induction.

Informed Consent in Labor

Once labor ensues, the intense physical and emotional feelings, including pain, suffering, and fear, become barriers to a woman's capacity to consent.[47(p384)] The laboring woman may not be able to clearly articulate her multitude of feelings, or to focus on a provider's questions or attempts to provide information for consent. Providers need to resist taking over decision making for women in the throes of labor. Since the middle of labor may be a difficult time to have an informed discussion, ideally some of the woman's ideas and choices would have been explored and documented prenatally.

Discussions about pain relief strategies for women in labor are especially problematic when a woman is already in distress about labor pain. As Surtees notes, "the seduction of sedation," when women are already vulnerable due to pain during labor, may lead to uninformed choices.[48(p173)] Additionally, providers may have strong biases either for or against different pain relief modalities such as epidurals. Natural birth proponents may label as a failure a labor in which a woman chooses to receive an epidural. In their view, offering or encouraging epidurals can be seen as colluding in the medicalization of childbirth, especially if a hospital or birthing site limits women's other choices of pain control by not having birthing balls or tubs or doula support readily available, or other patient-directed pharmacologic methods such as nitrous oxide. On the other hand, other providers and women alike may see relief of pain in labor, no matter the potential sequelae of intervention, as a way to help a laboring woman feel more in control over or indeed "emancipation from" her body's processes.[48(p180)] This option may be particularly important for women whose past experiences with sexual violence may significantly affect them during labor, as the case of Jen illustrates.

> Jen was a 17-year-old who had become pregnant after being gang-raped. With the support of her maternity provider late in the pregnancy, Jen admitted that every vaginal exam was excruciatingly difficult for her. She requested an epidural earlier rather than later in labor since she imagined that not being able to feel the exams would help her immensely.

For women whose daily lives are filled with oppression and emotional suffering, the informed choice to have a few hours of pain-free labor, even with a technology that affects control over other choices such as getting out of bed during labor, may offer the most empowering moments of their lives. For a survivor like Jen, this choice about how to cope with difficult physical examinations during labor may reduce her suffering and improve her overall birth experience and recovery.

Technology in Labor: Fetal Monitoring

The widespread, unquestioned use of electronic fetal monitoring also demonstrates how technology has dominated choices in normal birth. Rosa's story illustrates this.

> Rosa had given birth twice in Central America before coming to the US. Her third pregnancy, in the US, was complicated by concerns for slow fetal growth, resulting in extra ultrasounds and fetal monitoring. When she came to the hospital after her waters broke with only irregular contractions, she was not expecting to stay attached to a monitor throughout her labor. She worried that even though the labor felt a lot like her previous labors, this baby must have something wrong to need all this monitoring. Her nurse was busy with two patients and was not able to spend much time with Rosa at this stage.

Not only does the individual fetal monitor reinforce techno-maternity, so does the central monitoring process (remote surveillance) that many hospitals employ. This technology permits busy nurses to watch multiple fetal heart tracings remote from the laboring woman's room, leaving individual laboring women alone for longer periods while still being "monitored."

Given that continuous support in labor has been shown to reduce operative delivery and improve women's satisfaction with birth,[49] the ultimate effect of central monitoring intrudes upon the potential for healthier maternal and infant outcomes.

Dignity in Childbirth: Human Rights During Labor

In the last decade, growing awareness of disrespect and abuse toward women in childbirth has emerged as an international human rights and women's rights issue.[50] A landmark review in 2010 documented multiple accounts of behaviors toward laboring women in both the developed and developing world such as "physical abuse, non-consented care, non-confidential care, non-dignified care, discrimination based on specific patient attributes, abandonment of care, and detention in facilities."[51(p9)] This has led to statements defining respectful maternity care by international organizations such as the World Health Organization (WHO) and the International Federation of Gynecology and Obstetrics:

> Respectful Maternity Care (RMC) focuses on the interpersonal interactions that a woman encounters during labor, delivery, and postpartum. While RMC primarily emphasizes the absence of disrespect and abuse by health care providers and other staff, its definition also advocates positive and supportive staff attitudes and behaviors that increase a woman's satisfaction with her birth experience.[52(p1)]

To this end, the WHO now incorporates into its definition of quality maternity care both the provision of care and the experience of care (i.e., some assessment of the woman's experience of childbirth), making RMC not only a human rights issue but also a critical element in quality of care.[52]

Providers often resist believing that disrespect and abuse are occurring with any frequency and may view their own behaviors as "necessary or even life-saving."[52(p5)] Sometimes seemingly disrespectful care may not be about the provider's personal actions but about systemic issues such as inadequate staffing to allow time with women in labor.[52] However, lest those in higher-income countries think that lack of dignity and abuse during childbirth are limited to women giving birth in lower-resource countries, consider a more inclusive definition of dignity and human rights during childbirth and consider the stories of women of color or those from poorer neighborhoods who describe impersonal and disrespectful care during pregnancy and childbirth.

For example, Lazarus reports on interviews with poor women in a publicly funded clinic, where long wait times, rushed visits, and lack of continuity are the norm;[53] Esposito describes inner-city women's reports of hospital care that felt racist or impersonal.[54]

Dignity in childbirth means more than avoiding hurting or harming the woman with uncomfortable exams, pushing on her belly, or ignoring her painful cries. The fundamentals of WCC promote dignity in childbirth by seeking to understand the individual woman's context, her background story, and her current vulnerability. Emphasizing her rights during childbirth includes understanding systems issues that may be affecting her—the lack of an interpreter, the unfamiliar hospital, the busy labor ward without enough nurses, the obstetrical policy that insists on a specific but not evidence-based algorithm or technological safety bundle that may not apply best to her today. Respectful childbirth care clearly also includes addressing implicit bias and unconscious racism, with providers examining their frustrations or impatience that this teenager of color "got herself pregnant" and now struggles vocally and vociferously to cope with labor pain, or that this refugee woman is refusing what might be a medically indicated induction or cesarean.

Technological Considerations in Infant Feeding

> After a long induction, Pat develops a uterine infection, requires antibiotics, and finally has a cesarean delivery. Pat and Mike are knowledgeable about the benefits of breastfeeding and told their doctors from the beginning of the pregnancy that Pat intended to breastfeed. At the delivery, Pat's daughter is taken to the infant warmer in the operating room to be examined by the nurses and doctors, weighed, and given medicine. When Pat gets to hold her daughter in the recovery room they are both so tired they fall asleep with baby on mother's chest. Once in the postpartum room, the nurse declares that it is time to wake the baby up and feed. Pat fumbles with the squirmy little baby, who sucks hard on her nipple but keeps stopping to cry. Eventually they both rest again, and this pattern repeats itself a few times through the course of the night. The next morning when Pat tells her nurse about her struggles, the nurse returns with a breast pump on wheels, and says that if Pat can't nurse the baby she should at least pump so that the baby "gets something." Pat is so disheartened when she sees the few drops of colostrum in the bottle attached to the breast pump that when the nurse offers formula she agrees.

This case illustrates the breastfeeding challenges faced by women in a system embedded in values that may emphasize technological "solutions" and may even provide misinformation. While a woman may hear about the benefits of breastfeeding from multiple sources, like Pat she also receives complicated messages from media, family, and even health professionals about other feeding possibilities that can undermine her confidence in her body's ability to feed her baby. These messages may lead many women to internalize the belief that they are physically unable to breastfeed. Caregivers for women may themselves have limited belief in women's ability to breastfeed. In Pat's situation, the nurse, rather than reassuring her that her postpartum nursing/milk "production" course was normal, implied that the baby was not getting enough to eat. As clinicians caring for postpartum women, "I'm not making enough milk" is the most common concern that we hear. In research on breastfeeding women who supplement with formula immediately postpartum (64%), the most cited reason (36% in one study) is perception of inadequate milk supply.[55] Despite our efforts to educate women about normal breastmilk production—about how newborns need only tiny amounts of colostrum and about the importance of early suckling in long-term milk production—many women still say they "do not have enough milk." When they go home and tell their friends and family that they "had to" supplement or switch to formula because they "didn't make enough milk," they reinforce the cultural belief in this possibility. Seen from a cross-cultural perspective, most women around the world and throughout history have breastfed; being physiologically unable to produce milk is exceedingly rare, and the cultural belief in "not enough milk" is a recent development.

As woman-centered clinicians, our role is to listen to a woman's goals, values, and struggles and empower her to care for her infant in the way that she chooses. However, clarifying women's goals around breastfeeding is challenging. On the one hand, we may take the approach of MI, asking about their goals and dreams for the baby, and work our way toward talking about breastfeeding. On the other hand, we may assume that a woman will want to make the healthiest choice for her baby and therefore approach the conversation having concluded that the woman is going to breastfeed. We despair about how many women who, prenatally, voice plans to breastfeed and yet how few actually do. Patients often tell providers what they want to hear. A woman who decides not to breastfeed may feel that not only has she let down herself and her baby, but that she has disappointed her provider as well. We need to examine whether we allow women to voice their actual plans and feelings. How do we educate women about breastfeeding, enlighten them about the corporate marketing that has become internalized as culture, and reassure each woman about her body's capacity to feed her baby, without coming across as judgmental of person, family, or culture? We can listen at every stage. We can empower women to analyze cultural and advertising messages and rely on their own innate decision-making and physiologic capacity. We can learn to provide true support of breastfeeding and help systems do the same. We can educate families about how to support breastfeeding women. We can continue to support policies that limit medically inappropriate marketing. We can normalize struggle rather than viewing it as a failure.

Solutions Beyond Technology

Technology is an integral part of women's daily lives and of childbirth in the 21st century. Providers and women wanting to maximize healthy birth outcomes while avoiding the overuse of technology in pregnancy and labor need new strategies. Most importantly, we need to preserve human connection when we embrace technology. Strategies emphasizing relational care are key to reducing techno-maternity care. These include fostering choice in contraceptive methods and decision making about pregnancy, offering prenatal group visits, training women's friends or family members as lay doulas, putting doulas in every labor room, encouraging birth plans, and supporting women's infant feeding choices.

Recently in the US, a renewed, sustained, national call has emerged for reducing interventions in childbirth as a strategy to prevent unnecessary cesarean sections,[56-58] These expert guidelines emphasize shared, woman-centered communication; for instance, a "key strategy" in the California Maternal Quality Care Collaborative toolkit to promote vaginal birth is to "Improve Communication through Shared Decision Making."[57(p13)] The toolkit highlights literacy-appropriate decision aids and patient engagement that respects women's cultural and religious beliefs. Similar tools and guidelines in the UK emphasize normal birth practices for low-risk women.[59]

Incorporating technology in a woman-centered way could potentially lead to medical visits where "a medical practitioner and a woman could be jointly involved in the process of examination of her body or intervention on it, with the mediation of medical technology."[60(p7)] This strategy of always incorporating with technology the human elements of nursing and caring, connected always to the woman's lived contexts, could become a "model for person-centered care." Indeed, the fundamental principles of MI involve this kind of facilitative shared decision making between provider and woman.

Unfortunately, technology is seductive—yet another complicated blood test, the image on a screen or a squiggling line across a computer monitor or on a paper strip, grabbing our eyes and pulling us away from human eye contact or skin-to-skin contact with the laboring woman. Thus, the challenge here lies in keeping our own human, "high touch" skills fresh and active and not subsumed by technology.

References

1. Shields SG, Candib LM, eds. *Woman-Centered Care of Pregnancy and Birth*. Oxford, UK: Radcliffe Medical Press; 2010.
2. Mahjouri N. Techno-maternity: rethinking the possibilities of reproductive technologies. *Third Space*. 2004;4. http://journals.sfu.ca/thirdspace/index.php/journal/article/view/mahjouri/157. Accessed March 27, 2018.
3. World Health Organization. *Unsafe Abortion: Global and Regional Estimates of Incidence of Unsafe Abortion and Associated Mortality in 2008*. Geneva: 2011.
4. Gravett CA, Gravett MG, Martin ET, et al. Serious and life-threatening pregnancy-related infections: opportunities to reduce the global burden. *PLoS Med*. 2012;9(10):e1001324.
5. Regan L, Glasier A. The British 1967 Abortion Act—still fit for purpose? *Lancet* 2017; 390(10106):1936–1937.
6. Mendez JE. *Report of the Special Rapporteur on Torture and Other Cruel, Inhuman or Degrading Treatment or Punishment. A/HRC/22/53*. United Nations General Assembly, Human Rights Council; February 1, 2013.
7. Presser HB. The role of sterilization in controlling Puerto Rican fertility. *Populat Stud*. 1969;23(3):343–361.
8. Mass B. Puerto Rico: a case study of population control. *Latin Am Perspect*. 1977;4(4):66–81.
9. Stern AM. Sterilized in the name of public health: race, immigration, and reproductive control in modern California. *Am J Public Health*. 2005;95(7):1128–1138.
10. Grekul J. Sterilization in Alberta, 1928 to 1972: gender matters. *Can Rev Sociol*. 2008;45(3):247–266.
11. Grahn H. Clarifying statistics on percentage of First Nations people sterilized under Sexual Sterilization Act in Alberta. Grekul J, personal communication, January 14, 2018.
12. Reilly PR. Eugenics and involuntary sterilization: 1907–2015. *Ann Rev Genom Hum Genet*. 2015;16:351–368.
13. El Feki S, Avafia T, Fidalgo TM, et al. The Global Commission on HIV and the Law: recommendations for legal reform to promote sexual and reproductive health and rights. *Reprod Health Matt*. 2014;22(44):125–136.

14. California State Auditor. *Report 2013-120 summary—June 2014: sterilization of female inmates.* 2014. http://auditor.ca.gov/reports/summary/2013-120. Accessed March 27, 2018.
15. Gavin L, Moskosky S, Carter M, et al. Providing quality family planning services: recommendations of CDC and the U.S. Office of Population Affairs. *MMWR Recomm Rep.* 2014;63(RR-04):1–54.
16. ACOG Committee on Health Care for Underserved Women. Committee Opinion No. 654 summary: reproductive life planning to reduce unintended pregnancy. *Obstet Gynecol.* 2016;127(2):415.
17. Wilson RD. Choosing pre-conception planning for women/families: counselling and informed consent (part 2)—pre-conception reproductive planning, lifestyle, immunization, and psychosocial issues. *J Obstet Gynaecol Can.* 2017. https://doi.org/10.1016/j.jogc.2017.08.037. Accessed March 27, 2018.
18. Callegari LS, Aiken AR, Dehlendorf C, Cason P, Borrero S. Addressing potential pitfalls of reproductive life planning with patient-centered counseling. *Am J Obstet Gynecol.* 2017;216(2):129–134.
19. Whitaker AK, Quinn MT, Munroe E, Martins SL, Mistretta SQ, Gilliam ML. A motivational interviewing-based counseling intervention to increase post abortion uptake of contraception: a pilot randomized controlled trial. *Patient Educ Counsel.* 2016;99(10):1663–1669.
20. Ott M, Sucato G, Committee on Adolescence. Contraception for adolescents. *Pediatrics.* 2014;134(4):e1257–1281.
21. ACOG: Committee on Adolescent Health Care Long-Acting Reversible Contraception Working Group. Committee opinion no. 539: adolescents and long-acting reversible contraception: implants and intrauterine devices. *Obstet Gynecol.* 2012;120(4):983–988.
22. Tomlin K, Bambulas T, Sutton M, Pazdernik V, Coonrod DV. Motivational interviewing to promote long-acting reversible contraception in postpartum teenagers. *J Pediatr Adolesc Gynecol.* 2017;30(3):383–388.
23. Aiken ARA, Guthrie KA, Schellekens M, Trussell J, Gomperts R. Barriers to accessing abortion services and perspectives on using mifepristone and misoprostol at home in Great Britain. *Contraception.* 2018;97(2):177–183.
24. Shigesato M, Elia J, Tschann M, et al. Pharmacy access to ulipristal acetate in major cities throughout the United States. *Contraception.* 2018;97(3):264–269.
25. Office of the Secretary HHS. Regulation for the enforcement of federal health care provider conscience protection laws. Final rule. *Federal Register.* 2011;76(36):9968–9977.
26. Card R. Federal provider conscience regulation: unconscionable. *J Med Ethics.* 2009;35(8):471–472.
27. Alderman EM. Confidentiality in pediatric and adolescent gynecology: when we can, when we can't, and when we're challenged. *J Pediatr Adolesc Gynecol.* 2017;30(2):176–183.

28. Benn P, Chapman AR. Ethical and practical challenges in providing noninvasive prenatal testing for chromosome abnormalities: an update. *Curr Opin Obstet Gynecol.* 2016;28(2):119–124.
29. Farrell RM, Nutter B, Agatisa PK. Patient-centered prenatal counseling: aligning obstetric healthcare professionals with needs of pregnant women. *Women Health.* 2015;55(3):280–296.
30. Hoffmann TC, Del Mar C. Clinicians' expectations of the benefits and harms of treatments, screening, and tests: a systematic review. *JAMA Intern Med.* 2017;177(3):407–419.
31. Bramwell R, Carter D. An exploration of midwives' and obstetricians' knowledge of genetic screening in pregnancy and their perception of appropriate counselling. *Midwifery.* 2001;17(2):133–141.
32. Preloran HM, Browner CH, Lieber E. Impact of interpreters' approach on Latinas' use of amniocentesis. *Health Educ Behav.* 2005;32(5):599–612.
33. Browner CH, Preloran HM, Casado MC, Bass HN, Walker AP. Genetic counseling gone awry: miscommunication between prenatal genetic service providers and Mexican-origin clients. *Soc Sci Med.* 2003;56(9):1933–1946.
34. Healy S, Humphreys E, Kennedy C. A qualitative exploration of how midwives' and obstetricians' perception of risk affects care practices for low-risk women and normal birth. *Women Birth.* 2017;30(5):367–375.
35. Healy S, Humphreys E, Kennedy C. Midwives' and obstetricians' perceptions of risk and its impact on clinical practice and decision-making in labour: an integrative review. *Women Birth.* 2016;29(2):107–116.
36. Brody H, Thompson JR. The maxi-min strategy in modern obstetrics. *J Fam Pract.* 1981;12(6):977–986.
37. Sandall J, Soltani H, Gates S, Shennan A, Devane D. Midwife-led continuity models versus other models of care for childbearing women. *Cochrane Database System Reviews.* 2016;4:CD004667.
38. Fishbeyn B. Restricting choices of childbearing women. *Am J Bioeth.* 2016;16(2):1–2.
39. Vaginal birth after previous cesarean delivery. *Int J Gynecol Obstet.* 1999;66(2):197–204.
40. Roberts RG, Deutchman M, King VJ, Fryer GE, Miyoshi TJ. Changing policies on vaginal birth after cesarean: impact on access. *Birth.* 2007(34):316–322.
41. Leeman LM, Beagle M, Espey E, Ogburn T, Skipper B. Diminishing availability of trial of labor after cesarean delivery in New Mexico hospitals. *Obstet Gynecol.* 2013;122(Part 1):242–247.
42. ACOG Committee on Obstetric Practice. ACOG Committee Opinion No. 340. Mode of term singleton breech delivery. *Obstet Gynecol.* 2006;108(1):235–237.
43. Lawson GW. The term breech trial ten years on: primum non nocere? *Birth.* 2012;39(1):3–9.

44. Little MO, Lyerly AD, Mitchell LM, et al. Mode of delivery: toward responsible inclusion of patient preferences. *Obstet Gynecol.* 2008;112(4):913–918.
45. ACOG. Cesarean delivery on maternal request. Committee Opinion No. 559 *Obstet Gynecol.* 2013;121:904–907.
46. Laughon S, Zhang J, Grewal J, Sundaram R, Beaver J, Reddy U. Induction of labor in a contemporary obstetric cohort. *Am J Obstet Gynecol.* 2012;206(6):486.e481, 486.e489.
47. Rosenthal MS. Socioethical issues in hospital birth: troubling tales from a Canadian sample. *Sociol Perspect.* 2006;49(3):369–390.
48. Surtees R. Midwifery partnership with women in Aotearoa/ New Zealand: a poststructuralist feminist perspective on the use of epidurals in "normal" birth. In: Stewart M, ed. *Pregnancy, Birth and Maternity Care: Feminist Perspectives.* 2nd ed. Elsevier Science: Midwives, Edinburgh; 2004:169–183.
49. Bohren MA, Hofmeyr GJ, Sakala C, Fukuzawa RK, Cuthbert A. Continuous support for women during childbirth. *Cochrane Database System Rev.* 2017;7:CD003766.
50. Center for Reproductive Rights and Federation of Women Lawyers, Kenya. Failure to deliver: violations of women's human rights in Kenyan health facilities. 2007. https://www.reproductiverights.org/document/failure-to-deliver-violations-of-womens-human-rights-in-kenyan-health-facilities. Accessed March 27, 2018.
51. Bowser D, Hill K. *Exploring Evidence for Disrespect and Abuse in Facility-Based Childbirth.* USAID-TRAction Project Harvard School of Public Health University Research Co., LLC; September 20, 2010.
52. Hastings MB. Policy brief: pulling back the curtain on disrespect and abuse. Health Policy Project. 2015. http://whiteribbonalliance.org/wp-content/uploads/2016/03/Policy-Brief-Pulling-Back-the-Curtain-on-DR.pdf. Accessed March 27, 2018.
53. Lazarus ES. What do women want? Issues of choice, control, and class in pregnancy and childbirth. *Med Anthropol Q.* 1994;8(1):25–46.
54. Esposito NW. Marginalized women's comparisons of their hospital and free-standing birth center experiences: a contrast of inner-city birthing systems. *Health Care Women Int.* 1999;20(2):111–126.
55. Pierro J, Abulaimoun B, Roth P, Blau J. Factors associated with supplemental formula feeding of breastfeeding infants during postpartum hospital stay. *Breastfeed Med.* 2016;11:196–202.
56. Spong C, Berghella V, Wenstrom K, Mercer B, Saade G. Preventing the first cesarean delivery: summary of a joint Eunice Kennedy Shriver National Institute of Child Health and Human Development, Society for Maternal-Fetal Medicine, and American College of Obstetricians and Gynecologists Workshop. *Obstet Gynecol.* 2012;120:1181–1193.
57. Smith H, Peterson N, Lagrew D, Main E. *Toolkit to Support Vaginal Birth and Reduce Primary Cesareans: A Quality Improvement Toolkit.* Stanford, CA: California Maternal Quality Care Collaborative; 2016.

58. ACOG. Obstetric Care Consensus No. 1: safe prevention of the primary cesarean delivery. *Obstet Gynecol.* 2014;123(3):693–711.
59. National Institute for Health and Care Excellence (NICE). Intrapartum care for healthy women and babies: Clinical guideline CG190. https://www.nice.org.uk/guidance/cg190/chapter/Recommendations. Published December 2017. Updated February 2017. Accessed March 27, 2018.
60. Stankovic, B. Situated technology in reproductive health care: do we need a new theory of the subject to promote person-centred care? *Nurs Philos.* 2017;18:e12159.

13

WOMEN WITH DISABILITIES

ETHICS OF ACCESS AND ACCOMMODATION FOR INFERTILITY CARE

Leslie Francis, Anita Silvers, and Brittany Badesch

Women with disabilities who have difficulty becoming pregnant may face not only the typical challenges of infertility but also societal barriers relating to their disabilities. In this chapter, we describe barriers encountered by these women, including legal issues, training and attitudes of physicians, and insurance coverage and ability to pay. Moreover, structural issues encountered by these women include lack of adaptive equipment, inexperience of providers in treating these patient populations, and lack of access to health insurance coverage for infertility care. Further, common but erroneous perceptions—widely shared among not only providers but also the public more generally—are that women with disabilities are less interested in sexuality and less likely to flourish through motherhood. They may be stereotyped as less capable of carrying pregnancies or raising children, and as being riskier patients overall. Encountering expressions of such disability-targeting opposition to their pursuit of biologic reproduction may damage their determination that overcoming these problems to achieve a successful outcome to pregnancy will be worthwhile.

Some commentators claim that the current situation is not unjust, on several grounds: that infertility care for women with disabilities may raise medical or social issues that infertility care for other women does not, and that no one can justly claim infertility care as a basic healthcare need. In this chapter, we explore the assumptions that underlie problematic judgments about fertility treatment for women with disabilities and present an account of reasonable accommodation in infertility care for women with disabilities who seek to form families by experiencing biologic reproduction themselves. Our aim is to indicate how unnecessary barriers to their doing so can be reduced.

Women with Disabilities and Fertility Care: Experiences and Obstacles

Significant numbers of women with disabilities become pregnant each year. Estimates are that over 160,000 women with chronic physical disabilities become pregnant each year in the US[1] and that 9.4% of pregnant women in the UK are women with disabilities.[2] Reportedly, the first North American clinic offering specialty care for women with mobility impairments opened in Toronto in 2017.[3] These figures are at best estimates, however, and the interests and needs of this patient population may be far greater, as estimates are that 10% of women of reproductive age have disabilities.[2]

One of the significant problems in discussing reproductive care for women with disabilities is the limited evidence available about women with disabilities and their reproductive care. As of our writing of this chapter, this evidentiary gap is garnering significant attention. The US National Institute of Health (NIH) Eunice Kennedy Shriver National Institute of Child Health and Human Development has recently issued a call for proposals under the NIH small grants program, a call aimed to address the paucity of data on pregnancy in women with disabilities.[4] Researchers affiliated with the Lurie Institute for Disability Policy at Brandeis University are engaged in extensive study of reproductive care for women with disabilities.[5] Our analysis in this chapter, however, is perforce limited by the evidence currently available. Beyond limited knowledge, other barriers to reproductive care for women with disabilities include inadequate laws and enforcement of even these laws, attitudes of family and others who encounter them, physician knowledge and attitudes, and insurance coverage.

In the US under the Americans with Disabilities Act (ADA), physicians' offices and hospitals are public accommodations.[6] Such facilities serving the public are required not to discriminate against persons with disabilities "in the full and equal enjoyment of the goods, services, facilities, privileges, advantages, or accommodations" they provide.[7] It is discrimination to deny individuals with disabilities participation in or the benefit of these services on the basis of disabilities.[8] It is also discriminatory to afford, based on disability, disparate opportunities to benefit from services.[9] Such discrimination includes the imposition of eligibility criteria "that screen out or tend to screen out an individual with a disability from fully and equally enjoying any goods, services, facilities, privileges, advantages, or accommodations, unless such criteria can be shown to be necessary."[10] It is discrimination to fail "to make reasonable modifications in policies, practices, or procedures, when such modifications are necessary to afford such goods, services, facilities, privileges, advantages, or accommodations . . . unless the entity can demonstrate that making such modifications would fundamentally alter the nature of the good."[11] It is also discrimination to fail to take necessary steps to avoid differential treatment of people with disabilities because of the absence of auxiliary aids and services.[12]

These ADA standards are significant, and they have been enshrined in law since 1990. More recently, they have been joined by the Affordable Care Act § 4203,[13] which requires that standards be set for accessible medical equipment, including diagnostic equipment. Yet evidence remains that healthcare providers often fail to meet these antidiscrimination requirements.[14]

Physicians' lack of training, limited experience with women with disabilities, and discouraging attitudes also pose problems for women with disabilities who seek reproductive care. Studies from the UK, Sweden, and the US have begun to reveal the impact of experience and attitudes on the pregnancy experiences of women with different types of disabilities. For example, a UK study using data from 2015 indicates some significant differences in the care, birth, and postnatal experiences of women with disabilities.[15] Women with disabilities were less likely to feel involved in their care, less likely to have a choice about delivery location (although some of this variance was due to medical conditions), and less likely to receive help in breastfeeding. Women with disabilities were also more likely to report being spoken to in a way they could not understand; this was particularly true for women with learning disabilities or sensory impairments. Women with sensory disabilities also were less likely to access prenatal care before 12 weeks' gestation. This study emphasizes the importance of recognizing the differences in experiences of maternity care of women with different types of disabilities. To take another example, a qualitative study from Sweden indicates that women with intellectual disabilities encounter mixed reactions from partners and relatives who learn about their pregnancies, fear losing custody of their children, and may be reluctant to disclose their pregnancies because of these fears.[16]

Several recent US studies by a group from the Lurie Institute for Disability Policy at Brandeis look at a variety of aspects of the experience of women with disabilities in healthcare. One study examines perceptions of women with mobility impairments; these women report being met with curiosity, hostility, concerns about costs, and concerns about adequacy as a parent.[17] These women were often asked how they got pregnant, with questioners apparently assuming that they were either uninterested in sex, incapable of it, or the victims of exploitation or rape. Another study from the same group reports that when women with mobility impairments became pregnant, their family members expressed negative reactions, worried about their safety, and questioned their parenting capability.[18] This study recommends improved education of family members and support for women with physical disabilities during and after pregnancy.[18] In the case of genetic conditions, this study also reports family concerns that the condition would be transmitted to the offspring; the women reported taking offense when relatives celebrated the birth of an unaffected child.[18] Participants in a related study also reported the importance for women with disabilities of self-advocacy and peer support, including internet resources.[19]

Training and experience of healthcare providers is another issue faced by pregnant women with disabilities. A qualitative descriptive study by the Lurie Institute group (interviews with 14 clinicians) reported clinicians had no training in caring for obstetrical patients with mobility impairments.[20] Many of those interviewed had not planned to provide this kind of care but were led to do so by a request from someone they knew, because of partners, or because of expectations in their practice setting. Several stated that their patients were their best teachers. They also became teachers for other providers. They reported finding the experience of caring for this population deeply rewarding. Negative experiences involve not the patients themselves but systems issues: lack of equipment, tendency of others to view all of these patients as being at high risk, and lack of continuity with other providers.

Ability to pay for infertility care is a further issue. Estimates are that approximately 12% of US women of childbearing age have received infertility care.[21] Insurance payment for this care is variable, however, depending on the type of coverage. Medicaid is the source of coverage for 25 million adult women in the US today; roughly two-thirds of these women are between the ages of 19 and 49.[22] Medicaid typically covers contraceptive services and pregnancy; pregnant women come under one of the coverage categories even in states that have not participated in the ACA Medicaid expansion.[22] Medicaid pays for nearly half of all births in the US; coverage rates are highest in the states across the southern tier of the US.[22] According to a 2016 study, no state Medicaid programs provide fertility treatment for either women or men.[23] Although a number of states do cover diagnostic testing that can reveal the explanation for infertility, in some of these states the testing is only covered if it is for reasons other than infertility.[23]

For women with other forms of insurance coverage, the situation is somewhat better but far from ideal. Medicare, which may cover women or men who are permanently disabled if they meet eligibility criteria, covers "reasonable and necessary services associated with treatment for infertility."[24] Medicare currently covers just over 900,000 US women of reproductive age (19 to 44).[25] Employer-provided insurance, which is the coverage source for more than half of US women of childbearing age, is required to cover some forms of infertility treatment in 13 states, but some of these mandates do not include in vitro fertilization (IVF).[26] Coverage for veterans includes some infertility care; since 2017, IVF has been covered for certain veterans who have a service-connected disability that necessitates its use.[27]

Ethical Arguments

Providers may raise several different concerns about offering reproductive care to women with disabilities. These concerns include the provider's lack of education or competence to provide the care, potential risks to the woman of receiving particular types of care or of carrying a pregnancy and giving birth, the inability of the woman to give informed consent, potential risks to any offspring, costs of care, inability to pay for care, and the woman's ability to raise a child and especially to keep it safe. In this section, we argue that there is at best limited and partial justification for many of these concerns, especially in the context of background injustice. In analyzing these arguments, it is also critical to take into account differences among types of disabilities as well as differences among particular women.

A fundamental starting point of any discussion of justice and disability is the recognition that important aspects of disability are social.[28] Disability is a difference in the ability to function, but ability to function is as much a matter of the design of a world and its social organization as it is of the physical and mental differences among the people in that world. A woman with a spinal cord injury, for example, may be unable to climb onto an examining table that cannot be adjusted, when with adjustable heights she could easily move herself onto the table. A woman with intellectual disabilities may be able to manage aspects of parenting in structured social circumstances that she would not be able to manage in situations lacking these structures.[29] People with psychiatric disabilities may need mental health services that address their ability to function as parents.[29] How to take into account the interplay between bodies and minds and the social worlds they inhabit poses complex ethical questions that are core to the discussion in this section of the chapter.

Physician Competence

It is unethical for physicians to treat patients when they lack the ability to deliver care competently. However, this statement hides questions about whether it may be unethical for physicians to lack certain care competencies or skills in treating certain kinds of patients or in offering certain types of care. Whether this is so depends on factors that include the training reasonably available to physicians; data from the Lurie Institute described in the previous section[20] indicate that training programs for many physicians do not include disability-related education. A 2009 report on the status of healthcare for individuals with disabilities in the US identified lack of education of healthcare providers about disability as a root cause of existing disparities.[30] This deficiency is not confined to the US, as physicians in a UK-based study "admitted that they had relatively little exposure to adult disability in medical school or residency training."[31] The effects of this lack of training and experience in preparing providers to care for individuals with disabilities are also not limited to general medical practice. The paucity of training for medical professionals specifically in reproductive healthcare for women with disabilities often results in women encountering "providers who lack disability-related training or sensitivity and/or fail to recognize the woman as a person with sexual and reproductive health care needs."[32]

Research from the Lurie Institute, however, also indicates that despite a current gap in formal training experiences, many physicians do have the opportunity to learn from colleagues in their practice settings or from patients themselves.[20] Physicians should be expected to take advantage of these opportunities when they are readily available, especially when the absence of knowledge is widespread and adversely affects patients' ability to access needed care—that is, when they are providing care in a context of more general injustice. Fortunately, as the Lurie Institute study also indicates, physicians on the whole are willing to do so and find the ability to offer such care deeply satisfying.[20] Another study sounds a cautionary note, however. When researchers developed a curriculum on care for people with disabilities[33] and tested it, they found that although attitudes of medical students generally were improved by familiarity with patients with disabilities, a small proportion of male medical students exposed to the curriculum appear to have developed increasingly negative attitudes toward people with disabilities.[34] These negative attitudes included perceptions that people with disabilities expected special treatment, resented people without disabilities, and felt sorry for themselves.[34] Moreover, even if not all specialists in the various aspects of reproduction learn to treat women with disabilities, healthcare systems should be expected to provide referrals to experts who do. Finally, the medical education system also must work toward providing current and future trainees with educational experience that will equip them to provide just reproductive care to women with disabilities. We return to this need in the final section of the chapter.

Physician Choice

In the US at least, physicians are legally permitted to make choices about the patients they wish to treat. So long as they do not abandon patients, they are also legally permitted to discontinue care for particular patients. They are not, however, legally permitted to refuse to treat people in certain discriminatory ways—for example, because of their race, their sex, or their disability. Nor it is ethical for them to refuse to treat based on characteristics such as disability. Histories of injustice matter here; if all that were at stake in a particular physician choice was that one patient needed to get a different physician, although the patient might be disappointed, this is not an issue of systemic injustice. On the other hand, if no other physicians are available with the skills needed to treat the patient in question, or if more generally patients of that type have difficulty in accessing needed care because physicians refuse to treat them, there would be a significant problem of justice.

A major difficulty in determining whether there are issues of justice when physicians decline to treat patients lies in identifying reasons why the care was denied. In many cases, physicians might have mixed motives. For example, the physician might both sincerely believe that he or she is not capable of giving care to a particular patient and react to the patient based on negative stereotypes. One potentially important motive in the mix is fear of liability; physicians may express the concern that people with certain kinds of disabilities are more likely to have adverse outcomes of care and thus more likely to affect the physicians' care quality ratings or to sue for damages in the case of an adverse outcome.

Physician's attitudes toward persons with disabilities might also be influenced by lack of experience in caring for women with disabilities that results in a sense of unfamiliarity and potentially reduced willingness to care for this population. As we have discussed, there is a known deficiency in medical education in providing adequate experience and training related to disability. Tervo[35] evaluated the attitudes of both US and Canadian medical students toward individuals with disabilities and their comfort in difficult clinical scenarios involving disability. This study also examined what factors, including background in disability, were associated with more positive attitudes toward people with disabilities and more comfort with the clinical scenarios. One factor that stood out was gender: male medical students had poorer attitudes and more behavioral misconceptions about patients with disabilities than female medical students did.[35] Other studies have also demonstrated an association between lack of experience and more negative attitudes toward patients with disabilities, which could affect willingness to care for these patients.[36,37] A finding of particular relevance to our discussion is that physicians were less likely to perceive people with disabilities as sexually active and thus in need of reproductive care.[38]

In addition to unfamiliarity and fear of litigation, surveys have indicated that physicians perceive patients with disabilities to be more complex, and therefore to require greater time and more services than patients without disabilities.[38] Such perceptions pose a risk that providers will be less willing to treat patients with disabilities overall.

Risks to the Woman

Physicians ethically may decline to provide care when they believe doing so would be medically inappropriate. One reason why care might be deemed inappropriate is the judgment that the risks outweigh the benefits. The American Society for Reproductive Medicine (ASRM) advises physicians that they may decline to provide infertility care when they believe risks to the patient are too high for treatment to be ethical.[39] The same ASRM ethics opinion also makes clear that physicians may provide care for women at elevated risk, provided the women are fully informed and receive counseling if necessary.[39] The opinion also cautions that decisions should be made in a medically objective, firmly based, and unbiased manner. There is reason for concern in this respect, however, as evidence indicates that physicians are likely to inflate the risks of pregnancy for people with disabilities. Conversely, physicians also may be likely to underestimate the likelihood that women with disabilities might be desirous of sex, sexually active, or distressed by infertility.[38] This assumption is mistaken, however; Shandra[40] demonstrated that women with disabilities were equally likely to desire motherhood and to intend to have children as women without disabilities. Such data affirm that if physicians make assumptions surrounding patients' reproductive goals, the care they provide is at risk of not being congruent with patient priorities.

Inability to Give Informed Consent

Another concern about reproductive care and women with disabilities is whether they are able to give informed consent. These concerns may be particularly acute for women with intellectual disabilities or for women with mental illness. This is an area, however, in which it is especially important to be aware of the differences among types of individuals and among individual women.[41,42] One frequently raised concern is that women with intellectual disabilities may not fully understand the risks and benefits of treatment. However, depending on the extent and type of intellectual disability, these women may be able to understand and wish to pursue values that are important for them, such as the desire to have children. The sordid history of eugenics in the US and elsewhere[43–45] and the infamous never-overruled decision of the US Supreme Court upholding sterilization, *Buck v. Bell*,[46] are imperative cautionary reminders of the risks of too-ready assumptions of incapacity. When people do have limited understanding, the Convention on the Rights of Persons with Disabilities (CRPD) Article 12 asserts the full legal personhood of people with disabilities and requires that states parties provide appropriate measures of support to enable this achievement.[47] Although not without critics,[48] supported decision making is one important method for achieving legal personhood. Rather than substituting a guardian or other surrogate for the intellectually disabled individual, supported decision making advocates providing various kinds of assistance that help people with disabilities articulate their current values and choices.[49]

Risks to Offspring

Concern about risks to offspring is another reason why providers might decline to provide infertility care to women with disabilities. Some of these risks might be associated with the pregnancy itself and others with later childrearing ability. What data there are indicate that providers may overestimate risks of pregnancy in women with disabilities because of their lack of training and experience. On the other hand, some conditions, such as Turner syndrome, do increase the objective risk to both mother and child. In such cases, as described above, ASRM[39] advises that physicians may decline care if they believe the risk is too great. ASRM[50] also judges that providers may ethically decline care in the case of "well-grounded reasons that . . . patients will be unable to provide minimally adequate or safe care for offspring." This ethics opinion cautions that any such judgments must be made in a manner that is nondiscriminatory. Organizations such as the National Council on Disability[29] and commentators[51] have documented the history of misjudgments of the ability to parent among persons with disabilities. Cureton[52] points out that although people with disabilities may parent differently, this does not mean they parent less well. Misinformed judgments and physicians' ill-informed fears about a woman's ability to parent might influence the initial counseling she receives regarding pregnancy management and could even result in an "unwarranted recommendation for termination of a desired pregnancy."[53]

Also relevant here are the problems of justice raised by inadequate social arrangements and services that may threaten, or even result in, parents with disabilities losing custody of their children when they otherwise would have been able to care for them successfully.[29] Examples are extensive of failures to provide parenting instruction, counseling, assistive devices, or a variety of in-home services that could enable people with disabilities to parent successfully. Examples are also rife of child protective services failing to take into account arrangements with partners, family, or friends that also enable successful parenting in cases of disability.

Conscientious Objection

Some physicians may have personal objections to providing forms of healthcare such as contraception or abortion. These refusals are themselves controversial, especially when they involve failures to refer to other providers, when the situation is emergent, or when other providers are not available.[54] It is difficult to see, however, why these reasons of conscience would single out people with disability for refusal of care.

Ability to Pay

Another reason physicians may not offer infertility care to patients is their inability to pay. As we have described, insurance coverage for infertility is patchwork at best. The option of paying privately may be beyond the means of many people with disabilities; according to Census Bureau data, the poverty rate for people with disabilities is nearly 30%, and women with disabilities have the lowest labor force participation rate of any demographic group.[55]

ASRM[56] advises physicians that they should try to address and lessen barriers to reproductive care, but this advice is precatory only. While it seems reasonable to advise physicians to attempt to improve the situation with respect to access to care, and to attempt to lower the costs of care, it does not seem so to expect physicians to care for women who simply cannot pay.

Whether coverage for infertility treatment should be paid for through shared social costs—by one form of insurance or another—remains controversial. Politically, the US has a long history of refusing to pay for forms of care deemed objectionable, especially abortion;[57] this position has gained recent ascendancy for contraceptive care as well.[58] Others criticize sharing the costs of infertility by arguing that the desire to have children, while perhaps an important goal for many, is not a matter of health. The decision by the Veterans Health Administration to cover infertility care, including IVF for some veterans whose needs were service related, was lauded as expressing respect for the sacrifices these veterans had made.[59] On the other hand, ASRM[56] emphasizes the importance to many of family formation, even judging that the creation of a family "is a basic human right."

Reasonable Modifications and Accommodations

The concept of "reasonable modifications" comes from the specification of what constitutes discrimination in US law. Under the ADA, as we have described, it is discrimination for a public accommodation to fail to make reasonable modifications in policies, practices, or procedures needed to allow people with disabilities to enjoy the service on equal terms.[1] It is a defense to a discrimination claim if the entity can demonstrate that making such modifications would fundamentally alter the nature of the good.[60] These requirements apply to physicians' offices, offices of other healthcare providers, healthcare facilities, private home care agencies, adoption agencies, daycare centers and schools, places of entertainment, and many other private-sector facilities serving parents with disabilities or their children.[61] It is also discrimination for public services to fail to make such modifications.[62] And it is discrimination for employers to fail to make reasonable accommodations when requested by people with disabilities.[63] In this section, we detail some modifications and accommodations that should be instituted regarding reproductive care for people with disabilities.

Medical education is a public service when provided by state universities and a public accommodation when provided by private universities. Including the experience of caring for people with disabilities could be a reasonable modification in medical education. As discussed above, physician competence and physician choices augment barriers for women with disabilities seeking fertility and reproductive care. A lack of previous experience working with individuals with disabilities and inadequate training in medical education have been shown to correlate with physicians feeling less prepared, uncomfortable, and reluctant to provide care for this population.[33–37,64–66] Interventions to reduce these barriers could therefore be targeted at improving medical education surrounding care for individuals with disabilities. There is currently a lack of data supporting specific curricular models in medical education to address this gap in training, but it is an active area of research and one proposal has undergone initial evaluation.[33,34]

The accreditation agencies that determine eligibility for federal funding for medical education and residency training programs have core curriculum requirements that must be met by programs in order to receive accreditation and funding. Unfortunately, disability competency is not currently a core curriculum requirement mandated by the accreditation agencies for medical training programs.[30] One step to improve medical training and better equip physicians to care for women with disabilities would be for accrediting agencies to include disability competency in their requirements.

In addition to reducing barriers to competent care through improved medical training, the medical community should work to minimize physical barriers in clinical settings. There are straightforward steps that medical practices can take to comply with the ADA and accommodate patients with disabilities. General accommodations include ensuring adequate accessible parking and accessible pathways through the clinic and into the exam room, including an appropriately sized entry door with adequate width, as well as space once inside the exam rooms for transfers. Clinics and hospitals must also have accessible examination equipment available such as accessible exam tables and lifts. To provide women with disabilities adequate access to reproductive care and fertility treatments, clinics need to implement additional adaptations, such as having padded leg supports available instead of typical stirrups for gynecological exams. Detailed information about these adaptations and other necessary accommodations for patients with mobility disabilities can be found on the website of the US Department of Health and Human Services.[67] Providers should also have means of communicating physician recommendations that are accessible to persons with various disabilities. This might include having instructions available in Braille, large print, audiotape, and/or on a computer disk, instructions accessible to individuals with only primary-school-grade reading ability, and sign language interpretation for physician visits.

In reducing barriers to reproductive and fertility care for women with disabilities seeking pregnancy and motherhood, it is important not to forget that accessible care will be necessary not only during the preconception and prenatal periods but also longitudinally for the mother and child after birth. This has implications not only for adult medicine and obstetrics and gynecology clinics but also for pediatric practices so that mothers with disabilities can be active participants in their children's medical care. Reasonable accommodations for pediatric practices must go beyond physical adaptations to the clinic setting. Involvement of multidisciplinary professionals can optimize care and minimize barriers. For example, occupational therapists can work with families and recommend accessible equipment for parents such as accessible cribs for use by parents with disabilities. Social workers can connect women with resources for assistance with childcare and programs for parental training. This may be particularly important in supporting mothers with intellectual disabilities.

In their chapter "Supporting Parents with Disabilities and Their Families in the Community," the National Council on Disability[29] emphasizes aspects of disability as a societal construct. Recognition that parents without disabilities require and utilize many supports to raise children—among them daycare, tutoring, or grandparent involvement—on a regular basis calls into question why services that support the needs of parents with disabilities in caring for their children are not more readily available. Unfortunately, significant barriers exist in the US currently in terms of long-term support of parents with disabilities, as government-funded personal assistance services do not allow attendants who are assisting parents with disabilities with their own care to provide help in caring for their children.[29] This is not the case in other countries, including Canada and Sweden, where similar government-supported services for individuals with disabilities can be used to assist with the care of a child. The ADA likely would not be interpreted to mandate this change, as the change from care for the disabled person himself or herself to care for a dependent child could be considered a fundamental alteration in the service provided. On the other hand, assisting the parent with a disability to participate in his or her children's activities—such as by mobility assistance to enter a playground—could be considered a reasonable modification of a public service or public accommodation. Advocating for policy change in this area would be a step toward reducing barriers for not only mothers but also fathers with disabilities in the pursuit of family relationships. Such policy changes might inadvertently decrease the bias of medical providers toward providing fertility care to women with disabilities as well as encouraging women who desire pregnancy but are deterred by attitudes of providers and societal barriers to seek fertility care.

Uncertainty about their ability to keep custody of their children is an ongoing concern for parents with disabilities.[16,29] In one notorious recent case, blind parents had their two-day-old daughter taken into state custody on the basis of initial awkwardness at breastfeeding—hardly an unusual experience for any new parents. The state mistakenly presumed that the parents were unfit and only permitted supervised hour-long visits two or three times a week for the child's first 2 months, until the parents succeeded in challenging their daughter's placement in foster care.[68] In another recent case, an Oregon couple, both of whom have mild to moderate cognitive impairments, have been fighting the state for custody of their two sons; although they have regained custody of the younger boy, the older child remains in state custody because of concerns that he has needs beyond their parenting capabilities.[69,70] One important recent court decision has held that it is a violation of the ADA for the state to fail to give accommodations to parents with disabilities before instituting provisions to terminate parental rights.[71] While not within the immediate domain of healthcare, such modifications in child custody practices are critical adjuncts to the parenting experiences of people with disabilities.

The possibility of obtaining reasonable accommodations in employment may also be important for women with disabilities contemplating pregnancy and parenting. As least two pathways are available for women with disabilities to claim accommodations for pregnancy and parenting. First, she might need accommodations because of the nature of the pregnancy and birth process. Most courts hold that normal pregnancy and childbirth is not a disability for purposes of the ADA, because it is not a physical or mental impairment that substantially limits a major life activity. Complex pregnancies or births, however, may be impairments, for example if they require substantial time on bedrest or longer recovery times postpartum. Second, she might need accommodations for pregnancy or parenting because of the nature of her underlying disability.

In both of these types of cases, the woman may claim accommodations such as time off work, a modified schedule, or modified responsibilities. These accommodations must be reasonable and would be subject to the qualification that they not impose an undue hardship on the employer. Accommodations are not reasonable if the employee remains unable to perform essential job functions; an example might be a teacher who cannot be in a classroom for a significant portion of the school day. Requested accommodations would be an undue hardship if they would require other employees to take over responsibilities that would be a significant imposition on them. On the other hand, many courts have held that a reasonable period off work, with a clear plan for the employee's return, is not an undue hardship in many employment situations. Schedule adjustments that would give an employee with a disability additional time needed to fulfill parental responsibilities might also be judged reasonable accommodations under Title I of the ADA.

As we emphasized at the outset of this chapter, disability is importantly a matter of social context. Encouragingly, the social context is changing for parents with disabilities. Independent living organizations such as Through the Looking Glass have been catalysts for these changes. They have contributed to research on essential supports for physically disabled mothers of young children.[72] Universal design in equipment for children such as cribs, car seats, feeding devices, tracking devices, and play materials is increasingly available.[73,74] The modifications we have suggested should be enriched by these developments.

Conclusion

For women with disabilities and their partners, pregnancy and parenting may be as important goods as they are for nondisabled people. The capability of people with disabilities to parent continues to be underestimated and poorly accommodated. Providers who treat women with disabilities need improved education and improved facilities so that this population may realize their ambitions to form families. Improvements in social services and payment structures should follow as well.

Note

1. Under US law, "accommodations" are individualized adjustments to enable people with disabilities to receive the benefits of public services or to enjoy public accommodations on a par with others; "modifications" change policies or practices along lines that further access more universally.

References

1. Iezzoni LI, Yu J, Wint AJ, Smeltzer SC, Ecker JL. General health, health conditions, and current pregnancy among U.S. women with and without chronic physical disabilities. *Disabil Health J.* 2014;7(2):181–188.

2. Redshaw M, Malouf R, Gao H, Gray R. Women with disability: the experience of maternity care during pregnancy, labour and birth and the postnatal period. *BMC Pregnancy Childbirth.* 2013;13:174. doi: 10.1186/1471-2393-13-174
3. Sunnybrook Health Sciences Centre. New pregnancy clinic supports women with physical disabilities. https://sunnybrook.ca/media/item.asp?c=&i=1566&f=north-american-pregnancy-clinic-disabilities. Published May 10, 2017. Accessed March 22, 2018.
4. Department of Health and Human Services. Pregnancy in women with disabilities. https://grants.nih.gov/grants/guide/pa-files/PA-17-451.html. Published August 3, 2017. Accessed March 22, 2018.
5. Lurie Institute for Disability Policy. Current projects. http://lurie.brandeis.edu/research/projects.html. Published 2018. Accessed March 22, 2018.
6. 42 U.S.C. § 12181(7)(F) (2018).
7. 42 U.S.C. § 12182(a) (2018).
8. 42 U.S.C. § 12182(b)(1)(A)(i) (2018).
9. 42 U.S.C. § 12182(b)(1)(A)(ii) (2018).
10. 42 U.S.C. § 12182(b)(2)(A)(i) (2018).
11. 42 U.S.C. § 12182(b)(2)(A)(ii) (2018).
12. 42 U.S.C. § 12182(b)(2)(A)(iii) (2018).
13. 29 U.S.C. § 794(f) (2018).
14. Pendo E. Disability equipment barriers, and women's health: using the ADA to provide meaningful access. *SLU J Health Law Policy.* 2008;2:15–56.
15. Malouf R, Henderson J, Redshaw M. Access and quality of maternity care for disabled women during pregnancy, birth and the postnatal period in England: data from a national survey. *BJM Open.* 2017;7:e016757. doi:10.1136/bmjopen-2017-016757.
16. Höglund B, Larsson M. Struggling for motherhood with an intellectual disability—a qualitative study of women's experiences in Sweden. *Midwifery.* 2013;29(6):698–704.
17. Iezzoni LI, Wint AJ, Smeltzer SC, Ecker JL. "How did that happen?" Public responses to women with mobility disability during pregnancy. *Disabil Health J.* 2015;8:380–387.
18. Powell RM, Mitra M, Smeltzer SC, Long-Bellil LM, Smith LD, Iezzoni LI. Family attitudes and reactions toward pregnancy among women with physical disabilities. *Womens Health Iss.* 2017;27(3):345–350.
19. Iezzoni LI, Wint AJ, Smeltzer SC, Ecker JL. Recommendations about pregnancy from women with mobility disability to their peers. *Womens Health Iss.* 2017;27(1):75–82.
20. Smeltzer SC, Mitra M, Long-Bellil L, Iezzoni LI, Smith LD. Obstetric clinicians' experiences and educational preparation for caring for pregnant women with physical disabilities: a qualitative study. *Disabil Health J.* 2018;11:8–13.
21. Chandra A, Copen CE, Stephen EH. Infertility service use in the United States: data from the National Survey of Family Growth, 1982–2010. *National*

22. *Health Statistics Reports*. 2014;73. https://www.cdc.gov/nchs/data/nhsr/nhsr073.pdf.
22. Kaiser Family Foundation. Medicaid's role for women. https://www.kff.org/womens-health-policy/fact-sheet/medicaids-role-for-women/. Published June 22, 2017. Accessed March 22, 2018.
23. Walls J, Gifford K, Ranji U, Salganicoff A, Gomes I. 2016. Medicaid coverage of family planning benefits: results from a state survey. https://www.kff.org/report-section/medicaid-coverage-of-family-planning-benefits-results-from-a-state-survey-fertility-services/. Published September 15, 2016. Accessed March 22, 2018.
24. Centers for Medicare and Medicaid Services. Medicare Benefit Policy Manual, Ch. 15, 20.1. https://www.cms.gov/Regulations-and-Guidance/Guidance/Manuals/downloads/bp102c15.PDF. Published July 11, 2017. Accessed March 22, 2018.
25. Donovan MK. In real life: federal restrictions on abortion coverage and the women they impact. Guttmacher Institute. https://www.guttmacher.org/gpr/2017/01/real-life-federal-restrictions-abortion-coverage-and-women-they-impact. Published January 5, 2017. Accessed March 22, 2018.
26. National Conference of States Legislatures. State laws related to insurance coverage for infertility treatment. http://www.ncsl.org/research/health/insurance-coverage-for-infertility-laws.aspx. Published June 1, 2014. Accessed March 22, 2018.
27. Veterans Health Administration. Directive 1332. www.va.gov/vhapublications/viewpublication.asp?pub_id=5431. Published June 20, 2017. Accessed March 22, 2018.
28. Shakespeare T. The social model of disability. In: Davis LJ, ed. *The Disability Studies Reader*. New York, NY: Routledge; 2010:266–273.
29. National Council on Disability. Rocking the cradle: ensuring the rights of parents with disabilities and their children. https://www.ncd.gov/sites/default/files/Documents/NCD_Parenting_508_0.pdf. Published September 27, 2012. Accessed March 22, 2018.
30. National Council on Disability. The current state of health care for people with disabilities. https://www.ncd.gov/rawmedia_repository/0d7c848f_3d97_43b3_bea5_36e1d97f973d.pdf. Published September 30, 2009. Accessed March 22, 2018.
31. Claxton A. 1994. Teaching medical students about disability. *Br Med J.* 1994;308:805.
32. Mosher W, Bloom T, Hughes R, Horton L, Mojtabai R, Alhusen JL. Disparities in receipt of family planning services by disability status: new estimates from the National Survey of Family Growth. *Disabil Health J.* 2017;10:394–399.
33. Symons AB, McGuigan D, Aki EA. A curriculum to teach medical students to care for people with disabilities: development and initial implementation. *BMC Med. Educ.* 2009;9:78.

34. Symons AB, Morley CP, McGuigan D, Aki EA. A curriculum on care for people with disabilities: effects on medical student self-reported attitudes and comfort level. *Disabil Health J.* 2014;7(1):88–95.
35. Tervo RC, Azuma S, Palmer G, Redinius P. Medical students' attitudes toward persons with disability: a comparative study. *Arch Phys Med Rehabil.* 2002;83(11):1537–1542.
36. Goreczny AJ, Bender EE, Caruso G, Feinstein CS. Attitudes toward individuals with disabilities; results of a recent survey and implications of those results. *Res Develop Disabil.* 2011;32:1596–1609.
37. Chadd EH, Pangilinan PH. Disability attitudes in health care: a new scale instrument. *Am J Phys Med Rehabil.* 2011;90(1):47–54.
38. McColl MA, Forster D, Shortt SED, et al. Physician experiences providing primary care to people with disabilities. *Healthcare Policy.* 2008;4(1): e129–e147.
39. American Society for Reproductive Medicine. Provision of fertility services for women at increased risk of complications during fertility treatment or pregnancy: an Ethics Committee Opinion. *Fertil Steril.* 2016;106(6):1319–1323.
40. Shandra CL, Hogan D, Short S. Planning for motherhood: fertility attitudes, desires and intentions among women with disabilities. *Perspect Sexual Reprod Health.* 2014;46(4):203–210.
41. Hall DE, Prochazka AV, Fink AS. Informed consent for clinical treatment. *Can Med Assoc J.* 2012;184(5):533–540.
42. Appelbaum PS. Assessment of patients' competence to consent to treatment. *N Engl J Med.* 2007;357:1834–1840.
43. Cohen A. *Imbeciles: The Supreme Court, American Eugenics, and the Sterilization of Carrie Buck.* New York, NY: Penguin; 2016.
44. Lombardo PA, ed. *A Century of Eugenics in America: From the Indiana Experiment to the Human Genome Era.* Bloomington, IN: Indiana University Press; 2011.
45. Lombardo PA. *Three Generations No Imbeciles: Eugenics, the Supreme Court, and Buck v. Bell.* Baltimore, MD: Johns Hopkins University Press; 2008.
46. 274 U.S. 200 (1927).
47. United Nations Convention on the Rights of Persons with Disabilities. https://www.un.org/development/desa/disabilities/convention-on-the-rights-of-persons-with-disabilities/convention-on-the-rights-of-persons-with-disabilities-2.html. Published 2007. Accessed March 22, 2018.
48. Scholten M, Gather J. Adverse consequences of article 12 of the UN Convention on the Rights of Persons with Disabilities for persons with mental disabilities and an alternative way forward. *J Med Ethics.* 2018;44(4):226–233.
49. Bach M, Kerzner L. A new paradigm for protecting autonomy and the right to legal capacity: advancing substantive equality for persons with disabilities through law, policy and practice. Law Commission of Ontario. https://www.lco-cdo.org/

wp-content/uploads/2010/11/disabilities-commissioned-paper-bach-kerzner.pdf, Published October 2010. Accessed March 22, 2018.
50. American Society for Reproductive Medicine. Child-rearing ability and the provision of fertility services: an Ethics Committee opinion. *Fertil Steril.* 2017;108(6):944–947.
51. Powell R. Parents with disabilities face an uphill battle to keep their children. *Pacific Standard.* January 3, 2018. https://psmag.com/social-justice/parents-with-disabilities-face-an-uphill-battle-to-keep-their-children Accessed March 22, 2018.
52. Cureton A. Parents with disabilities. In: Francis L, ed. *The Oxford Handbook of Reproductive Ethics.* New York, NY: Oxford University Press; 2017:407–426.
53. Signore C, Spong CY, Krotoski D, Shinowara NL, Blackwell SC. Pregnancy in women with physical disabilities. *Obstet Gynecol.* 2011;117(4):935–947.
54. Antommaria A. Conscientious objection in reproductive health. In: Francis L, ed. *The Oxford Handbook of Reproductive Ethics.* New York, NY: Oxford University Press; 2017:209–225.
55. US Department of Labor. Issue brief: key characteristics of working women with disabilities. https://www.dol.gov/wb/resources/women_with_disability_issue_brief.pdf. Published July 2015. Accessed March 22, 2018.
56. American Society for Reproductive Medicine. Disparities in access to effective treatment for infertility in the United States: an Ethics Committee opinion. *Fertil Steril.* 2015;104(5):1104–1110.
57. *Harris v. McRae*, 448 U.S. 297 (1980).
58. Goldstein A, Eilperin J, Wan W. Trump administration narrows Affordable Care Act's contraception mandate. *Washington Post.* October 6, 2017. https://www.washingtonpost.com/national/health-science/trump-administration-could-narrow-affordable-care-acts-contraception-mandate/2017/10/05/16139400-a9f0-11e7-92d1-58c702d2d975_story.html?utm_term=.074c4e29e84d. Accessed March 22, 2018.
59. Shane L. VA to start offering IVF services to veterans this spring. *Military Times.* January 19, 2017. https://www.militarytimes.com/veterans/2017/01/19/va-to-start-offering-ivf-services-to-veterans-this-spring/. Accessed March 22, 2018.
60. 42 U.S.C. § 12182(b)(2)(A)(ii) (2018).
61. 42 U.S.C. § 12181(7) (2018).
62. 42 U.S.C. § 12131(2) (2018).
63. 42 U.S.C. § 12112(b)(5)(A) (2018).
64. Burge P, Cleaver S, Isaacs B, Lunsky Y, Jones J, Hastie, R. Attitude of medical clerks toward persons with intellectual disabilities. *J Coll Family Phys Can.* 2012;58(5):282–288.
65. Delucia LM, Davis EL. Dental students' attitudes toward the care of individuals with intellectual disabilities: relationship between instruction and experience. *J Dental Educ.* 2009;73(4):445–453.

66. Ruedrich S, Dunn J, Schwartz S, Nordgren L. Psychiatric resident education in intellectual disabilities: one program's ten years of experience. *Acad Psychiatry*. 2007;31(6):430–434.
67. Department of Health and Human Services, Office for Civil Rights. 2010. Access to medical care for individuals with mobility disabilities. https://www.ada.gov/medcare_ta.htm. Published July 22, 2010. Accessed March 22, 2018.
68. Powell R. Can parents lose custody simply because they are disabled? *GPSolo*. 2014;31(2). https://www.americanbar.org/publications/gp_solo/2014/march_april/can_parents_lose_custody_simply_because_they_are_disabled.html. Accessed March 22, 2018.
69. Powell R. Parents with disabilities face an uphill battle to keep their children. *Pacific Standard*. January 3, 2018. https://psmag.com/social-justice/parents-with-disabilities-face-an-uphill-battle-to-keep-their-children. Accessed March 22, 2018.
70. Swindler S. *In re Hicks*, 890 N.W.2d 696 (Mich. App. 2016). Judge rules Oregon parents with low IQs can take youngest son home. *The Oregonian*. December 24, 2017. http://www.oregonlive.com/pacific-northwest-news/index.ssf/2017/12/judge_rules_oregon_parents_wit.html. Accessed March 22, 2018.
71. *In re Hicks*, 890 N.W.2d 696 (Mich. App. 2016).
72. Jacob J, Kirshbaum M, Preston P. Mothers with physical disabilities caring for young children. *J Soc Work Disabil Rehabil*. 2017;16(2):95–115.
73. Through the Looking Glass. Baby care equipment on the market. https://www.lookingglass.org/pdf/Baby-care-products-chart-TLG-9-2016.pdf. Published 2016. Accessed March 22, 2018.
74. Disabled Parenting Project. Links to adaptive parenting products. http://www.disabledparenting.com/marketplace/links-to-adaptive-parenting-products/ Published 2018. Accessed March 22, 2018.

14

RESEARCH WITH PREGNANT WOMEN

A FEMINIST CHALLENGE

Margaret Olivia Little, Marisha N. Wickremsinhe, Elana Jaffe, and Anne Drapkin Lyerly

Introduction

The 1990s ushered in an era of reforms for the clinical research enterprise.[1,2] In response to the increasing concern that medical research was predominantly conducted with adult white male subjects,[2] legislative and other changes prompted a steady shift toward broader representation of other populations—specifically women, racial and ethnic minorities, and children—in medical research. Progress with women's health has been particularly remarkable. The 1993 NIH Revitalization Act mandated women's and minorities' inclusion in clinical research[3] and marked a key step forward in advancing the health interests of women; today over half of clinical research participants are women,[4] though gaps remain with regard to specific diseases.

But one key group of women has been left out: those who are pregnant. Each year, millions of women face serious illness during pregnancy. In the US alone, more than 500,000 women will face diabetes or hypertension during their pregnancies;[5] an estimated 20% of pregnant women in the US experience psychiatric disorders such as generalized anxiety or alcohol dependence.[6] Globally, the issue is yet more dire. For example, an estimated 13 million pregnant women worldwide experience a mental disorder,[7] at least 1.5 million women who give birth each year are living with HIV,[8] an estimated 28 million women are at risk for malaria,[9] and over 200,000 experience active tuberculosis during pregnancy.[10]

Left untreated, such diseases can have significant consequences for women's own health: pregnant women with malaria, for example, face a nearly 50% chance of dying from the disease.[11] A hiatus in treatment during pregnancy can also have effects on a woman's health long after the pregnancy is over and the baby is delivered: pausing treatment for a pregnant woman with multiple sclerosis can cause irreversible disability.[12] Untreated maternal disease can also have dire consequences for her future child: untreated diabetes in early pregnancy can lead to serious birth defects;[13] untreated depression is associated with growth restriction and preterm delivery;[14] untreated maternal HIV infection can lead to transmission of infection to the fetus;[15] untreated malaria is associated with miscarriage as well as in utero growth restriction that can lead to neonatal death.[16,17] Access to preventive medicines, too, can be critical for pregnant women. For instance, pregnant women living in areas with high rates of HIV transmission are among those who most need access to preventives (e.g., pre-exposure prophylaxis)—because the physiology of pregnancy appears to actually *increase* a woman's susceptibility to HIV infection.[18–20]

Yet, the evidence base for the use of treatments and preventives during pregnancy is shockingly sparse.[21,22] In fact, pregnant women have been called "the last therapeutic orphans."[23] Few pharmaceuticals are approved by the US Food and Drug Administration (FDA) specifically for use during pregnancy.[24] Though FDA officials have advised that drugs approved for adult populations are implicitly approved for use in pregnant adults,[25] nearly 98% of drugs approved by the FDA between 2000 and 2010 have "undetermined" teratogenic risk; the average lag between drug approval and determination of fetal safety is 27 years.[26] The vast majority of medications used to treat numerous illnesses during pregnancy—whether chronic disease that precedes pregnancy, or infection or other conditions that arise during pregnancy—rely on a poor evidence base for the compound's safety, dosing, or efficacy in the pregnant body. The result is guesswork—and anxiety—for women, their families, and healthcare providers as they try to make decisions about how best to prevent or treat illness in the context of pregnancy.

The reason for this lack of evidence is a simple one: pregnant women and their health needs have been excluded from the social investment in clinical research. This exclusion is systematic: the health needs of pregnant women are not addressed in activities that shape the research agenda; reproductive toxicology studies that facilitate an understanding of fetal safety are often not performed in a timely fashion; pregnant women are routinely excluded from trials that offer the prospect of direct benefit; and when women become pregnant while participating in clinical trials, they are typically removed from the study medication regardless of whether they or their future child may stand to benefit from medication continuation or may experience harm from study removal. As a result, pregnant women are often left behind from novel advances. Those who are treated tend to be given older drugs that are less effective or have worse side effect profiles.[27] And all too often, given the poor evidence base, they are not treated at all. Pregnant women, in short, are an afterthought in the drug/vaccine development life cycle.

This inattention occurs despite the fact that regulations governing human subjects research permit such research. In the US, for instance, the regulations governing research conducted with pregnant women and fetuses—Subpart B of the Department of Health and Human Services (HHS) Policy for the Protection of Human Research Subjects (45 CFR 46)[28]—were changed in 2001 to clarify the permissibility of such research as long as certain protections are in place: that preclinical studies have been conducted to inform assessment of the research's potential risks and benefits, for instance, and specific risk standards are met.[29]

But the culture of clinical research with pregnant women lags far behind what the regulations allow. For one, pharmaceutical companies have few incentives to conduct research in pregnant women—indeed, liability concerns give them every reason not to.[30] More broadly, even where researchers and those who fund them are highly motivated to address pregnant women's health concerns, misunderstandings about the regulations governing such research persist.[31]

But another issue, we suspect, is more foundational. One of the key reasons for the lack of research with pregnant women may have less to do with operationalizing such research as it does with conceptualizing it. There is a continued confusion and unease around foundational ethical questions about such research. A variety of stakeholders in the research enterprise, including policymakers, Institutional Review Boards (IRBs), and researchers themselves, remain profoundly unclear about how to morally frame research during pregnancy.[1]

In this chapter, we articulate three models that have been advanced for morally framing research with pregnant women: an unfettered protectionist model, in which pregnant women are categorized as a "vulnerable population" for purposes of clinical research; a model of unrestricted deference to the pregnant woman's autonomy; and a model that construes the fetus as a pediatric research subject. Each, we argue, is critically flawed. As in other arenas, pregnancy presents a specific context that deserves a theory of its own.

With lessons learned from their respective limitations, we point toward ways in which research during pregnancy must be given unique consideration, and toward progressive work beginning development of an adequate model.

Unfettered Protectionism: Pregnant Women as a "Vulnerable Population"

The first model for morally framing research with pregnant women categorizes them as a "vulnerable population" for purposes of clinical research. For example, and importantly, US regulations governing human subjects research (Subpart A, also known as the Common Rule) have historically listed pregnant women as a vulnerable population.[32] Though the designation is far from universal,[33] it has exerted a powerful framing in many jurisdictions, including countries whose human subjects research guidelines have been influenced by US regulations and training programs. More broadly, at the 2016 Global Forum on Bioethics in Research meeting on the ethics of research in pregnancy, which drew participants from over 40 countries, the persistence of the assumption that pregnant women are "vulnerable" was identified as a critical barrier to research by many attendees.[34] For many research contexts, it seems, the state of pregnancy is perceived as one that renders women in need of a protectionist orientation.

While presumably well intentioned, the categorization of pregnant women as a vulnerable population for purposes of research has had two deep problems.

First, the regulatory category is increasingly acknowledged to be offensive to pregnant women.[35,36] The other populations classified as vulnerable in the US regulations are children, prisoners, "mentally disabled persons," and those "economically or educationally disadvantaged."[32] These, note, are populations that are inherently at risk for exploitation, or are, by capacity or by context, compromised in their ability to provide valid consent to research. For the mentally disabled, constrained voluntariness is due to compromise in decisional capacity; for prisoners, it is due to power dynamics that inherently impinge on the voluntariness of participation.

But none of these scenarios applies to pregnant women as a category. To state the obvious, pregnancy does not itself limit the ability to reason. And while there are some cultures in which pregnancy meaningfully constrains women's free decision making around matters such as research participation, or places them in conditions ripe for exploitation, this is highly contextual and not something that redounds to the category of pregnancy in its own right.

Second, the designation of pregnant women as a "vulnerable population" has ended up having a profoundly chilling effect when it comes to research—even highly responsible research—into the health needs of pregnant women and the children they bear.[37] Such a designation has led to a regulatory culture that regards the ethical imperative it oversees to be exclusion of pregnant women in research, rather than responsible inclusion in carefully designed trials. This culture is so strong, indeed, that it can lead to the exclusion of pregnant women even in research that carries *no* theoretical risk to the fetus. For example, a lifestyle intervention trial to prevent diabetes in women in India excluded pregnant women, even though no scientific complexity or theoretical risk was attributed to use of that intervention during pregnancy.[38]

This stance of unfettered protectionism has a paradoxical effect: it leads to a *lack* of protection for pregnant women and the children they bear.[2] The 2013–2016 Ebola crisis in West Africa offers a particularly instructive example of this at the individual level. During the Ebola virus disease (EVD) epidemic, pregnant women were at extraordinarily high risk of death: infection carried a high likelihood of death, estimated between 89% and 93%.[39] The implications of fetal infections were even worse, with almost 100% fetal or neonatal mortality.[39] No mother–baby pair has ever survived.[39] At the time of the epidemic, there were no approved treatments or vaccines against EVD. Given the especially significant consequences of infection during pregnancy, pregnant women were among those with the greatest stake in having access to trials where new preventives and therapeutics were being tested. Nevertheless, the paradigm of exclusion prevailed. Despite recommendations and multiple ethics committee requests (notably citing that the relevant "vulnerability" here for pregnant women and fetuses was to the disease, due to high mortality rates from infection), pregnant women had a tremendously difficult time getting access to the experimental interventions.[39,40] The fear of harming the woman and her fetus through such interventions meant that, ultimately, they were put directly in harm's way. As Gomes and colleagues describe the case, pregnant women were, in fact, "protected to death."[39]

The lack of research with pregnant women also leads to greater harm at the population level. Overprotectionism in the sphere of clinical research has the effect of *shifting* and *expanding* risk in the sphere of clinical care. The lack of carefully structured safety research leaves us without data to guide decisions about which medicines are safest to use during pregnancy. Yet medicines *are* prescribed and used during pregnancy: indeed, the average number of medications (over-the-counter or prescription) used by American women during the course of pregnancy is 4.2.[41] The risks associated with a particular intervention, for both the woman and the child she bears, are thus shifted from a controlled research setting to an uncontrolled clinical setting, where outcomes may not be systematically measured or reported. For instance, after nearly 30 years on the market, researchers indicated that if pregnant women take a commonly prescribed hypertension medication during the first trimester, their newborns were potentially more likely to be born with heart and nervous system problems.[42] While the association has since been debated due to a lack of confirmatory studies (and some indicating no risk), the rub has been that if researchers had studied the drug in pregnancy earlier on, congenital anomalies that may have resulted from three decades of pregnant women's use of the medication since the approval could have been prevented by use of alternative medications. Other examples highlight the risks for women. For instance, a full decade went by before the oral medication that replaced insulin as the mainstay of treatment for gestational diabetes was studied to determine its pharmacokinetics during pregnancy. The result of the study, when finally performed, was distressing: at equivalent doses, drug concentrations in pregnant women were only *half* that of non-pregnant women.[43] Earlier research to inform proper dosing may have led to better control of blood sugar and fewer treatment failures.

The critical need for more equitable inclusion of pregnant women's health interests in clinical research has now been acknowledged and promoted by several leading health organizations, including the American College of Obstetricians and Gynecologists (ACOG),[44] the Pan American Health Organization (PAHO),[45] the Office of Research on Women's Health of the US's National Institutes of Health (ORWH NIH),[46] and the Council for International Organizations of Medical Sciences (CIOMS)—a nongovernmental organization established by the World Health Organization (WHO) and the United Nations Educational, Scientific and Cultural Organization (UNESCO) that seeks to advance public health through guidance on health research.[47] CIOMS has explicitly urged that pregnant women not be regarded as a vulnerable population (indeed, they urge dropping the category in general, due to its chilling effect on research needed for the very populations it is meant to protect).

And in an encouraging sign of progress, recent revisions to the US regulations included the very welcome announcement that pregnant women will no longer be listed in the category of vulnerable populations (the revisions are required to be implemented as of January, 2019).[48,49] This is an important step forward. Pregnant women, and the children they bear, need to be protected in the research enterprise, but they also need to be protected *through* the research enterprise.

Deferring to Pregnant Women's Autonomy

The previous section has argued that there is a moral imperative to pursue clinical research during pregnancy, for the sake of both pregnant women and the children they may bear, and that pregnant women should not be categorized as a vulnerable population. Of course, to say that they are not vulnerable is not to say they are simply like any other research participant: pregnant women carry a fetus that can be harmed by exposure to the compounds and biologics being studied. How should we morally frame inclusion of pregnant women in research, given that their participation carries the potential to harm a fetus that cannot consent to participation?

Here, some have argued that the hard-fought lessons on women's reproductive rights point to the right model. If we have learned anything, one might think, it is that decisions around the pregnant woman's body and health, as well as around the fetus, are ones that should be left to the pregnant woman herself. Pregnant women should have strong decisional authority when it comes to making decisions about how best to incorporate the fact of pregnancy into their decision making. It would not be appropriate to constrain the opportunities pregnant women have to participate in clinical research based on third-party judgments about which risks are acceptable to take during pregnancy. Decisions involving the fetus, it is argued, should defer to the individual pregnant woman.[2]

Certainly, pregnant women's autonomy needs to be respected in the context of clinical research, no less than any other. But the issues raised by the conduct of research during pregnancy are specific and unique: addressing them requires construction of public and transparent standards of allowable fetal risk.

First, an important clarification: the key ethical issue presented by clinical research during pregnancy is different from the (important) issue of women's autonomy around abortion. Sometimes concern is raised that standards of allowable fetal risk in research perforce attribute strong moral status to the fetus in a way that is troublesome. After all, fetal protection standards in research apply throughout gestation, even at very early stages of pregnancy, when the law protects—or should protect—women's right to abort.

It is certainly true, we would concur, that the clinical research enterprise should not opine on the moral status of the early fetus. But the central issue in clinical research in fact sidesteps this contentious issue. Most research with pregnant women is conducted with pregnancies that would continue to term.[3] What happens in utero to the fetus can profoundly affect the welfare of the child who will be born. Whatever one believes about the contemporaneous moral status a fetus carries at a given stage of gestation—an issue on which reasonable people will disagree—for pregnancies that are continued, the impact of research done prior to birth is a critical consideration. That is, in establishing standards for allowable fetal risk in research, even at early stages of gestation, the clinical research enterprise need not assert that the fetus at that stage has full moral status; indeed, it could be highly supportive of pregnant women's rights to determine whether or not the pregnancy continues. Rather, it must take account of the very real possibility that the pregnancy will continue, including the potential risks and benefits of the protocol to that prospective child. The central concern about fetal risk in research, in short, is concern for the fetus as a future child.

Of course, the prospective child's well-being is something that pregnant women continuing their pregnancies care deeply about. As legal scholar Vanessa Merton puts it, there are few who can be better trusted than pregnant women to make good decisions for their fetuses.[50] Further, it is important that pregnant women have broad discretion and authority to decide how best to navigate the needs and interests of their future child, including in contexts that may involve tradeoffs to their own needs or those of other family members, given the embodied nature of pregnancy. Noting this, defenders of a model of full deference to a pregnant woman's autonomy as a moral frame for the research context may still urge that, while a pregnant woman needs to be given relevant information on evidence about potential fetal risks, the only constraints on allowable fetal risks in research should be the ones she determines.

Pregnant women do need and deserve strong deference in decisions taken on behalf of their future child. That said, it is inappropriate to defer to pregnant women's individual decision making for determining acceptable fetal risk in clinical research. The reason has to do with the distinctive nature of the research enterprise itself.

Clinical research is an arena that is—appropriately—highly regulated. It has extensive standards and strong oversight of a great many issues, including standards for valid consent and the like, but especially, and critically, formal standards of allowable harms that may be incurred by research participation. For *any* research population, even so-called healthy volunteers, there are standards of risk that must be met before participants are ever allowed an opportunity to enroll. The reasons for this are several. For one, understanding the potential risks is no easy matter. The structure of clinical research is highly complex and technical: a very high degree of expertise would be needed to understand and interpret risk assessments in this context, especially given the varying levels of evidence and inference being made in the different stages of research. Further, there is ample empirical evidence that prospective participants are subject to the "therapeutic misconception"—the mistaken impression that research protocols are designed to advance their individual health interests when they are not.[51] In addition, the clinical research enterprise carries potential for—and indeed a specific history of—abuses.[52] Even if a given individual is in no danger of misunderstanding the risks of a given trial, regulatory structures are needed to establish strong guardrails as disincentives to potential bad actors, both to protect participants in the aggregate and to maintain the public trust that is a critical prerequisite of clinical research proceeding. Further, some studies may exclude individuals for scientific reasons such that inclusion of certain individuals would be a problematic use of resources or inconsistent with risk/benefit profiles deemed appropriate for the study. Finally, *ex ante* risk standards are needed to inform decisions about who may safely participate and to determine "stopping rules" that data and safety monitoring boards—groups set up to monitor incoming evidence around safety during the course of the trial—must enforce.

For all of these reasons, it is critical that there be clear, transparent, and generalized standards of allowable research-related risks to the fetus as well as the pregnant woman herself. Indeed, pregnant women will also want to know that an opportunity to join a trial has been vetted by rigorous screening about the potential harms the trial might bring. And it is not just for the sake of the pregnant woman. As in public health, when we fund prenatal medical care, or in clinical care, when we have guidelines informing which medications physicians should prescribe during pregnancy, we are doing this for the sake of the pregnant woman and for the benefit of the child who will be born. The fetus as a future child is an independent and consensus object of beneficent concern. So, too, the clinical research enterprise must have consensus standards of about what fetal risks are acceptable. In all of these contexts, such standards will perforce embed values-based decisions about which risks are reasonable. It will, of course, still be up to the individual pregnant woman to decide whether trials that meet those standards are acceptable to her given her own risk tolerances. But we cannot simply defer to individual pregnant women's autonomy as the standard for acceptable risk—for the sake of the pregnant woman, for the sake of the future child, and for the viability of the clinical research enterprise itself.

Assimilating to Pediatric Research

The previous section has argued that clinical research guidance must include consensus standards on allowable fetal risk based on the fetus as a prospective child. Given the connection to children, some have argued that the standards for fetal risk in research should be modeled on those used for pediatric research subjects. After all, if the fetus is an object of concern as a future child, then we can use standards developed *for* children. Bioethicist Carson Strong suggests that the standards governing research-related risk to the fetus should be in parity with the risk standards governing research with children—not because of any claim about fetal status, but because "injuries to the fetus can impact the child."[53] A third model for morally framing research with pregnant women—more specifically, for framing the difference made by the presence of the fetus as a future child—is to treat the fetus *as* a child now for purposes of fashioning allowable risks.

It is certainly true that comparing fetal and pediatric protections can be instructive. Indeed, as Strong also points out, there are places in the regulations where fetuses are actually *over*-protected in research relative to what we tolerate for born children—something that deserves interrogation.[4] That said, there is a critical danger in simply assimilating fetal standards of risk to those fashioned for children. Even if we are considering the fetus under the guise of a future child, there is an important difference between research in pregnancy and research in pediatrics. In pediatric research, the child is physically separated; in pregnancy, the fetus is physically attached and physiologically interconnected with the woman. And this has important implications for fashioning standards around risk—in particular, for standards of risk in trials that offer the prospect of medical benefit.

As a general matter, clinical trials can be divided according to whether or not the trial in question carries the prospect of medical benefit to its participants. While early stage trials, for instance, may lack sufficient evidence to justify any responsible attribution of potential benefit, or indeed may intentionally use subtherapeutic doses to minimize exposure, later-stage trials testing the efficacy of the intervention may provide important medical benefits to their participants, ranging from the benefits of new medication to the healthcare that is provided as part of responsible study implementation.

US regulations governing pediatric research—Subpart D of the HHS Policy for the Protection of Human Research Subjects (45 CFR 46)—are clear about the standards for acceptable risk to child subjects. For research that carries the prospect of direct medical benefit to the child, research-related risks must be justified by the anticipated benefit to the participant.[54] For research that carries no prospect of medically benefiting the child, risk to the child is capped at a *de minimis* standard. Depending on other details, that standard is either "minimal risk" or a "minor increase over minimal"; technical details aside, both are extremely low and function as absolute ceilings on risk.[5]

Based on this structure, Strong proposes an analysis of risks that research can impose on the fetus when it involves the prospect of medical benefit. He divides his analysis into two scenarios: research directed toward a medical condition of the fetus, and research directed toward a medical condition of the pregnant woman. In the former, he argues, risk to the fetus can be above the *de minimis* standards so long as it is proportionate to the prospective benefits the trial holds out for the fetus. In the latter, he argues, fetal risk must be capped at the pediatric *de minimis* standards.

But this is a very problematic approach, and in two directions. On the one hand, it *over-separates* the risks and benefits to the woman and the fetus; on the other hand, it oblates adequate attention to pregnant women's health needs when they *are* separate.

Take first the over-separation. In saying that fetal risk cannot rise above the *de minimis* standards when research is directed at a medical condition of the pregnant woman, Strong clearly assumes that such research could not carry the potential to benefit the fetus *as well as* the woman. Notably absent from his view is the possibility of fetal benefit consequent on improvement of maternal disease. But this, as we have seen, can be a significant and often expected occurrence. Maternal disease—whether infectious or metabolic—can have deeply harmful effects on fetal development; put simply, maternal illness can be teratogenic.[55] For instance, diabetes has been called one of the "most challenging" medical conditions to adequately treat in pregnant women.[56] Pregnancy itself can exacerbate diabetes-related complications for the woman; in addition, unmanaged diabetes is especially toxic to fetal health: uncontrolled maternal blood sugar levels during the first trimester of pregnancy increase the rate of major congenital abnormalities from around 3% to 20% to 25%.[57] Beyond the issue of teratogenesis, maternal health can affect fetal growth and duration of gestation—both predictors of infant health. For instance, when left untreated, maternal diseases such as asthma are associated with premature delivery and growth problems in the fetus; yet, the effective treatment of asthma during pregnancy is associated with neonatal outcomes similar to those of healthy pregnant women.[58] Even if research is aimed at improving the medical condition of the pregnant woman herself, success at that mission can bring specific and quantifiable medical benefits to the fetus—namely, by reducing the effects of maternal disease on fetal health. The pregnant woman's participation in research designed to intervene on maternal illness, that is, may offer a clear net benefit to the fetus. Using risk standards designed with born children in mind for the context of pregnancy can hide the interconnections that mark the physiology of pregnancy and the social and biologic interface between maternal and child health. To cap fetal risk at the *de minimis* ceiling, in these cases, rather than at least retaining a ratio standard for its own risks and benefits, is problematic.

Take next the issue of oblating the pregnant women's own medical interests. Even if we include a ratio standard for fetal risks and benefits in research aimed at the pregnant woman's condition, a problem remains. To say that fetal research-related risks that are greater than *de minimis* can be justified only by the fetus's own medical benefit inappropriately and unfairly limits pregnant women's access to research that may provide critically important benefit to them. We can tolerate a bit more fetal risk for the sake of maternal benefit.

Tradeoffs between strong maternal benefit and fetal risk are familiar in the clinical context. Pregnant women and their providers make decisions all the time about responsible tradeoffs that sometimes include some measure of fetal risk for a critical maternal benefit. To give just one example, pregnant women with epilepsy will usually need medication that carries modest but real risks to the fetus. If the woman could spare the fetus the effects of medication needed for her health, as parents of born children can do, she would; but she cannot. And the willingness or fact of continuing a pregnancy does not mean that pregnant women forfeit all right to take care of their own critical health needs. The healthcare of pregnant women continuing their pregnancies, in short, paradigmatically includes standards of responsible medical treatment that decidedly do not—and should not—hold the woman's own health hostage in order to avoid anything over the most minimal of risks to the fetus.

Of course, the clinical research context is not the same as the context of delivering healthcare to a patient, even when it carries the prospect of medical benefit. It is, by definition, less evidenced (though it has been argued that this is in fact not the case for pregnancy, where clinical care entails such profound evidence gaps), and its potential for abuse requires stronger protective hedges. Further, unlike healthcare, there is no unconditional right to access clinical research participation given that clinical research is, first and foremost, an evidence-gathering enterprise. That said, the whole point of the research is to find a preventive or treatment that can be responsibly used in the clinical setting. If "responsibly used" includes scenarios in which some fetal risk is justified because an intervention is needed for the health of the gestating woman, it is problematic to rule such tradeoffs out of court in research. The goal of such research is to find medication that satisfies responsible medical treatment of pregnant women, where all parties want to minimize fetal risk to the lowest required; but the measure of what is required includes the pregnant woman's critical health needs. While it is appropriate in the research context to be more conservative in risk tolerance to the fetus as we consider which tradeoffs for maternal benefit are acceptable, it should not, in principle, remove the category of such a justifying tradeoff.[59,60]

As such, assimilating fetal risk standards to those developed for born children is deeply problematic. As in other areas of policy and regulation around pregnancy, the embodied nature of gestation is essentially, not just accidentally, relevant to developing an appropriate framework. And indeed, both US regulations and CIOMS guidance tacitly allow tradeoffs of fetal risk for maternal benefit. They do so, though, by remaining extremely vague. The "prospect of benefit" category is simply described as a category of potential benefit to either woman *or* fetus, and the standard says only that risks should be justified by those benefits, without naming to whom the benefits and to whom the risks redound.[28,47]

Helpful in one sense, as a nod to the highly interconnected physiologies of the pregnant woman and fetus, the lack of specificity about how to think about tradeoffs is also highly limiting. Maternal and fetal risks and benefits are not isomorphic, and presumably there are limits—on both sides—about when benefit to one can justify risk to the other. Without consensus guidelines, individual IRBs are left to make their own decisions, with dangers of erring in both directions—of over- or under-protecting both fetus and woman, or simply turning down research that is too ethically complex to feel confident approving. Up against this likelihood, researchers too, unsure of the parameters their IRBs will allow, may opt out of pursuing research critical to advancing the evidence base.

Guidance specific to pregnancy is needed. The fetus as a future child is an independent and consensus object of concern—for pregnant women, paradigmatically, but also for researchers contemplating the implications of inclusion, and IRBs responsible for research oversight. At the same time, finding the standard for which risks are acceptable for researchers to contemplate imposing during gestation is something that must take into account the distinctive context *of* gestation.

Toward a Feminist Framework

Largely excluded from the research agenda, pregnant women are currently second-class medical citizens. This has led to tremendous harm to them, as well as to their children, whose health can be seriously compromised by maternal illness during gestation. Advocates for women's health must take up the banner to advance responsible research in the context of pregnancy.

If the mandate to achieve equitable consideration in the research agenda is in itself a challenge for feminists working in health research, though, the challenge also presents other ethical questions around what the feminist approach should be. Of critical concern, there currently exists no comprehensive framework for responsible research that accounts for all of the complexities inherent to pregnancy. Instead, the clinical research community appears divided as to how to understand the pregnant research subject, and how, by extension, to adequately protect and address the health needs of this unique population. As the research community increasingly recognizes the need to address pregnant women's health, this conceptual gap becomes more urgent. We must develop a framework adequate to the distinctive context of pregnancy.

Work toward a more progressive foundation and framework is only now beginning in earnest. Thus we have endorsement of the idea that risk standards for a fetus, at a minimum, should not be *more* conservative than those for a born child, as they actually are at present in US regulations.[61,62] We have calls to end requirements for additional paternal consent for a pregnant woman's participation in research—currently required in the scenario of research that may be beneficial to the fetus but not the woman.[44,63,64] We have endorsement of the idea that the prospect of maternal benefit can itself justify some measure of fetal risk,[59,60] even as we urgently need a framework to provide guidance on when or how much risk can be thusly justified. We have theories of fair access for pregnant women that urge a rethinking of summary exclusion simply because a woman is pregnant,[65,66] even as we urgently need criteria for when exclusion *is* reasonable.

At the end of the day, addressing the research community's residual ethical unease with research during pregnancy will require the development of a more complete and unified ethical framework. Without assurances about what is ethical and appropriate when conducting clinical research with pregnant women, even those researchers willing in principle to conduct such research can experience profound uneasiness about the permissibility of conducting studies needed to treat the populations they serve. Much good work has begun; much more is needed. Pregnant women—and the children they may bear—deserve nothing less.

Acknowledgments

This work was supported by the National Institute of Allergy and Infectious Diseases of the National Institutes of Health under award number R01AI108368. The content is solely the responsibility of the authors and does not necessarily represent the official views of the National Institutes of Health.

Notes

1. Through our work on the Pregnancy and HIV/AIDS: Seeking Equitable Study (PHASES) project, we have consulted over 140 researchers, clinicians, regulators, community advisory board members, and policymakers regarding their perspectives on ethical concerns related to conducting and approving research with pregnant women.
2. The paradox of over-protectionism is a historical thread in feminist theory. For example, early 20th-century laws mandating the exclusion of women from serving on juries were often invoked to "protect" women from hearing gruesome details of criminal trials.[67] However, the consequences of such mandates, in addition to being simply offensive and discriminatory on the basis of gender (with no legitimate reason to exclude on such basis), were that women defendants were not guaranteed the right to be tried by a jury of their peers.
3. As Dr. Lisa Harris has noted, however, women seeking abortion may be appropriate participants in research, particularly in studies that require fetal or embryonic tissue, studies with high risk of fetal loss, or studies designed to improve abortion methods. These research scenarios raise a distinct set of issues that are beyond the scope of this paper. See: Harris LH. Clinical research involving pregnant women seeking abortion services. In: Baylis F, Ballantyne A, eds. *Clinical Research Involving Pregnant Women*. Research Ethics Forum, Vol. 3. Cham, Switzerland: Springer; 2016.
4. For example, in research that does not carry the prospect of direct medical benefit, pediatric research subjects can be subjected to a slightly higher allowable risk called "minor increase over minimal risk,"[54] while fetuses can be subjected only to "minimal risk."[28]
5. There is also a provision to allow "research not otherwise approvable" in both Subpart B (pertaining to research with pregnant women) and Subpart D (pertaining to research with children), in which research can be approved, through a rigorous review process, by the Secretary of the Department of Health and Human Services.[28,54] With respect to studies with children, research that is not directly beneficial to

participants but that poses greater than a minor increase over minimal risk may be approvable in certain cases, as bioethicist Dave Wendler notes.[68]

References

1. Mastroianni A, Kahn J. Swinging on the pendulum: shifting views of justice in human subjects research. *Hastings Cent Rep.* 2001;31(3):21–28.
2. Institute of Medicine (US) Committee on Ethical and Legal Issues Relating to the Inclusion of Women in Clinical Studies. In: Mastroianni AC, Faden R, Federman D, eds. *Women and Health Research: Ethical and Legal Issues of Including Women in Clinical Studies: Volume I.* Washington, DC: National Academies Press; 1994.
3. National Institutes of Health (NIH). NIH guidelines on the inclusion of women and minorities as subjects in clinical research. 1994. https://grants.nih.gov/grants/guide/notice-files/not94-100.html
4. Office of Research on Women's Health. *Report of the Advisory Committee on Research on Women's Health, Fiscal Years 2015–2016.* Office of Research on Women's Health and NIH Support for Research on Women's Health. 2017. NIH Publication No. 17 OD 7995.
5. Hamilton BE, Martin JA, Osterman MJ, Curtin SC, Mathews TJ. Births: final data for 2014. *Nat Vital Stat Rep.* 2015;64(12):1–63.
6. Vesga-Lopez O, Blanco C, Keyes K, Olfson M, Grant BF, Hasin DS. Psychiatric disorders in pregnant and postpartum women in the United States. *Arch Gen Psychiatry.* 2008;65(7):805–815.
7. World Health Organization (WHO). Maternal mental health. 2018. http://www.who.int/mental_health/maternal-child/maternal_mental_health/en/.
8. UNAIDS. *The Gap Report: Children and Pregnant Women Living with HIV.* 2014. http://www.unaids.org/sites/default/files/media_asset/09_Childrenandpregnantwomenlivingwithhiv.pdf
9. World Health Organization (WHO). *World Malaria Report.* 2015. https://www.who.int/malaria/publications/world-malaria-report-2015/report/en/
10. Sugarman J, Colvin C, Moran AC, Oxlade O. Tuberculosis in pregnancy: an estimate of the global burden of disease. *Lancet Glob Health.* 2014;2(12):e710–716.
11. Schantz-Dunn J, Nour NM. Malaria and pregnancy: a global health perspective. *Rev Obstet Gynecol.* 2009;2(3):186.
12. Portaccio E, Moiola L, Martinelli V, et al. Pregnancy decision-making in women with multiple sclerosis treated with natalizumab: II: Maternal risks. *Neurology.* 2018;90(10):e832–839.
13. Correa A, Gilboa SM, Besser LM, et al. Diabetes mellitus and birth defects. *Am J Obstet Gynecol.* 2008;199(3):237.
14. Grote NK, Bridge JA, Gavin AR, Melville JL, Iyengar S, Katon WJ. A meta-analysis of depression during pregnancy and the risk of preterm birth, low birth weight, and intrauterine growth restriction. *Arch Gen Psychiatry.* 2010;67(10):1012–1024.
15. World Health Organization (WHO). Maternal mental health. 2018. http://www.who.int/hiv/topics/mtct/about/en/.

16. McGready R, Lee SJ, Wiladphaingern J, et al. Adverse effects of falciparum and vivax malaria and the safety of antimalarial treatment in early pregnancy: a population-based study. *Lancet Infect Dis.* 2012;12(5):388–396.
17. Luxemburger C, McGready R, Kham A, et al. Effects of malaria during pregnancy on infant mortality in an area of low malaria transmission. *Am J Epidemiol.* 2001;154(5):459–465.
18. Gray RH, Li X, Kigozi G, et al. Increased risk of incident HIV during pregnancy in Rakai, Uganda: a prospective study. *Lancet.* 2005;366(9492):1182–1188.
19. Mugo NR, Heffron R, Donnell D, et al. Increased risk of HIV-1 transmission in pregnancy: a prospective study among African HIV-1 serodiscordant couples. *AIDS.* 2011;25(15):1887–1895.
20. Thomson KA, Hughes JP, Baeten J, et al. Female HIV acquisition per sex act is elevated in late pregnancy and postpartum. 25th Conference on Retroviruses and Opportunistic Infections (CROI 2018), Boston, abstract 45, 2018.
21. Giacoia GP. Introduction: Report of NICHD Workshop on Use of Drugs and Pregnancy (September 23–24, 2000). *Semin Perinatol.* 2001;25(3):115–119.
22. Mattison D, Zajicek A. Gaps in knowledge in treating pregnant women. *Gend Med.* 2006;3:169–182
23. Wisner KL. The last therapeutic orphan: the pregnant woman. *Am J Psychiatry.* 2012;169(6):554–556.
24. Haire D. *FDA-Approved Obstetrics Drugs: Their Impact on Mother and Baby.* National Women's Health Alliance. 2001. https://asanfranciscodoula.com/resources/Preview%20of%20%E2%80%9CFDA%20Approved%20Obstetric%20Drugs-%20Their%20Effects%20on%20Mother%20and%20Baby%E2%80%9D.pdf
25. Yao LP. Communicating information about risks of prescription products and vaccines used during pregnancy. Risk Communication Advisory Meeting, Food and Drug Administration, March 5, 2018. https://www.fda.gov/downloads/AdvisoryCommittees/CommitteesMeetingMaterials/RiskCommunicationAdvisoryCommittee/UCM599983.pdf.
26. Adam MP, Polifka JE, Friedman JM. Evolving knowledge of the teratogenicity of medications in human pregnancy. *Am J Med Genet C Semin Med Genet.* 2011;157C(3):175–182. doi:10.1002/ajmg.c.30313
27. World Health Organization (WHO). Technical update on treatment optimization: use of efavirenz during pregnancy: a public health perspective. 2012. http://www.who.int/iris/handle/10665/70920
28. Subpart B, 45 CFR 46, 2009.
29. Final rule, 45 CFR Part 46. Rules and regulations. *Federal Register.* 2001;66(219). https://www.gpo.gov/fdsys/pkg/FR-2001-11-13/pdf/01-28440.pdf.
30. Mastroianni AC, Henry LM, Robinson D, Bailey T, Faden RR, Little MO, Lyerly AD. Research with pregnant women: new insights on legal decision-making. *Hastings Cent Rep.* 2017;47(3):38–45.
31. Krubiner CB, Faden RR, Cadigan RJ, et al. Advancing HIV research with pregnant women: navigating challenges and opportunities. *AIDS.* 2016;30(15):2261–2265.

32. Subpart A, 45 CFR 46, 2009.
33. Ells C, Lyster C. Research ethics review of drug trials targeting medical conditions of pregnant women. In: Baylis F, Ballantyne A, eds. *Clinical Research Involving Pregnant Women*. Research Ethics Forum, Vol. 3. Cham, Switzerland: Springer; 2016.
34. Hunt A, Banner N, Littler K. The global forum on bioethics in research meeting, "Ethics of Research in Pregnancy": emerging consensus themes and outputs. *Reprod Health*. 2017;14(3):158.
35. Hurst SA. Vulnerability in research and health care; describing the elephant in the room? *Bioethics*. 2008;22(4):191–202.
36. Wild V. How are pregnant women vulnerable research participants? *Int J Fem Approaches Bioeth*. 2012;5(2):82–104.
37. Schonfeld T. The perils of protection: vulnerability and women in clinical research. *Theor Med Bioeth*. 2013;34(3):189–206.
38. Mathews E. Should pregnant women be excluded from a community-based lifestyle intervention trial? A case study. *Reprod Health*. 2017;14(3):165.
39. Gomes MF, de la Fuente-Núñez V, Saxena A, Kuesel AC. Protected to death: systematic exclusion of pregnant women from Ebola virus disease trials. *Reprod Health*. 2017;14(3):172.
40. Caluwaerts S. Nubia's mother: being pregnant in the time of experimental vaccines and therapeutics for Ebola. *Reprod Health*. 2017;14(3):157.
41. Mitchell AA, Gilboa SM, Werler MM, Kelley KE, Louik C, Hernández-Díaz S. Medication use during pregnancy, with particular focus on prescription drugs: 1976–2008. *Am J Obstet Gynecol*. 2011;205(1):51.e1–8.
42. Cooper WO, Hernandez-Diaz S, Arbogast PG, et al. Major congenital malformations after first-trimester exposure to ACE inhibitors. *N Engl J Med*. 2006;354(23):2443–2451.
43. Hebert M, Ma X, Naraharisetti S, et al. Are we optimizing gestational diabetes treatment with glyburide? The pharmacologic basis for better clinical practice. *Clin Pharmacol Ther*. 2009;85(6):607–614.
44. Committee on Ethics. The American College of Obstetricians and Gynecologists (ACOG) Committee Opinion No. 646: Ethical considerations for including women as research participants. *Obstet Gynecol*. 2015;126(5):e100–107.
45. Pan American Health Organization (PAHO). Zika ethics consultation: ethics guidance on key issues raised by the outbreak. 2016. http://iris.paho.org/xmlui/handle/123456789/28425
46. Foulkes MA, Grady C, Spong CY, Bates A, Clayton JA. Clinical research enrolling pregnant women: a workshop summary. *J Womens Health*. 2011;20(10):1429–1432.
47. *International Ethical Guidelines for Health-Related Research Involving Humans*. 4th ed. Geneva: Council for International Organizations of Medical Sciences (CIOMS); 2016.
48. Final rule, 45 CFR Part 46. Rules and regulations. *Federal Register*. 2017;82(12). https://www.gpo.gov/fdsys/pkg/FR-2017-01-19/pdf/2017-01058.pdf.

49. US Department of Health and Human Services (HHS). The final rule to further delay the general compliance date of the 2018 Requirements to January 21, 2019, while permitting the use of three burden-reducing provisions of the 2018 Requirements during the delay period. https://www.govinfo.gov/content/pkg/FR-2018-06-19/pdf/2018-13187.pdf
50. Merton V. Ethical obstacles to the participation of women in biomedical research. In: Wolf S, ed. *Feminism and Bioethics: Beyond Reproduction*. New York, NY: Oxford University Press; 1996.
51. Lidz CW, Appelbaum PS, Grisso T, Renaud M. Therapeutic misconception and the appreciation of risks in clinical trials. *Soc Sci Med*. 2004;58(9):1689–1697.
52. Beecher HK. Ethics and clinical research. *N Engl J Med*. 1966;274(24):1354–1360.
53. Strong C. How should risks and benefits be balanced in research involving pregnant women and fetuses? *IRB*. 2011;33(6):1.
54. Subpart D, 45 CFR 46. 2009.
55. Wilson RD, Johnson JA, Summers A, et al. Principles of human teratology: drug chemical and infectious exposure. *J Obstet Gynaecol Can*. 2007;29(11):911–917.
56. American College of Obstetricians and Gynecologists (ACOG). ACOG practice bulletin #60: pregestational diabetes mellitus. *Obstet Gynecol*. 2005;105(3):675–685.
57. Allen VM, Armson BA, SOGC Genetics Committee. SOGC clinical practice guideline: teratology associated with pre-existing and gestational diabetes. *J Obstet Gynaecol Can*. 2007;29(11):927–944.
58. Tan KS, Thomson NC. Asthma in pregnancy. *Am J Med*. 2000;109(9):727–733.
59. Little MO, Lyerly AD, Mastroianni AC, Faden RR. Ethics and research with pregnant women: lessons from HIV/AIDS. In: Baylis F, Ballantyne A, eds. *Clinical Research Involving Pregnant Women*. Research Ethics Forum, Vol. 3. Cham, Switzerland: Springer; 2016.
60. Little M, Wickremsinhe M, Lyerly A. Research in pregnancy: the ethics of risk-benefit tradeoffs between woman, fetus, and future child. *Obstet Gynecol*. 2017;129:76S–77S.
61. Little M. Minimal risk and research with pregnant women. Task Force on Research Specific to Pregnant and Lactation Women meeting, November 6, 2017. https://www.nichd.nih.gov/sites/default/files/2017-11/7-LITTLE_Minimal_risk_110617.pdf.
62. Summary presentation. Task Force on Research Specific to Pregnant and Lactation Women meeting, November 6, 2017. https://www.nichd.nih.gov/sites/default/files/2017-11/Spong_TF2_summary_presentation.pdf.
63. Lyerly A. Consent requirements in research with pregnant women. Task Force on Research Specific to Pregnant and Lactation Women meeting, November 6, 2017. https://www.nichd.nih.gov/sites/default/files/2017-11/5-Consent_Requirements_Lyerly.pdf.

64. Minkoff HL, Moreno JD. Paternal consent for fetal research. *N Engl J Med*. 1993;329(4):278.
65. Ballantyne A, Rogers W. Pregnancy, vulnerability, and the risk of exploitation in clinical research. In: Baylis F, Ballantyne A, eds. *Clinical Research Involving Pregnant Women*. Research Ethics Forum, Vol. 3. Cham, Switzerland: Springer; 2016.
66. van der Graaf R, van der Zande IS, den Ruijter HM, et al. Fair inclusion of pregnant women in clinical trials: an integrated scientific and ethical approach. *Trials*. 2018;19(1):78.
67. McDonald L. A jury of one's peers. 2011. https://www.aclu.org/blog/mass-incarceration/jury-ones-peers?redirect=blog/womens-rights/jury-ones-peers/.
68. Wender D. Do U.S. regulations allow more than minor increase over minimal risk pediatric research? Should they? *IRB*. 2013;35(6):1–8.

INDEX

abjection, 140–41
ableism, 5, 136, 170
abortion, 2, 14, 15, 234–36, 238, 241–42
   abortion providers/provision, 190–201, 205–6
   anti-abortion, 189–93, 201
   anti-choice/Pro-life, 191–92, 202–3
   ethics of, 190–91
   pro-choice, 190–92, 199–203
   right to, 199–200, 205, 235, 285–86
Acquired Immune Deficiency Syndrome (AIDS), 107–8, 112, 122
agency, 2, 14, 113, 120–22, 139–40, 190, 202, 205–6, 216, 227
aging, 12, 109, 115, 121–22
American Academy of Pediatrics (AAP), 240
American College of Obstetrics and Gynecology (ACOG), 97, 240, 245, 284
American Society for Reproductive Medicine (ASRM), 266–69
Americans with Disabilities Act (ADA), 260–61, 269, 270–73
asylum seekers, 45–58
   children or adolescents, 47, 52
   United Nations, 46, 49, 58
   United Nations High Commission for Refugees (UNHCR), 47–48
autonomy, 88, 93, 99–101, 109–10, 133–34, 214–217, 221–22
   feminist interpretation of, 109–10, 227

HIV children or adolescents, 113, 115–16, 242
HIV family planning, 116–18
   optimizing, 120
   pregnant women, 285–87
   relational, 3–4, 6, 110, 122, 142, 210, 215–16, 219–23, 227

Beauchamp, T.L. and Childress, J.F., 9, 109–10
Behar, R., 9
beneficence, 88, 93, 96–98, 102, 109, 129–30, 133–36, 214
   feminist interpretation, 109–10
   violence, 133–34
British Columbia First Nations Health Authority, 35
British Columbia Tripartite Framework, 35

Canada Health Act, 29–30
Canadian Centre for Refugee and Immigrant Health Care (CCRIHC), 51–53, 55, 58
Canadian HIV Women's Sexual and Reproductive Health Cohort Study (CHIWOS), 123
Canadian Task Force on Preventive Health Care, 140
capacity, 3, 24, 216–17, 220–22, 247, 251–52, 282
capitalism, 133

case finding, 2, 12–13, 142–43, 145
Charter on Medical Professionalism, 57
childbirth, 244–46, 250, 252
  dignity, 249–50
  labor, 246–50
children or adolescents
  asylum seekers, migrants, refugees, 47–52, 56–57
  HIV, living with, 112–16, 119–20
  HIV, aging out, 115
  violence, 136, 144
cisgender, 13–14, 167–69, 172–73, 178, 182
cisnormativity, 13–14, 167–68, 170–74, 183
  cissexism, 174
  institutionalized, 175–77, 180–82
  learned, 172–73
classism, 5, 136, 150–51, 170
clitoris, 91
  clitoral hood, 88–89
  clitoral hood size reduction, 87–88
Coleman, P., 204
colonial, 21–22, 24, 119
  colonialism, 27–28, 36–37
  colonization, 21–22, 27–28, 143
  colonized, 36
community, 63–68, 70, 74–76, 151–52
  value of, 68–72, 77–78
confidentiality, 76, 110, 133–34
conflict of interest, 88, 97, 101
conscience, 193, 195–97, 199
conscientious objection, 193, 195–97, 268
conscientious provision, 190–91, 193–98, 201, 205
consent
  childbirth, 244, 247
  informed, 88, 94–95, 101, 215, 263, 267
  parental, 238
  paternal, 292

violation of, 237, 249
women with disabilities, 263, 267
cosmetic surgery, 87, 91–92
Council for International Organization of Medical Sciences (CIOMS), 284, 291
cultural humility, 181
cultural safety, 26–29, 35, 143–44

danger talk, 200–1
defibulation, 87–88, 95
Diagnostic and Statistical Manual of Mental Disorders (DSM), 174–75
disability, 15
  access to care structural barriers, 259, 261–64, 268–69
  access to care structural improvements, 267, 270–71, 273
  attitudes towards, 265–66
  children, 261, 268, 271–73
  competency/competent care, 270–71
  discrimination, 260–61, 269
  infertility, 259
  infertility care, 260–71
  infertility care justice/injustice, 259–60, 263–65, 268
  infertility care reasonable accommodation, 259–60, 272–73
  infertility care reasonable modifications, 269–70
  lack of provider training, 264–66, 269–70
  negative attitudes, 264–66
  pregnancy experience, 261–62
  refusal of care, 265–68
  reproductive care, 260–71
discrimination, 182, 265
  disability, 260–61, 269
  gender-based, 119–20
  HIV, 121–22
  reproductive, 249
  sex workers, 151–52, 154–55, 160–62

displaced, 48–49
    internally displaced people
        (IDP), 46–47
    persons, 46
    population, 47

equality/inequality, 6, 49, 111, 131–32,
    181, 214
equity, 10, 30–31, 34–35, 56–57,
    111, 138–39

Farmer, P., 6
female genital cosmetic surgery
    (FGCS), 2, 12, 87–92,
    94–95, 97–102
female genital mutilation/cutting,
    87–88, 94–95
feminist bioethics, 1–2, 4, 9, 292
feminist epistemology, 67
feminist standpoint theory, 67
First Nations, 21–24, 28–30, 33–34
    First Nations Health Governance, 35
    First Nations Regional Health Survey,
        22, 26
Food and Drug Administration
    (FDA), 280

gender, 2–3, 8–9, 12, 22, 63, 67, 74,
    76–78, 115, 130, 137, 143–44
    analysis, 11, 77–78, 133–34, 137, 145
    gender and sex distinctions, 8–9
    gender-based, 49–50, 119–20
    gendered, 36, 70, 72, 77, 132, 137
    gendered language, 180–81
    gendered spaces, 177, 179
    identity, 13–14, 108, 114–15, 167–69,
        171–80, 183
    research, 8–9
    roles, 65–67, 73, 75, 131–33, 137
genetic screening
    prenatal, 243–44
Greater Involvement of People Living
    with HIV/AIDS (GIPA), 108–9

harm reduction, 110–11, 115–16
health insurance, 45–46, 51–52, 57–58,
    117, 259–60
health literacy, 10–11, 76
    reproductive care, 239, 243–44, 252
hegemony/hegemonic, 134–36, 153
heteronormativity, 13–14, 167–68,
    170–73, 183
    institutionalized, 175–77, 180–82
heterosexism, 129, 136
heterosexuality, 173
homophobia, 173–76
    conversion therapy, 174–75
    egodystonic homosexuality, 174–75
Human immunodeficiency virus (HIV),
    2, 6, 12, 26, 107–9
    aging, 121–22
    Canadian HIV Women's Sexual and
        Reproductive Health Cohort Study
        (CHIWOS), 123
    children or adolescence aging out, 115
    children or adolescence living
        with, 112–16
    harm-reduction, 110–11, 115–16
    HIV family planning, 116–18
    newborn living with, 118–20
    policy, 122–24
    pregnancy living with, 116–18, 279
    principles, 109–11
    surveillance, 118, 119–21
human rights, 46–47, 94, 109, 136,
    198–99, 249–50
hymen, 93–94, 96
hymenoplasty, 87–88, 93–94, 101–2

immigrants, 10–11, 45–48, 50–52, 56, 58
    barriers to healthcare access, 45–46,
        49–50, 52–55
    children and adolescents, 48
    host country obligations, 45–46
    LGBTQ, 49–50
    undocumented, 45–47, 52–53, 56
    uninsured, 45–46, 51, 54–55

Indigenous, 21–22
　children, 23, 33, 119
　colonialism, 27–28, 36–37
　colonization, 21–22, 24, 27–28, 35–36, 119, 143
　First Nations, 21–24, 27–30, 33–34
　First Nations Health Governance, 35
　First Nations Regional Health Survey, 22, 26
　health/healthcare inequity for women, 10, 21–24, 26–30, 32–34, 36–37, 108–9, 119
　Inuit, 22–23, 27–28, 29–30, 35
　Métis, 22–23, 27–28
　Mid-wifery and perinatal care, 23, 31–33, 36
　people, 21–22, 26–27, 29–30, 32–34
　racism, 26–27, 30–31, 37
　stigma, 27–29, 32–33, 37
　violence, 23, 36, 137–38
　world view, 22, 29
　Xpey' Relational Environments Framework, 10, 21, 24–26f
inequity, 5, 24, 36–37, 58, 129, 136–37, 150, 153, 156
　gender, 107–9, 111, 120–21, 123, 129, 145
　health/healthcare for women, 10, 21, 22–24, 26–30, 32–34, 36–37, 108–9, 119
infertility, 15, 259
infertility care
　disability, 260–71
　disability justice/injustice, 259–60, 263–65, 268
　reasonable accommodation for disability, 259–60, 272–73
　reasonable modifications for disability, 269–70
　injustice, 108–9, 111, 227, 263–65
　systemic, 5, 37, 119, 136
Institute of Medicine (IOM), 6

integrity, 100, 192
internally displaced people (IDP), 46–47
International Federation of Gynecology and Obstetrics (FIGO), 97, 249
International Organization for Migration (IOM), 46
intersectionality, 4, 10, 12, 109, 111, 162
　violence, 137–39
Inuit, 22–23, 27–30, 35
Inuulitsivik Health Centre, 31

Joffe, C., 190
justice, 4–5, 109–10, 111, 117, 129–30, 133–36, 140–41, 195–96
　equality/inequality, 6, 49, 111, 131–32, 181, 214
　equity, 10, 30–31, 34–35, 56–57, 111, 138–39
　horizontal, 111
　infertility care and women with disabilities, 259–60, 263–65, 268
　injustice, 108–9, 111, 227, 263–65
　reproductive, 204–5
　social, 1, 5, 111, 136–37, 210, 226
　vertical, 111

labia, 90
　hypertrophy, 97
　labiaplasty, 87–91, 93, 97–100, 101
　majora, 88–89, 92, 95, 98–99
　minora, 88–92, 94, 98–99
LGBTQ+, 13–14, 49–50, 168–69, 176
Ludlow, J., 201

marginalization/marginalized, 2, 4–5, 7, 10, 32, 108, 111, 114–15, 137–39, 169–72, 174–75, 182, 198, 237
Meaningful Involvement of People Living with HIV (MIPA), 108–9
Métis, 22–23, 27–28
migrants, 46–48, 50–55, 56, 58
　children, 47–48

International Organization for Migration, 46
moral agency, 2

National Inquiry into Missing and Murdered Indigenous Women and Girls, 137–38
non-maleficence, 88–89, 93, 96, 98–101, 109–11
　feminist interpretation, 110–11
　harm reduction, 110–11
　supports violence, 129–30, 133–34, 135–36
Nunavik, 31

Office of Research on Women's Health (ORWR) (US), 284
oppression, 4–5, 13–14, 32, 111, 123, 132, 162, 248
　Indigenous, 21–22, 32, 36
　institutionalized, 167–68, 182–83
　marginalization/marginalized, 2, 4–5, 7, 10, 32, 108, 114–15, 137–39, 169–72, 174–75, 182, 198, 237
　people with disabilities, 5
　queer women and transgender, 167–72, 182–83
　violence, structural, 131–32, 137–39, 142, 143
　violence, gendered patterns of 132–33, 137

Pan American Health Organization (PAHO), 284
Parker, W., 194
paternalism, 34, 120, 155–56, 162
　paternalistic practices, 1, 110, 119
patient-centered care, 6–7, 13–14, 75–76, 204–5
　woman-centered care, 6–7, 15, 122–24, 233–34, 237–39, 250–53
patient-health professional relationship
　healthcare provider neutrality, 181–83

queer and trans patients, 177
shaped by oppression, 167–68
trust, 13–14, 177, 183
perinatal care, 30–31
perinatal mental health, 2, 14–15, 209–15, 218–19, 225, 227
perinatal outcomes, 54–55, 112–13, 218–19
perineoplasty, 87–88
place, 11, 63–67, 74–77
　value of, 67–72, 75, 77–78
policy
　cultural safety, 143–44
　public health insurance, 45–46, 51–52, 57–58, 117
　public health policy, 110–11, 119–20
　trauma informed, 110–11, 124, 129–30, 139, 141–45
　violence informed, 139, 141–45
Poppema, S., 194
power, 1, 3–4, 236–37, 244, 282
　distribution, 36
　empower, 248, 251–52
　gendered distribution, 3
　role of, 30–31
pregnant women, 15–16
　autonomy, 285–87
　Ebola, 283
　equitable inclusion-research, 281–84, 292–93
　exclusion from research, 280–81, 292
　health/healthcare inequity, 280–81
　HIV, 116–20
　illness, 279–80
　research models, 282–85, 287–92
　research with, 15–16, 281
　reasons for lack of research, 280–81
　right to abort, 285
　risk, clinical, 280, 283–84, 291
　risk, fetal, 285–91
　therapeutic orphans, 280
　"vulnerable," 282–85
prenatal testing, 243–44

principle-based theory, 9, 12, 109–10, 213–15
privacy, 29, 73, 76, 142, 178, 242
    right, 110
private pay/service, 88, 101, 157, 160–61, 268–70
public health, 50, 56–58, 101, 110, 113–14, 149, 194, 198–99, 213, 226, 284, 287
    insurance coverage, 45–46, 51–52, 57–58, 117
    policy, 110–11, 119–20
Purcell, E., 5
Puri, L., 49

queer, 2, 13–14
    accessing healthcare, 176–70
    definition, 168–69
    inclusion, 178, 180
    marginalization, 169–71, 175
    primary healthcare conceptualized, 167
    primary healthcare gender-affirming, 180–81
    safe clinics, 177–78, 180, 182–83
    safe providers, 176–77
    structural-physical changes, 176–78, 183

racism, 26–27, 30–32, 35, 37, 129, 136, 143, 167–68, 170, 250
reasonable accommodation, 259–60, 272–73
reasonable modifications, 269–70
reciprocity, 68
refugees, 2, 10–11, 45–48, 50–56, 58, 108–9
    barriers to healthcare access, 45–46, 49–55
    children and adolescents, 48, 50, 52
    defined, 46
    gender-based violence, 50

    host country obligations, 45–46
    insurance programs, 51–53
    LGBTQ+, 49–50
    pregnant, 52, 54–56
    smuggling, 52, 56
    trafficking in persons, 48–50, 52, 56
    undocumented, 45–47, 52–53, 55–56, 58
    uninsured, 45–46, 51, 54–55
    vulnerable, 45–46, 49
re-infibulation, 87–88, 95, 101–2
relational autonomy, 3–4, 6, 110, 122, 142, 210, 215–16, 219, 227
relational ethics, 14–15, 129–30, 135–37, 140, 144–45, 215–17
    violence, and response to, 135–36, 140–41, 144, 145
relational theory, 3–4, 6, 10, 14–15, 225, 227
reproductive care, 15
    access, 235
    breastfeeding, 251–52
    consent, 247
    contraception, 238, 240–42
    contraception long lasting, 240–41
    midwife/midwifery/doula, 245, 252
    motivational interviewing, 240–41
    preconception planning, 239
    reproductive ethics, 233–36
    respectful maternity care (RMC), 249
    sterilization, 236–37
    subjectivity, 234
    technology, 233–34, 244–49, 251–53
    techno-maternity, 234, 244–45, 252
    woman-centered, 234, 237, 239, 250, 251–53
    women with disabilities, 15
reproductive justice, 204–5
reproductive life plan, 239–41
reproductive rights, 204–5
research, clinical/medical
    exclusion, 279, 280–81, 283, 292

fetal risk, 285–86, 288–92
  fetal safety, 280–81
  inclusion, 279, 284
  Institutional Review Board (IRB), 281, 291
  Office of Research on Women's Health (ORWR) (US), 284
  pregnant women, 279, 280–81, 284–85
  risks, 286–87, 291
  therapeutic misconception, 286–87
research models for pregnant women
  assimilating pediatric research, 288–91
  feminist framework, 292
  protectionism-vulnerable population, 282–85
  respecting pregnant women's autonomy, 285–87
respect, 26–27, 32, 68, 133, 158, 249, 252
  for autonomy, 101, 110, 115–18, 133–34, 215–16, 219, 221, 223, 242
  disrespect, 13, 154–56, 249–50
  for persons, 28, 99–100, 110, 129–30, 133–36
rights, 47, 111, 151–52, 236–37
  abortion, 199–200, 205, 235, 285–86
  conscience and religious freedom, 195–96
  disability, 267, 272
  during childbirth, 249–50
  human, 46–47, 94, 109, 136, 198–99, 249–50
  reproductive, 204–5, 285
  United Nations Declaration on the Rights of Indigenous People (UNDRIP), 35
  women, 7, 93–94, 109, 123, 152, 154, 198–99, 249
Romanow Commission on Canadian Health Care, 34
Royal Australian and New Zealand College of Obstetricians and Gynaecologists (RANZCOG), 97

Royal College of Obstetricians and Gynaecologists (RCOG), 97, 101
Rural women
  access to healthcare, 11, 63–64, 66, 68–78
  "good" rural woman stereotype, 63–67, 69–75, 77–78
  intimate partner violence, 73–74
  rural health ethics, 63–64, 67, 70–72, 75–77
  rurality, 64–65, 70, 76
rural life stereotype, 63–72, 74–75, 77–78

sex, 7–9
  assigned at birth, 13–14, 167–69, 171, 173–74, 175, 178, 180
Sex and Gender Equity in Research (SAGER) Guidelines, 8–9
sex work, 2, 13, 156–57, 161–62
  definition, 149
  structural conditions, 150
  violence, 150–51, 161
sex workers, 2, 13, 120, 149, 159–60
  HIV, STIs, 149–51, 155–56, 158–62
  ideologies of deviance, 152, 154, 162
sexual violence, 12–13, 33–34, 52, 136, 247–48
social determinants of health, 24–25, 113–15, 123, 161
Society of Obstetricians and Gynaecologists of Canada (SOGC), 97
solidarity, 68
stereotypes
  abortion, 192, 196–97
  "good" rural women, 63–67, 69–75, 77–78
  rural life, 63–67, 69–72, 74–75, 77–78
  sex work, 149, 155–56, 159
  women with disabilities, 259, 265
sterilization, 195
  forced, 15, 195–96, 236–37, 240, 244, 267

stewardship, 100
stigma, 5, 13–15, 129
   abortion providers, 14, 189, 194, 196–97
   HIV, 109, 112–22
   Indigenous women/people, 27, 28–33, 37
   mental illness, 14–15, 225–27
   rural, 74–75
   sex workers, 13, 151–57, 159–62
Strong, C., 288
surveillance, 234, 244–45, 248–49
   HIV, 116, 118–21

taxonomy
   Penchansky R. and Thomas J., 63–64, 69–78
tension of opposites, 202–6
trafficking, 48–51
transgender, 2, 13–14
   accessing healthcare, 176
   dead naming, 179
   definition, 169
   exoticization, 179, 183
   gender-affirming medical care, 175–76, 181
   gender dysphoria, 175
   gender identity disorder, 175
   inclusion, 178, 180
   marginalization, 169–71, 175
   medical transition, 170–71, 179
   oppression in healthcare, 167
   social transition, 170–71
   structural-physical changes, 177–78, 183
   transphobia, 173, 175–76
   violence, 173, 179
transparency/transparent, 100–1, 285, 287
trust, 13–14, 27–28, 36, 58, 115–16, 120–21, 143, 286–87

patient-health professional relationship, 13–14, 177, 183
Truth and Reconciliation Commission, 27–28, 34–35

United Nations, 46, 49, 58, 235
   United Nations Declaration on the Rights of Indigenous People (UNDRIP), 35
   United Nations Educational, Scientific and Cultural Organization (UNESCO), 284
   United Nations High Commission for Refugees (UNHCR), 47–48
universal precautions, 141–42
universal screening, 139–141
US Centers for Disease Control and Prevention (CDC), 107–8, 239
US Department of Health and Human Services (DHHS), 195–96
US Food and Drug Administration (FDA), 280

vaginal rejuvenation, 87–88, 95–96
vaginoplasty, 87–88
veracity, 93, 96–98, 100
violence, 2, 12–13, 48–49, 108, 110–11, 113–15, 123, 130, 142–43
   against women, 48–49, 129–37, 139–41, 143–45, 241–42
   against women feminist perspective, 129–30, 136–37
   against women unchallenged, 136–37
   against queer/transgender, 49–50, 173, 179
   case-finding, 139, 143
   domestic, 70, 130
   family, 130
   gender-based, 49–50, 130–33, 137
   gender roles, 137

Indigenous people, 23, 36, 131–32,
   137–39, 142–143
interpersonal, 129, 135–40, 143
intimate partner violence (IPV),
   12–13, 73–74, 129–30
   safe disclosure, 143–44
   screening not effective, 139–40
   sexual, 12–13, 33–34, 52, 136,
      247–48
   sex workers, 150–51, 161
   structural, 5–6, 131–32, 134–39, 143
vulva, 89, 91, 95, 97–99, 101

woman-centered care, 6–7, 237–38
   HIV care, 122–24
   reproductive care, 15, 233–53
Woodman, M., 202–3
World Health Organization (WHO),
   24–25, 50–51, 108, 123, 140,
   143–44, 249, 284

Xpey' Relational Environments
   Framework, 10, 21, 24–26f

Young, I.M., 4–6, 111

www.ingramcontent.com/pod-product-compliance
Ingram Content Group UK Ltd.
Pitfield, Milton Keynes, MK11 3LW, UK
UKHW021317180426
11947UKWH00015B/1278